Robert K. Stoelting, M.D.

Professor and Chair
Department of Anesthesia
Indiana University School of Medicine
Indianapolis, Indiana

HANDBOOK OF
Pharmacology and Physiology in Anesthetic Practice

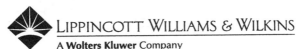
LIPPINCOTT WILLIAMS & WILKINS
A **Wolters Kluwer** Company
Philadelphia • Baltimore • New York • London
Buenos Aires • Hong Kong • Sydney • Tokyo

Library of Congress Cataloging-in-Publication Data

Stoelting, Robert K.
    Handbook of pharmacology and physiology in anesthetic
practice / Robert K. Stoelting.
        p.   cm.
    Companion v. to: Pharmacology and physiology in anes-
thetic practice / Robert K. Stoelting.
    Includes index.
    ISBN 0-397-51498-0
    1. Anesthetics—Physiological effect—Handbooks, manu-
als, etc.   I. Stoelting, Robert K.   Pharmacology and physiology on anesthetic practice.   II. Title.
    [DNLM: 1. Anesthetics—pharmacology—handbooks.
2. Physiology—handbooks.   QV 39 S872h   1995]
RD82.2.S686   1995
615'.781—dc20
DNLM/DLC
for Library of Congress   95-14253
                                                               CIP

PREFACE

The *Handbook of Pharmacology and Physiology in Anesthetic Practice* is intended to provide the reader with pertinent and concise details related to the pharmacology of drugs used during anesthesia and the perioperative period and principles of physiology relevant to understanding the patient's medical condition. Organization of the *Handbook* follows the same chapter and section headings as the parent textbook, *Pharmacology and Physiology in Anesthetic Practice,* thus providing the reader with a rapid link to more detailed information. Liberal use of figures and tables enhances the presentation of facts in an easy to recognize format for application in the operating room. The *Handbook* is intended to serve another useful function—a source of new information that was not available at the time of the publication of the parent textbook in 1991. In this regard, each *Handbook* chapter has been updated and revised to reflect current knowledge and understanding of pharmacology and physiology relevant to anesthetic practice.

I believe the *Handbook for Pharmacology and Physiology in Anesthetic Practice* can serve as a ''pocket ready'' and current reference source for the student and practitioner.

I wish to thank my secretary Deanna Walker for timely and conscientious preparation of the manuscript; and Lisa McAllister, Medical Editor, Lippincott-Raven, Paula Callaghan, Associate Editor, Lippincott-Raven, and P. M. Gordon Associates for guiding this new book through the development and publication process.

ROBERT K. STOELTING, M.D.

CONTENTS

PHARMACOLOGY

Chapter

1

Pharmacokinetics and Pharmacodynamics of Injected and Inhaled Drugs

Pharmacokinetics and pharmacodynamics of injected and inhaled drugs are reflected by the patient's physiologic and pharmacologic response to drugs administered during anesthesia (Updated and revised from Stoelting RK. Pharmacokinetics and pharmacodynamics of injected and inhaled drugs. In: Pharmacology and Physiology in Anesthetic Practice. 2nd ed. Philadelphia, JB Lippincott, 1991: 1–32.)

I. INTRODUCTION

A. **Pharmacokinetics** is the quantitative study of the absorption, distribution, metabolism, and excretion of injected and inhaled drugs and their metabolites **(what the body does to a drug).**
   1. Variability in drug responses may reflect individual differences in the pharmacokinetics of the drug.
   2. Selection and adjustment of drug dosage schedules are determined by the pharmacokinetics of the drug.
B. **Pharmacodynamics** is the study of the intrinsic sensitivity or responsiveness of receptors to a drug and the mechanisms by which these effects occur **(what the drug does to the body).**
   1. Intrinsic sensitivity of receptors is determined by measuring the plasma concentrations of a drug required to evoke specific pharmacologic responses.
   2. Variability in the intrinsic sensitivity of receptors among patients results in different pharmacologic responses to drugs despite similar plasma concentrations of drug.

C. Stereoselectivity

1. Biologically active materials (neurotransmitters, hormones) exhibit inherent stereoselectivity with specific receptor sites.

   a. Because most biochemical processes are stereoselective, natural products are usually obtained in an optically active form.

   b. Synthesis of drugs usually results in racemic mixtures containing 50% of each of the dextrorotatory (*d*) and levorotatory (*l*) isomers. (Racemic mixtures [*dl*] do not rotate polarized light.)

2. In medical practice, it is often erroneously assumed that only one compound is administered when, in fact, racemic mixtures are being utilized.

   a. **Stereoisomers** are nonsuperimposable mirror images of the same molecule **(enantiomers).**

   b. Enantiomers may have different affinities for receptors such that racemic mixtures may have different pharmacologic effects than a specific (*l* or *d*) enantiomer alone.

3. Stereoselectivity in drug action implies that only one isomer is active; the other isomer (50%) should be regarded as an impurity which could contribute to side effects.

   a. d-Propranolol acts as a beta antagonist while both isomers contribute to the local anesthetic effect.

   b. d-Ketamine is predominantly hypnotic and analgesic, whereas l-ketamine is the main source of unwanted side effects (see Chapter 6).

4. In the study of drugs, it is preferable to use a single isomer.

   a. Pharmacologic data (drug action, effects and side effects, metabolism, excretion), as described in the literature, are often based on racemic mixtures.

   b. Data based on racemic mixtures are often presented as if only one compound (the active isomer) were involved.

II. DESCRIPTION OF DRUG RESPONSE (Table 1-1)

III. PHARMACOKINETICS OF INJECTED DRUGS

A. Compartmental Models

1. Pharmacokinetics of injected drugs have been simplified by considering the body to be composed of a

Table 1–1
Description of Drug Response

Hyperactive—Unusually low dose produces the expected pharmacologic effect

Hypersensitivity—Allergy to a drug

Hyporeactivity—Unusually large dose is required to produce the expected pharmacologic effect

Tolerance—Hyporeactivity owing to chronic exposure to a drug; cross-tolerance is common between drugs that produce similar pharmacologic effects (alcohol and inhaled anesthetics)

Tachyphylaxis—Tolerance that develops acutely; reflects cellular tolerance

Additive—Two drugs (inhaled anesthetics) interact to produce an effect (MAC) equal to algebraic summation

Synergistic—Two drugs interact to produce an effect greater than algebraic summation

Agonist—A drug that activates a receptor by binding to the receptor

Partial agonist—A drug that binds only weakly to receptors and produces minimal pharmacologic effect

Antagonist—A drug that binds to the receptor without activating the receptor and, at the same time, prevents an agonist from stimulating the receptor

Competitive antagonism—Occurs when increasing concentrations of an agonist (acetylcholine) can overcome the effects of an antagonist (nondepolarizing muscle relaxant)

Noncompetitive antagonism—Occurs when increasing concentrations of an agonist cannot overcome the effects of an antagonist

number of compartments representing theoretical spaces with calculated volumes.

2. A **two-compartment model** can be used to illustrate basic concepts of pharmacokinetics that also apply to more complex models (Fig. 1–1).

   a. A drug is injected intravenously into the **central compartment** and subsequently distributes to the **peripheral compartment,** only to return eventually to the central compartment where clearance from the body occurs.

   b. Any residual drug present in the peripheral compartment at the time of repeat intravenous injection will diminish the effect of redistribution on the decrease in plasma concentration and result in

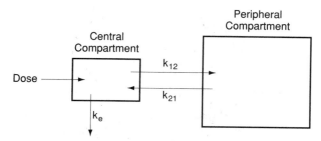

FIGURE 1–1. A two-compartment pharmacokinetic model as derived from a biexponential plasma decay curve (see Fig. 1–2). K_{12} and K_{21} are the rate constants that characterize intercompartmental transfer of drugs, and k_e is the rate constant for overall drug elimination from the body. (From Stanski DR, Watkins WD. Drug disposition in anesthesia. New York, Grune and Stratton, 1982; with permission.)

exaggerated (**cumulative**) effects of the repeat dose.

- B. **Plasma Concentration Curves.** A graphic plot of the plasma concentration of a drug (logarithms permit plotting a large range) vs. time following its rapid intravenous injection characterizes the **distribution phase** (passage of the drug from the central compartment to peripheral compartments) and **elimination phase** (drug clearance from the central compartment, principally by renal and hepatic mechanisms) of that drug (Fig. 1–2).
  1. **Elimination half-time** is the time necessary for the plasma concentration of a drug to decrease 50% during the elimination phase.
  2. **Context-sensitive half-time** describes the time necessary for the plasma concentration to decrease 50% after terminating an infusion of a particular duration. In contrast to elimination half-time, which reflects only elimination from the central compartment, the context-sensitive half-time describes multicompartment pharmacokinetics.
     - a. As the duration of continuous intravenous infusion increases, the context-sensitive half-time increases (thiopental and fentanyl more than propofol) reflecting the influence of duration of administration on passage of drug into peripheral compartments that can subsequently reenter the circulation (central compartment) and maintain the plasma concentration.

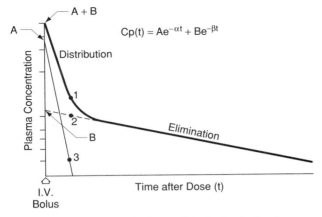

FIGURE 1–2. Schematic depiction of the decline in the plasma concentration of drug with time following rapid intravenous injection into the central compartment (see Fig. 1-1). Two distinct phases (biexponential) that characterize this curve are designated as the distribution (alpha) and elimination (beta) phases. (From Stanski DR, Watkins WD. Drug disposition in anesthesia. New York, Grune and Stratton, 1982; with permission.)

      b. Elimination half-time may be of no value in characterizing disposition of intravenous anesthetic drugs during dosing periods relevant to anesthesia.

  C. Route of Administration and Systemic Absorption of Drugs (Table 1-2). Systemic absorption, regardless of the route of drug administration, largely depends on the drug's solubility.

  D. Distribution of Drugs Following Systemic Absorption

    1. Following systemic absorption of a drug, the highly perfused tissues (heart, brain, lungs, kidneys, liver) receive a disproportionately large amount of the total dose (Table 1-3).

      a. As the plasma concentration of drug decreases below that in highly perfused tissues, the drug leaves these tissues to be **redistributed** to less well-perfused sites, such as skeletal muscles and fat (manifests as prompt awakening after a single dose of a drug).

      b. Repeated or single large doses of drug may saturate

Table 1–2
Route of Administration and Systemic Absorption of Drugs

Route	Absorption Characteristics
Oral	Large surface area of the small intestine provides principal site of absorption; first-pass effect at the liver may decrease the amount of drug delivered to the systemic circulation
Oral transmucosal (sublingual, buccal, nasal mucosa)	Hepatic first-pass effect does not occur
Transdermal	Provides sustained therapeutic plasma concentrations
Rectal	
Parenteral (subcutaneous, intramuscular, intravenous)	Rapid and precise drug delivery is best achieved by intravenous administration

Table 1–3
Body Tissue Compartments

	Body Mass (percent of 70-kg adult)	Blood Flow (percent of cardiac output)
Vessel-rich group	10	75
Muscle group	50	19
Fat group	20	6
Vessel-poor group	20	<1

inactive tissue sites, thus negating the role of these tissues in providing an inactive site for redistribution. When this occurs, the duration of action of drugs, such as thiopental and fentanyl, is likely to be prolonged as waning of drug effect now depends on metabolism rather than redistribution.

2. **Central nervous system distribution** of drugs is restricted by limited permeability characteristics of brain capillaries (blood–brain barrier).

3. **Volume of distribution (Vd)** of a drug is a mathematical expression (dose of drug administered intravenously divided by the resulting plasma concentration) that depicts the distribution characteristics of a drug in the body.
   a. Binding to plasma proteins and poor lipid solubility limit passage of a drug to tissues, thus maintaining a high concentration in the plasma and a small calculated Vd (nondepolarizing neuromuscular blocking drugs).
   b. A lipid-soluble drug that is highly concentrated in tissues with a resulting low plasma concentration will have a calculated Vd that exceeds total body water (thiopental, diazepam).
4. Solubility characteristics of **ionized and nonionized molecules** determine the ease with which drugs may diffuse through lipid components of cell membranes (Table 1–4).
5. **Ion trapping** reflects a concentration difference of total drug on two sides of a membrane that separates fluids with different pHs (ionized fraction cannot freely cross and is trapped) (Fig. 1–3).
6. **Protein binding** has an important effect on distribution of drugs because only the unbound fraction is readily available to cross cell membranes (large Vd), gain access to hepatic microsomal enzymes, and undergo renal clearance.
   a. Most acidic drugs bind to albumin, whereas basic drugs are more likely to bind to alpha-1 acid glycoprotein.

Table 1–4
Characteristics of Nonionized and Ionized Drug Molecules

	Nonionized	*Ionized*
Pharmacologic effects	Active	Inactive
Solubility	Lipids	Water
Cross lipid barriers (gastrointestinal tract, blood–brain barrier, placenta)	Yes	No
Renal excretion	No	Yes
Hepatic metabolism	Yes	No

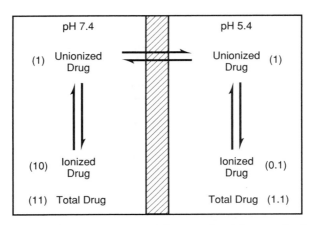

FIGURE 1–3. A concentration difference of total drug can develop on two sides of a membrane that separates fluids with different pHs. At steady state, the nonionized (unionized) drug concentration on both sides of the membrane is similar, but the concentration of ionized drug differs. (From Hug CC. Pharmacokinetics of drugs administered intravenously. Anesth Analg 1978;57:704–23; with permission.)

   b. The extent of protein binding parallels lipid solubility.
   E. Clearance of Drugs from the Systemic Circulation
   1. Clearance is the volume of plasma cleared of drug by renal excretion and/or metabolism in the liver or other organs.
      a. First-order kinetics is clearance of the drug in proportion to the amount of drug present in the plasma.
      b. Zero-order kinetics is clearance of a constant amount of drug from the plasma per unit of time.
   2. Clearance is one of the most important pharmacokinetic variables to be considered when defining a constant drug infusion regimen. To maintain an unchanging plasma concentration of drug, the intravenous infusion rate must be equal to the rate of drug clearance.
   3. Hepatic clearance may depend principally on hepatic blood flow (**perfusion-dependent elimination**) or hepatic enzyme activity (**capacity-dependent elimination**).

    4. Renal clearance of water-soluble compounds is more efficient than for compounds with high lipid solubility (hepatic metabolism converts lipid-soluble drugs to water-soluble metabolites).

      a. Drug elimination by the kidneys is inversely related to the serum creatinine concentration.

      b. The magnitude of increase in the serum creatinine concentration provides an estimate of the necessary downward adjustment in drug dosage.

F. Metabolism of Drugs

    1. The role of metabolism is to convert pharmacologically active, lipid-soluble drugs into water-soluble and often (not always) pharmacologically inactive metabolites.

    2. Microsomal enzymes responsible for metabolism of many drugs are located in the liver (principal site), kidneys, gastrointestinal tract, lungs, brain, vascular endothelium, and adrenal cortex.

      a. Microsomal enzymes include an iron-containing protein termed **cytochrome P-450.**

      b. Increased microsomal enzyme activity produced by drugs or chemicals is known as **enzyme induction.**

      c. If drug metabolism occurs at sites in addition to the liver, the clearance rates are likely to exceed hepatic blood flow.

G. Dose Response Curves (Fig. 1–4)

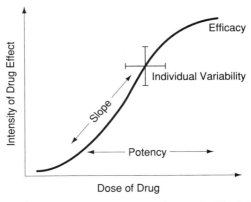

FIGURE 1–4. Dose-response curves are characterized by differences in potency, slope, efficacy, and individual responses.

Table 1–5
Events Responsible for Variations in Drug Responses Between Individuals

Pharmacokinetics
Bioavailability
Renal function
Liver function
Cardiac function
Patient age

Pharmacodynamics
Enzyme activity
Genetic differences

Drug Interactions

1. The **potency** of a drug makes little difference as long as the effective dose of the drug can be administered conveniently.
2. The **slope** of the dose-response curve is influenced by the number of receptors that must be occupied before a drug effect occurs.
   a. The slope is steep if a drug must occupy the majority of receptors before a drug effect occurs (a characteristic of neuromuscular blocking drugs and inhaled anesthetics).
   b. When the slope is steep, small increases in dose evoke intense increases in drug effect (see Section VIA4).
3. The **efficacy** of a drug (intrinsic activity) may be limited if the dose needed to achieve desirable effects is similar to that which produces undesirable effects (narrow therapeutic index).
4. **Individual responses** to a drug may vary as a reflection of differences in pharmacokinetics and pharmacodynamics among patients (Table 1-5).
   a. In **elderly patients,** variations in drug response most likely reflect decreased cardiac output, increased fat compartment, decreased protein binding, and decreased renal function.
   b. **Genetic differences** may be manifested as variations in drug responses owing to altered receptor sensitivity, changes in metabolic pathways (rapid vs. slow acetylators) and pharmacogenetics (atypical cholinesterase, malignant hyperthermia).

IV. PHARMACODYNAMICS OF INJECTED DRUGS

A. **Receptors** are often protein macromolecules in the lipid bilayer of cell membranes that exist for endogenous regulatory substances, such as hormones and neurotransmitters (see Chapter 39, Section V).

   1. A drug administered as an exogenous substance is an **incidental "passenger"** for these receptors.

   2. Receptors are often **classified** on the basis of effects of specific antagonists and by the relative potencies of known agonists (alpha, beta, mu, nicotinic).

   3. The concentration of receptors in the cell membrane is dynamic, either increasing **(up-regulation)** or decreasing **(down-regulation)** in response to specific stimuli (see Chapter 39, Section VB).

B. **Plasma drug concentrations** are a reliable monitor of therapy only when interpreted in parallel with the clinical course of the patient.

   1. Typically, there is a direct relationship between the dose of drug administered, the resulting plasma concentration, and the intensity of drug effect (receptor concentration).

   2. An initial loading dose is necessary to establish promptly a therapeutic plasma concentration of drug; this is then followed by a lower maintenance dose to match clearance of drug from the plasma.

      a. Intermittent doses result in abrupt increases, followed by decreases, in the plasma concentrations of drug such that a therapeutic plasma level is not sustained.

      b. Continuous variable-rate intravenous infusion of a drug is more likely than intermittent drug injections to match clearance of the drug, thus maintaining the plasma concentration in a therapeutic range, without the wide oscillations characteristic of intermittent administration.

V. PHARMACOKINETICS OF INHALED ANESTHETICS

A. Pharmacokinetics of inhaled anesthetics describes their absorption (uptake from alveoli into pulmonary capillary blood), distribution in the body, metabolism, and elimination, principally via the lungs.

   1. A series of partial pressure gradients beginning at the anesthetic machine serve to propel the inhaled anesthetic across various barriers (alveoli, capillaries, cell

Table 1–6
*Factors Determining Partial Pressure Gradients Necessary for
Establishment of Anesthesia*

***Anesthetic Input (Transfer of Inhaled Anesthetic from
Anesthetic Machine to Alveoli)***
Inspired partial pressure
    Concentration effect
    Second-gas effect
Alveolar ventilation
Characteristics of anesthetic breathing system

***Anesthetic Loss (Transfer of Inhaled Anesthetic from Alveolar
to Arterial Blood)***
Solubility (blood:gas partition coefficient)
Cardiac output
Alveolar-to-venous partial pressure difference

***Anesthetic Loss (Transfer of Inhaled Anesthetic from Arterial
Blood to Tissues)***
Solubility (brain:blood partition coefficient)
Cerebral blood flow
Arterial-to-venous partial pressure difference

---

    membranes) to their sites of action in the central nervous system (Table 1–6).
2. The principal objective of inhalation anesthesia is to achieve a constant and optimal brain partial pressure of the inhaled anesthetic.
3. The alveolar partial pressure (PA) of an inhaled anesthetic mirrors the brain partial pressure (Pbr) (Fig. 1–5).
    a. As a result, the PA is an indirect measurement of the Pbr.
    b. This is the reason that PA is used as an index of

$$P_A \rightleftharpoons P_a \rightleftharpoons P_{br}$$

FIGURE 1–5.   The alveolar partial pressure (*PA*) of an inhaled anesthetic is in equilibrium with the arterial blood (*Pa*) and brain (*Pbr*). As a result, the PA is an indirect measurement of anesthetic partial pressure at the brain.

the depth of anesthesia, recovery from anesthesia, and anesthetic equal potency (MAC).

B. Determinants of Alveolar Partial Pressure

1. The PA and, ultimately, the Pbr of an inhaled anesthetic are determined by **input (delivery) into alveoli minus uptake (loss)** of the drug from alveoli into arterial blood (Table 1-6).

2. **Inhaled partial pressure (PI)** is high during initial administration of anesthetic to offset uptake from alveoli into the arterial blood; it is then decreased during maintenance of anesthesia to match the decreased uptake as tissues accumulate anesthetic.

   a. **Concentration effect** is the principle that the higher the PI, the more rapidly the PA approaches the PI (more input to offset uptake).

   b. A range of PI sufficient to produce a concentration effect is possible only with nitrous oxide.

   c. **Second-gas effect** is the ability of high-volume uptake of one gas (the first gas, which is always nitrous oxide) to accelerate the rate of increase of the PA of a concurrently administered companion gas (second gas, such as oxygen and/or volatile anesthetics).

3. **Alveolar ventilation,** like PI, promotes input of anesthetics to offset uptake.

4. **Anesthetic breathing system** characteristics that influence the rate of increase of the PA are the volume of the external breathing system (acts as a buffer to slow achievement of the PA) and the gas inflow from the anesthetic machine (high gas flow rates [5-10 L·min^{-1}] negate the buffer effect of nonanesthetic gases in the anesthetic breathing system).

5. **Solubility** of inhaled anesthetics in blood and tissues is denoted by the partition coefficient (distribution ratio describing how the inhaled anesthetic distributes itself between two phases at equilibrium [when the partial pressures of the anesthetic in these two phases are identical]) (Table 1-7).

   a. **Blood:gas partition coefficients** determine the rate of increase of the PA (induction of anesthesia) relative to a constant PI (Fig. 1-6).

   b. Blood can be considered a pharmacologically inactive reservoir, the size of which is determined by the solubility of the anesthetic in blood.

(text continues on page 18)

Table 1-7
Comparative Solubilities of Inhaled Anesthetics

	Blood: Gas Partition Coefficient	Brain: Blood Partition Coefficient	Muscle: Blood Partition Coefficient	Fat: Gas Partition Coefficient	Oil: Gas Partition Coefficient
Soluble					
Methoxyflurane	12	2.0	1.3	48.8	970
Intermediate Solubility					
Halothane	2.4	1.9	3.4	51.1	224
Enflurane	1.8	1.3	1.7	36.2	98
Isoflurane	1.4	1.6	2.9	44.9	98
Poorly Soluble					
Nitrous oxide	0.46	1.1	1.2	2.3	1.4
Desflurane	0.42	1.3	2.0	27.2	18.7
Sevoflurane	0.65	1.7	3.1	47.5	55

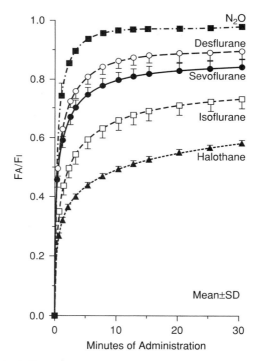

FIGURE 1–6. The pharmacokinetics of inhaled anesthetics during induction of anesthesia is defined as the ratio of end-tidal anesthetic concentration (F_A) to the inspired anesthetic concentration (F_I). Consistent with their relative blood:gas partition coefficients, the F_A/F_I of poorly soluble anesthetics (nitrous oxide, desflurane, sevoflurane) increases more rapidly than that of anesthetics with greater solubility. A decrease in the rate of change in the F_A/F_I after 10 to 15 minutes (three time constants) reflects decreased tissue uptake of the anesthetic as the vessel-rich group tissues become saturated. (From Yasuda N, Lockhart SH, Eger EI, et al. Comparison of kinetics of sevoflurane and isoflurane in humans. Anesth Analg 1991;72:316–24; with permission.)

    c. When blood solubility is low (as with nitrous oxide, desflurane, or sevoflurane), minimal amounts of an inhaled anesthetic must be dissolved in the blood before equilibrium is reached; thus, the induction of anesthesia (rate of increase of the PA) is rapid (Fig. 1–6).

    d. Tissue : blood partition coefficients determine uptake of anesthetic into tissues and the time necessary (three time constants) for equilibration of tissues with the arterial blood (Pa).

    e. Nitrous oxide transfer to closed gas spaces reflects the greater solubility (34 times) of nitrous oxide relative to nitrogen. As a result, nitrous oxide can leave the blood to enter an air-filled cavity 34 times more rapidly than nitrogen can leave the cavity to enter blood. Depending on the compliance of the walls surrounding the air cavity, there is an increased volume (gastrointestinal tract, pneumothorax, air bubbles) or pressure (middle ear) in the air cavity.

    f. Despite the ability of nitrous oxide to diffuse rapidly into an air bubble, there is no evidence that 50% inhaled nitrous oxide has a measurable effect on the incidence or severity of venous air embolism if the administration of nitrous oxide is discontinued immediately upon Doppler ultrasound detection of the venous air embolism.

    g. The volume of venous air embolism necessary to elicit a positive response with precordial Doppler ultrasound and transesophageal echocardiography is not different in the presence or absence of nitrous oxide.

6. Cardiac output influences uptake and, therefore, PA by carrying away more or less anesthetic from alveoli.

    a. Decreased cardiac output speeds the rate of increase of the PA (induction of anesthesia) because there is less uptake to oppose input.

    b. Left-to-right tissue shunts offset the dilutional effect of **right-to-left shunts** on the Pa.

7. Alveolar-to-venous partial pressure differences reflect tissue uptake of the inhaled anesthetic.

    a. After about three time constants, approximately 75% of the returning venous blood is at the same partial pressure as the PA.

    b. For this reason, uptake of a volatile anesthetic is

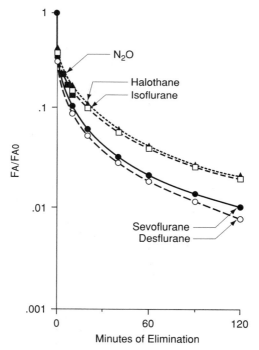

FIGURE 1–7. Elimination of inhaled anesthetics is defined as the ratio of the end-tidal anesthetic concentration (F_A) to the FA immediately before the beginning of elimination (F_{AO}). The rate of decrease (awakening from anesthesia) in the F_A/F_{AO} is most rapid with the anesthetics that are least soluble (nitrous oxide, desflurane, sevoflurane). (From Yasuda N, Lockhart SH, Eger EI, et al. Comparison of kinetics of sevoflurane and isoflurane in humans. Anesth Analg 1991;72:316–24, with permission.)

decreased greatly, as reflected by a narrowing of the inspired-to-alveolar partial pressure difference (Fig. 1–6).

C. **Recovery from anesthesia** is depicted by the rate of decrease in the Pbr as reflected by the PA (similar but not identical to induction of anesthesia) (Fig. 1–7).

1. Failure of certain tissues to reach equilibrium with the PA of the inhaled anesthetic during maintenance of

anesthesia (influenced by the duration of administration and tissue solubility of the inhaled anesthetic) means that the rate of decrease of the PA during recovery from anesthesia will be more rapid than the rate of increase of the PA during induction of anesthesia.

a. Metabolism of anesthetics with high blood and tissue solubility (halothane) speeds the rate of decrease in the PA, whereas the rate of decrease of the PA of less blood-soluble inhaled anesthetics (isoflurane, desflurane, sevoflurane) during recovery from anesthesia is entirely dependent on alveolar ventilation.

b. As predicted from its low blood gas solubility, the initial emergence and postoperative recovery of mental function (also the patient's presumed ability to maintain a patent upper airway) from desflurane anesthesia are more rapid than with isoflurane (although, depending on hospital policy, the time to discharge from the Postanesthesia Care Unit may not be shorter).

c. Emergence and early recovery after maintenance of anesthesia with sevoflurane/nitrous oxide (with or without intravenous induction of anesthesia with propofol) are more rapid than in patients anesthetized with isoflurane/nitrous oxide (Fig. 1–8).

d. Duration of anesthesia has a decreased impact on recovery from desflurane compared with other volatile anesthetics, reflecting the low tissue solubility of desflurane.

e. The solubility properties of desflurane and sevoflurane in blood and tissues permit more precise control of anesthetic depth and more rapid recovery from anesthesia than do volatile anesthetics with greater solubility.

f. The **awakening concentration** of anesthesia (end-tidal concentration present when patients open their eyes on request) decreases as patient age increases.

g. Aging delays elimination of inhaled anesthetic and increases the apparent volume of distribution at steady state (compatible with decreased tissue perfusion and an increase in the ratio of fat to lean body weight in the elderly).

2. Diffusion hypoxia reflects dilution of the PAO_2 (decrease in PaO_2 by about 10%) by the outpouring of

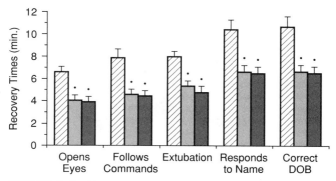

FIGURE 1–8. Times (mean ± SEM) from discontinuation of the maintenance anesthetic (*hatched bars:* propofol, isoflurane, nitrous oxide; *light shaded bars:* propofol, sevoflurane, nitrous oxide; *solid bars:* sevoflurane, nitrous oxide) until patients could open their eyes, follow commands, undergo tracheal extubation, respond to their names, and give their correct date of birth (DOB). (From Smith I, Ding Y, White PF. Comparison of induction, maintenance, and recovery characteristics of sevoflurane-N_2O and propofol-sevoflurane-N_2O with propofol-isoflurane-N_2O anesthesia. Anesth Analg 1992;74:253–9; with permission.)

nitrous oxide from the blood into the alveoli at the conclusion of anesthesia when the PI of nitrous oxide is abruptly decreased to zero. Filling the lungs with oxygen at the end of anesthesia will ensure that arterial hypoxemia will not occur as a result of the dilution of the PAO_2 by nitrous oxide.

VI. PHARMACODYNAMICS OF INHALED ANESTHETICS

A. Minimum Alveolar Concentration (MAC)

1. MAC of an inhaled anesthetic is defined as that concentration at 1 atmosphere that prevents skeletal muscle movement in response to a supramaximal painful stimulus (surgical skin incision) in 50% of patients (Table 1–8).

   a. MAC is age-dependent, being lowest in newborns, reaching a peak in infants 6 to 12 months of age, and then decreasing progressively with increasing age (Fig. 1–9).

Table 1–8
*Comparative Minimum Alveolar Concentration (MAC)
of Inhaled Anesthetics*

	MAC (30 to 55 years old, 37 C, PB 760 mmHg)
Nitrous oxide*	104%
Desflurane	6.3%
Sevoflurane	2.0%
Halothane	0.74%
Enflurane	1.68%
Isoflurane	1.15%
Methoxyflurane	0.16%

*Determined in a hyperbaric chamber in males 21 to 35 years old.

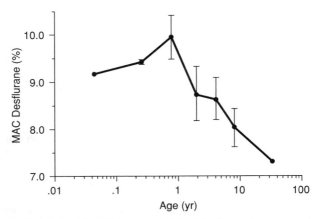

FIGURE 1–9.   The MAC (mean ± SD) of desflurane in neonates, infants, children, and adults. (From Taylor RH, Lerman J. Minimum alveolar concentration of desflurane and hemodynamic responses in neonates, infants, and children. Anesthesiology 1991;75:975-9; with permission.)

    b. MAC is decreased following a single dose of fentanyl, 3 $\mu g \cdot kg^{-1}$ IV, but increasing the dose to 6 $\mu g \cdot kg^{-1}$ IV produces little further decrease in MAC (Fig. 1–10).

    c. The MAC for skin incisions cannot be used to predict concentrations of anesthetic necessary to suppress motor responses to other noxious stimuli (tracheal intubation requires higher concentrations) (Fig. 1–11).

    d. MAC BAR is the anesthetic concentration that prevents the adrenergic response to skin incision in 50% of patients.

    e. A volatile anesthetic alone is unable to suppress hemodynamic responses (blood pressure and heart rate) in response to painful stimuli, such as tracheal intubation. A "normal" blood pressure following such stimulation can be achieved only if prestimulation blood pressure is depressed to levels that may be clinically unacceptable.

    f. Although it has been assumed that duration of anesthesia has no influence on MAC, there is evidence that MAC (based on motor response to electrical tetanic stimulation) decreases during the administration of anesthesia and the performance of surgery (Fig. 1–12).

2. The fact that the alveolar concentration reflects the partial pressure at the site of anesthetic action (brain) has made MAC the most useful index of anesthetic equal potency.

    a. Similar MAC concentrations of inhaled anesthetics produce equivalent depression of the central nervous system (one point on the dose-response curve), whereas effects on other organ systems (cardiopulmonary parameters) may be different for each drug, emphasizing that dose-response curves for effects of different inhaled anesthetics on organ systems other than the brain are not parallel (see Chapter 2).

    b. Use of MAC allows a quantitative analysis of the effect, if any, of various pharmacologic and physiologic factors on anesthetic requirements (Table 1–9).

3. MAC values for inhaled anesthetics are additive (0.5 MAC nitrous oxide plus 0.5 MAC isoflurane has the same effect on the central nervous system as 1-MAC isoflurane).

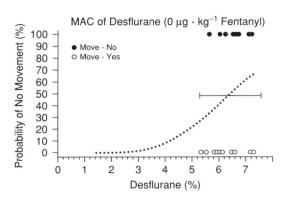

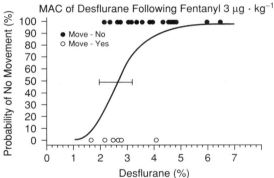

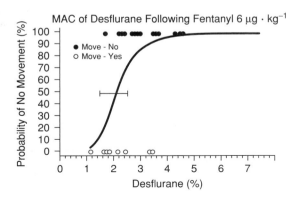

   a. In adults, MAC for a volatile anesthetic is decreased about 1% for every 1% alveolar nitrous oxide that is administered concomitantly.

   b. The MAC-reducing effect of nitrous oxide in children is attenuated in the presence of less soluble anesthetics (60% nitrous oxide decreases MAC 60%, 40%, 20%, and 24% for halothane, isoflurane, desflurane, and sevoflurane, respectively).

4. The steep nature of the dose-response curves for inhaled anesthetics is emphasized by the fact that 1 MAC prevents movement in 50% of patients, whereas a modest increase to 1.3 MAC prevents movement in at least 95% of patients. Likewise, there may be small differences between the doses of volatile anesthetics that produce desirable degrees of central nervous system depression and undesirable degrees of cardiac depression.

B. Mechanisms of Anesthesia

1. **Meyer-Overton Theory (Critical Volume Hypothesis)**

   a. Correlation between lipid solubility of inhaled anesthetics and MAC suggests that anesthesia occurs when a sufficient number of molecules dissolve in lipid cell membranes.

   b. Conceptually, expansion of cell membranes by dissolved anesthetic molecules could distort channels necessary for sodium ion flux and the subsequent development of action potentials necessary for synaptic transmission.

2. **Protein Receptor Hypothesis**

   a. Evidence for protein receptors in the central nervous system as a site and mechanism of action of inhaled anesthetics is suggested by the steep dose-response curve (MAC) for inhaled anesthetics (crucial degree of receptor occupancy).

   b. The stereospecificity of the MAC-reducing effects of dexmedetomidine suggests the presence of a homeogenous receptor population (activation of

◄ **FIGURE 1–10.** The probability of movement versus the desflurane concentration with or without fentanyl (3 or 6 μg · kg⁻¹ IV). (From Sebel PS, Glass PSA, Fletcher JE, Murphy MR, Gallagher C, Quill T. Reduction of MAC of desflurane with fentanyl. Anesthesiology 1992; 76:52–9; with permission.)

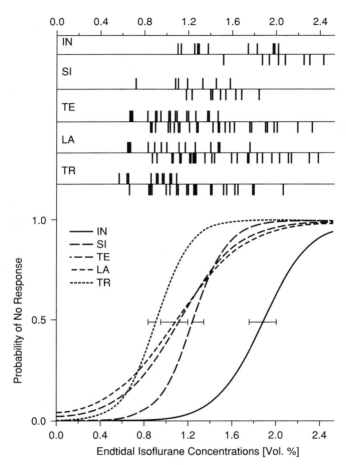

FIGURE 1–11.   Responses (movement [horizontal line above] or no movement [horizontal line below]) to preoperative stimulation represented by tracheal intubation (*IN*), skin incision (*SI*), response to a continuous (tetanus) electrical stimulation (*TE*), direct laryngoscopy (*LA*), and trapezious squeeze (*TR*). The probability of response versus endtidal isoflurane concentration is plotted. (From Zbinden AM, Maggiorini M, Petersen-Felix S, Lauber R, Thomson DA, Minder CE. Anesthetic depth defined using multiple noxious stimuli during isoflurane/oxygen anesthesia. I. Motor reactions. Anesthesiology 1994;80:253–60; with permission.)

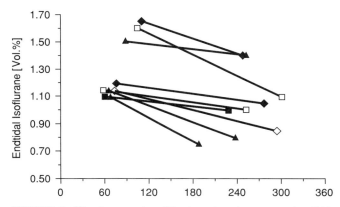

FIGURE 1–12. Preoperative (60 minutes) and postoperative (180 to 300 minutes) individual MAC determinations using continuous electrical stimulation (MAC tetanus). Each line represents an individual patient. (From Petersen-Felix S, Zbinden AM, Fischer M, Thomson DA. Isoflurane minimum alveolar concentration decreases during anesthesia and surgery. Anesthesiology 1993;79:959–65; with permission.)

an inhibitory guanine [G] protein to increase potassium ion conductance with resulting hyperpolarization of cell membranes).

3. Activation of Gamma-Aminobutyric Acid (GABA$_A$) Receptors
   a. Volatile anesthetics and injected anesthetics may activate GABA$_A$ channels (hyperpolarize cells), inhibit certain calcium channels (prevents release of neurotransmitters) and inhibit glutamate channels (Fig. 1–13) and Table 1–10.
   b. As such, volatile anesthetics share common cellular actions with sedative-hypnotics (GABA$_A$ receptors) and analgesics (calcium channels) (Fig. 1–13).
   c. Evidence of stereoselectivity is evidence for a direct anesthetic action on specific protein receptors and not a generalized bilayer effect (nevertheless, phospholipids of the membrane bilayer are all one stereoisomer).

4. Neurobiologic Basis for Anesthesia
   a. A neurobiologic basis for the hypnotic and sedative effects of anesthetic drugs (volatile anesthetics, bar-
   (text continued on page 30)

Table 1–9
Impact of Physiologic and Pharmacologic Factors on Minimum Alveolar Concentration (MAC)

Increase in MAC
Hyperthermia
Hypernatremia
Drug-induced increases in CNS catecholamine stores

Decrease in MAC
Hypothermia
Hyponatremia
Pregnancy
Lithium
Lidocaine
Opioids (intravenous, ?neuraxial)
PaO_2 <38 mmHg
Systemic blood pressure <40 mmHg
Increasing age
Preoperative medication
Drug-induced decreases in CNS catecholamine stores
Alpha-2 agonists
Acute alcohol ingestion
Cardiopulmonary bypass (?)
Increasing duration of anesthesia (?)

No Change in MAC
Hyperkalemia or hypokalemia
Anesthetic metabolism
Chronic alcohol abuse
Thyroid gland dysfunction
Gender
$PaCO_2$ of 15–95 mmHg
PaO_2 >38 mmHg
Blood pressure >40 mmHg

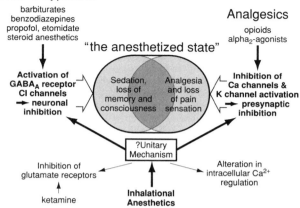

FIGURE 1–13. The major pathways for sedative-hypnotics and analgesics in generating the anesthetized state considered to be characteristic of volatile anesthetics. (From Lynch C, Pancrazio JJ. Snails, spiders and stereospecificity—Is there a role for calcium channels in anesthetic mechanisms? Anesthesiology 1994;81:1–5; with permission.)

Table 1–10
Anesthetics Enhance Gamma-aminobutyric Acid (GABA) Inhibition by Different Mechanisms

Drugs	*Mechanism*
Benzodiazepines	Enhance inhibition by increasing binding of endogenously released GABA
Barbiturates Etomidate Propofol Volatile anesthetics	Enhance inhibition by modifying the receptor/chloride channel such that it remains open longer after binding endogenously released GABA
Volatile anesthetics	Inhibit GABA disposal
Alpha-adrenergic agonists	Enhance presynaptic release of GABA

(Adapted from Tanelin DL, Kosek P, Mody I. MacIver MB. The role of the GABA$_A$ receptor/chloride channel complex in anesthesia. Anesthesiology 1993;78:757–75.)

biturates, benzodiazepines, propofol, etomidate) is their ability to activate $GABA_A$ chloride channels, resulting in cell hyperpolarization (preventing depolarization and thereby inhibiting neuronal activity) (Fig. 1–13).

b. Actions at the $GABA_A$ receptor may account for drug-induced unconsciousness.

c. Sedative-hypnotics or analgesics alone do not produce a complete anesthetic state, whereas a combination of a benzodiazepine, propofol, or barbiturate with an opioid or alpha-2 agonist can produce an anesthetic state equivalent to that achieved by a volatile anesthetic alone (Fig. 1–13).

Chapter

2

Inhaled Anesthetics

Inhaled anesthetics currently used clinically include the inorganic gas nitrous oxide and the volatile liquids halothane, enflurane, isoflurane, desflurane, and sevoflurane (Fig. 2-1 and Table 2-1). (Updated and revised from Stoelting RK. Inhaled anesthetics. In: Pharmacology and Physiology in Anesthetic Practice. 2nd ed. Philadelphia, JB Lippincott, 1991:33-69.)

I. INTRODUCTION

A. Volatile anesthetics are halogenated methyl ethyl ether derivatives, with the exception of halothane, which is a halogenated alkane derivative.
1. Halogenation provides nonflammability (fluorine) and molecular stability (trifluorocarbon atom).
2. When fluorine is the only halogen present (desflurane), there is often an associated decrease in blood solubility and potency, an increase in vapor pressure, and a resistance to metabolism.
3. Volatile anesthetics exist as clear, nonflammable liquids at room temperature and are delivered to the patient as a vapor.
B. Low blood : gas solubility characteristic of nitrous oxide, desflurane, and sevoflurane contributes to the rapid onset of (alveolar partial pressure [PA]) and recovery from the effects of these inhaled anesthetics (see Table 1-7 and Figs. 1-6 and 1-7).

II. COMPARATIVE PHARMACOLOGY

A. Inhaled anesthetics often evoke differing pharmacologic effects at comparable MAC concentrations (dose-response curves may not be parallel).
B. Measurements obtained from healthy volunteers exposed to equal potent concentrations of inhaled anesthetics have provided the basis of comparison for pharmacologic effects of these drugs on various organ

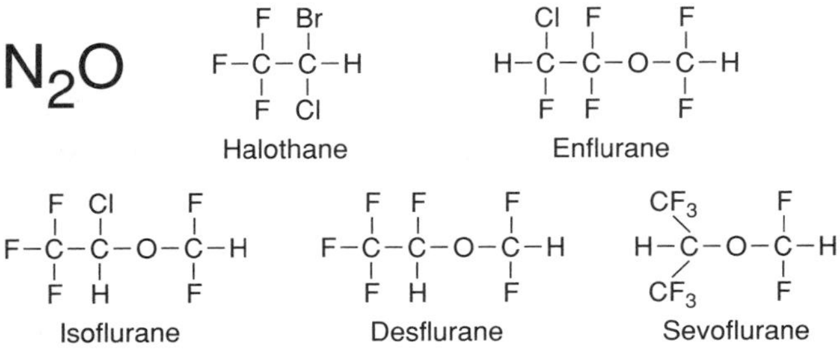

FIGURE 2–1. Inhaled anesthetics.

systems. In this regard, it is important to recognize that surgically stimulated patients who have other confounding variables may respond differently than healthy volunteers (Table 2–2).

III. CENTRAL NERVOUS SYSTEM EFFECTS

A. **Electroencephalogram (EEG).** As the dose of volatile anesthetic approaches 1 MAC, the frequency on the EEG decreases and maximum voltage occurs.

  1. **Seizure activity** may accompany the administration of enflurane, especially if the dose is higher than 2 MAC or when hyperventilation of the lungs decreases the $PaCO_2$ to lower than 30 mmHg.

  2. **Evoked potentials** are decreased in amplitude and the latencies are increased in a dose-dependent manner by volatile anesthetics.

B. **Cerebral Blood Flow**

  1. Volatile anesthetics that are administered in concentrations higher than 0.6 MAC produce dose-dependent increases in cerebral blood flow (halothane > enflurane, isoflurane, desflurane, sevoflurane) despite concomitant decreases in cerebral metabolic oxygen requirements (Fig. 2–2).

  2. Nitrous oxide also increases cerebral blood flow, but its restriction to concentrations lower than 1 MAC may limit the magnitude of this change (there is also evidence that nitrous oxide is a more potent cerebral vasodilator than isoflurane in an equivalent dose).

(text continues on page 35)

Table 2–1
Physical and Chemical Properties of Inhaled Anesthetics

	Nitrous Oxide	Halothane	Enflurane	Isoflurane	Desflurane	Sevoflurane
Molecular weight	44	197	184	184	168	200
Specific gravity (25 C)		1.86	1.52	1.50	1.47	1.53
Boiling point (C)		50.2	56.5	48.5	22.8	58.6
Vapor pressure (mmHg, 10 C)	Gas	244	172	240	669	170
Odor	Sweet	Organic	Ethereal	Ethereal	Ethereal	Ethereal
Pungency	None	None	Moderate	Moderate	Moderate	None
Antioxidant necessary	No	Yes (thymol)	No	No	No	No
Stability						
Soda lime	Yes	No	Yes	Yes	Yes	No
Sunlight	Yes	No	Yes	Yes	Yes	Yes
Reacts with metal	No	Yes	No	No	No	No

Table 2–2
*Variables that Influence the Pharmacologic Effects
of Inhaled Anesthetics*

Anesthetic concentration

Spontaneous vs. controlled ventilation

Variations from normocapnia

Surgical stimulation

Patient age

Coexisting disease

Concomitant drug therapy

Intravascular fluid volume

Preoperative medication

Injected drugs to induce and/or maintain anesthesia or skeletal
  muscle relaxation

Alterations in body temperature

Rate of increase in the alveolar concentration

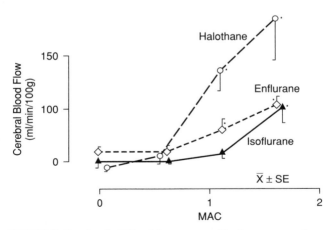

FIGURE 2–2. Cerebral blood flow measured in the presence of nor-
mocapnia and in the absence of surgical stimulation. $P < 0.05$. (From
Eger EI. Isoflurane [Forane]: a compendium and reference. 2nd ed.
Madison, WI, Ohio Medical Products, 1985:1–110; with permission.)

3. Anesthetic-induced increases in cerebral blood flow occur within minutes and are independent of blood pressure changes, emphasizing the cerebral-vasodilating effects of these drugs. Subsequent normalization of cerebral blood flow (which, in animals, occurs within 30 to 150 minutes) reflects a concomitant increase in cerebral vascular resistance.

4. Autoregulation of cerebral blood flow may be impaired by inhaled anesthetics (halothane > isoflurane).

5. Inhaled anesthetics do not alter the responsiveness of the cerebral circulation to changes in $PaCO_2$.

C. **Cerebral Metabolic Oxygen Requirements**

1. Inhaled anesthetics produce dose-dependent decreases in cerebral metabolic oxygen requirements (isoflurane > halothane) that are maximal when the EEG becomes isoelectric.

2. The greater decrease in cerebral metabolic oxygen requirements produced by isoflurane may explain why cerebral blood flow is not predictably increased by this anesthetic at concentrations lower than 1.1 MAC (less carbon dioxide is produced, which opposes any increase in cerebral blood flow).

3. **Cerebral protection** is not predictably provided by volatile anesthetics, although isoflurane may favorably alter the global cerebral oxygen supply-demand balance (as a result of unchanged cerebral blood flow and decreased cerebral metabolic oxygen requirements).

D. **Intracranial Pressure**

1. Inhaled anesthetics produce increases in intracranial pressure that parallel the increases in cerebral blood flow produced by these drugs.

2. Patients with space-occupying intracranial lesions are most vulnerable to drug-induced increases in intracranial pressure.

3. Hyperventilation of the lungs to decrease the $PaCO_2$ to about 30 mmHg opposes the tendency for inhaled anesthetics to increase intracranial pressure (institute hyperventilation before introduction of halothane and at the same time as introduction of isoflurane).

E. **Cerebrospinal fluid production** is increased by enflurane but not by nitrous oxide or isoflurane.

F. **Conscious memory** is suppressed by volatile anesthetics (0.45 MAC isoflurane) and nitrous oxide (0.6 MAC). These concentrations are similar to **MAC awake.**

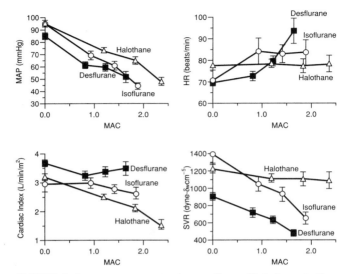

FIGURE 2–3. Comparative circulatory effects of halothane, isoflurane, and desflurane as determined in healthy adult male volunteers. *MAP,* mean arterial pressure; *HR,* heart rate; *SVR,* systemic vascular resistance. (Modified from Weiskopf RB, Cahalan MK, Eger EI, et al. Cardiovascular actions of desflurane in normocarbic volunteers. Anesth Analg 1991;73:143–56; with permission.)

IV. CIRCULATORY EFFECTS

A. Blood Pressure

1. Volatile anesthetics produce dose-dependent and similar decreases in blood pressure, whereas nitrous oxide produces either no change or modest increases in blood pressure (Fig. 2-3).
2. Surgical stimulation and substitution of nitrous oxide for a portion of the volatile anesthetic decreases the magnitude of blood pressure decrease produced by volatile anesthetics (Fig. 2-4).
3. The decrease in blood pressure produced by halothane and enflurane is attributable principally to decreases in myocardial contractility, whereas decreases produced by isoflurane, desflurane, and sevoflurane are principally the result of decreases in systemic vascular resistance.

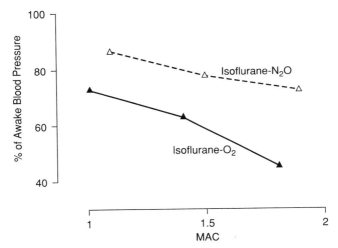

FIGURE 2–4. The substitution of N_2O for a portion of isoflurane produces less depression of blood pressure than the same dose of volatile anesthetic alone. (From Eger EI. Isoflurane [Forane]. A compendium and reference. 2nd ed. Madison, WI, Ohio Medical Products, 1985;1–110; with permission.)

4. Preoperative increases in blood pressure owing to apprehension may be followed by decreases in blood pressure that exceed the true pharmacologic effect of the volatile anesthetic.

B. Heart Rate
1. Halothane and sevoflurane are not associated with changes in heart rate despite decreases in blood pressure, suggesting depression of the carotid sinus (baroreceptor) reflex response by the volatile anesthetic (Fig. 2–3). Junctional rhythm and associated decreases in blood pressure most likely reflect suppression of sinus node activity by halothane.
2. In contrast to halothane and sevoflurane, heart rate tends to increase during isoflurane- or desflurane-induced decreases in blood pressure, suggesting improved preservation of the carotid sinus reflex response.
   a. Heart rate increases are dose-dependent, occurring at low doses of isoflurane and high doses of desflurane.

      b. Opioids and advanced age may be associated with blunting of the heart rate response.

      c. Enhanced heart rate responses may occur in young patients and in the presence of drugs with vagolytic effects.

C. Cardiac Output and Stroke Volume

    1. Halothane and enflurane produce dose-dependent decreases in cardiac output owing to decreases in myocardial contractility; by contrast, isoflurane, desflurane, and sevoflurane are not associated with significant decreases in cardiac output despite concomitant decreases in blood pressure (Fig. 2–3).

    2. Cardiac output is modestly increased by nitrous oxide, possibly reflecting a mild sympathomimetic effect of this drug.

    3. In addition to improved maintenance of heart rate (offsetting decreased stroke volume), the minimal depressant effects of some volatile anesthetics on cardiac output could reflect activation of homeostatic mechanisms that obscure direct cardiac depressant effects (all volatile anesthetics are direct myocardial depressants in vitro).

    4. Another possible explanation for the decreased impact of isoflurane, desflurane, and sevoflurane on myocardial contractility may be the greater anesthetic potency of these drugs relative to halothane or enflurane (more readily depress the brain and thus, at a given MAC value, appear to spare the heart).

D. Right Atrial Pressure

    1. Inhaled anesthetics produce dose-dependent increases in right atrial pressure.

    2. Increased right atrial pressure during administration of nitrous oxide most likely reflects increased pulmonary vascular resistance owing to sympathomimetic effects of this drug.

E. Systemic (Peripheral) Vascular Resistance

    1. Isoflurane, desflurane, and sevoflurane produce dose-dependent decreases in calculated systemic vascular resistance that parallel decreases in blood pressure produced by these drugs (Fig. 2–3).

      a. Substitution of nitrous oxide for a portion of the volatile anesthetic decreases the magnitude of decrease in systemic vascular resistance produced by these drugs.

      b. Decreases in systemic vascular resistance during administration of isoflurane, but not desflurane, reflect substantial (up to fourfold) increases in **skeletal-muscle blood flow.**

2. Failure of calculated systemic vascular resistance to decrease during administration of halothane does not mean that this drug lacks vasodilating effects on some organ systems (cerebral vasodilation, cutaneous vasodilation). These vasodilating effects of halothane are offset by absent changes or vasoconstriction in other vascular beds such that the overall effect is an unchanged calculated systemic vascular resistance.

3. The increase in **cutaneous blood flow** produced by all volatile anesthetics arterializes peripheral venous blood, providing an alternative to sampling arterial blood for evaluation of pH and $PaCO_2$.

F. Pulmonary Vascular Resistance

1. Volatile anesthetics appear to exert little or no predictable effect on pulmonary vascular smooth muscle.

2. Nitrous oxide may produce increases in pulmonary vascular resistance, especially in patients with preexisting hypertension.

G. Duration of Administration

1. Administration of a volatile anesthetic for 5 hours or longer is accompanied by recovery from depressant circulatory effects (return of cardiac output toward a normal level, increased heart rate, peripheral vasodilation) compared with measurements at 1 hour.

   a. Blood pressure is unchanged with time as increases in cardiac output are offset by decreases in systemic vascular resistance.

   b. Evidence of recovery from cardiovascular effects with time is most apparent during administration of halothane and least apparent during administration of isoflurane (a predictable outcome since cardiac output is not significantly decreased and heart rate is increased at 1 hour).

2. The return of cardiac output toward predrug levels with time, in association with an increase in heart rate and peripheral vasodilation, resembles a beta-agonist response.

H. Cardiac Dysrhythmias

1. The ability of volatile anesthetics to decrease the dose of epinephrine necessary to evoke ventricular cardiac dysrhythmias is greatest with halothane (consistent with its alkane structure) and least with en-

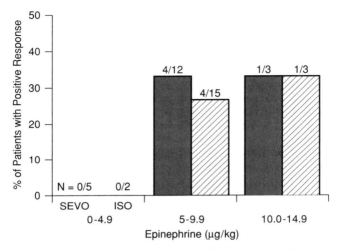

FIGURE 2–7. Responses to submucosally injected epinephrine in 40 patients receiving sevoflurane (SEVO) or isoflurane (ISO) anesthesia. (From Navarro R, Weiskopf RB, Moore MA, et al. Humans anesthetized with sevoflurane or isoflurane have similar arrhythmic response to epinephrine. Anesthesiology 1994;80:545–9; with permission.)

creased incidence of myocardial ischemia during administration of isoflurane compared with other volatile anesthetics or opioids.

a. More important than the anesthetic drug selected in the subsequent development of myocardial ischemia is the prevention of sustained and excessive decreases in blood pressure and/or increases in heart rate (higher than 110 beats·min^{-1} seems to be particularly undesirable in patients with coronary artery disease).

b. It is estimated that as many as two thirds of the episodes of perioperative myocardial ischemia are unrelated to hemodynamic abnormalities (**silent ischemia**).

J. Spontaneous Breathing

1. Circulatory effects produced by volatile anesthetics during spontaneous breathing are different from those observed during normocapnia and controlled ventilation of the lungs.

2. This difference may reflect the impact of sympathetic

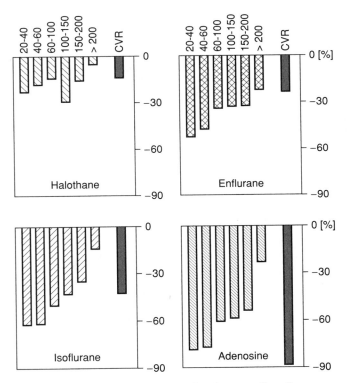

FIGURE 2–8. Changes in segmental resistances of small coronary arterial vessels and of total coronary vascular resistance (CVR) are depicted in the presence of volatile anesthetics and adenosine. The drugs were administered to a canine model in doses sufficient to maintain the mean arterial pressure at 60 mmHg. (From Conzen PF, Habazettl H, Vollmar B, Christ M, Baier H, Peter K. Coronary microcirculation during halothane, enflurane, isoflurane, and adenosine in dogs. Anesthesiology 1992;76:261–70; with permission.)

Table 2–3
*Preexisting Diseases and Drug Therapy Affecting the
Circulatory Effects of Inhaled Anesthetics*

Diseased cardiac muscle in which contractility is decreased even
  before administration of depressant anesthetics

Aortic stenosis and possible adverse effects of peripheral
  vasodilation

Prior drug therapy that alters sympathetic nervous system activity or
  decreases myocardial contractility

nervous system stimulation owing to accumulation of
carbon dioxide and improved venous return during
spontaneous breathing.

  K. Preexisting Disease and Drug Therapy. The signifi-
     cance of circulatory effects produced by inhaled anes-
     thetics (Table 2-3) may be influenced by preexisting
     diseases and drug therapy.
  L. Mechanisms of Circulatory Effects
     1. There is no single mechanism that explains the de-
        pressant circulatory effects of volatile anesthetics in
        all situations (Table 2-4).
     2. Plasma catecholamine concentrations typically do
        not increase during administration of volatile anes-
        thetics, providing evidence that these drugs do not
        activate, and may even decrease, activity of the cen-
        tral and peripheral sympathetic nervous system.
        a. Nitrous oxide produces signs of mild sympatho-
           mimetic stimulation (mydriasis, diaphoresis, in-
           creased body temperature, cutaneous vasocon-
           striction) associated with increases in the plasma
           concentrations of catecholamines.
        b. Isoflurane (and possibly desflurane and sevo-

Table 2–4
Mechanisms of Circulatory Effects from Inhaled Anesthetics

Direct myocardial depression

Inhibition of central nervous system sympathetic outflow

Peripheral autonomic ganglion blockade

Attenuated carotid sinus reflex activity

Decreased formation of cyclic adenosine monophosphate

Decreased influx of calcium ions through slow channels

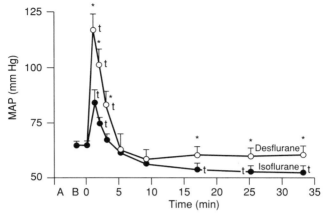

FIGURE 2–9. An abrupt and sustained increase in the concentration of desflurane from 0.55 MAC to 1.66 MAC (0) resulted in a substantial but transient increase in mean arterial pressure (MAP). A similar increase in isoflurane MAC produced an increase in MAP that was substantially less than that observed in patients receiving desflurane. Within 5 minutes after increasing the anesthetic concentration, the MAP had decreased below awake (A) and baseline values at 0.55 MAC (B) reflecting the greater depth of anesthesia present at this time. (From Weiskopf RB, Moore MA, Eger EI, et al. Rapid increase in desflurane concentration is associated with greater transient cardiovascular stimulation than with rapid increase in isoflurane concentration in humans. Anesthesiology 1994;80:1035–45; with permission.)

flurane) may possess mild beta-agonist properties evidenced by maintenance of cardiac output, increased heart rate, and decreased systemic vascular resistance.

M. Rate of Change in Delivered Concentration

1. A rapid increase in the MAC of desflurane increases sympathetic nervous system activity (catecholamine release), heart rate, and blood pressure more than does an equivalent increase in the MAC of isoflurane (Figs. 2–9 and 2–10).

2. Small increases in desflurane concentration to greater than 6% are more likely to cause transient increases in heart rate, blood pressure, and plasma epinephrine concentration than are similar 1% increases in desflurane concentration below 5%.

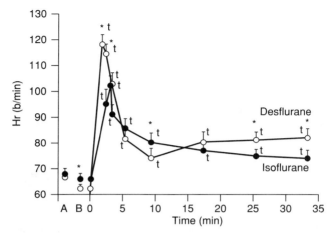

FIGURE 2–10. An abrupt and sustained increase in the concentration of desflurane from 0.55 MAC to 1.66 MAC (0) resulted in a substantial but transient increase in heart rate (HR). A similar increase in isoflurane MAC produced an increase in HR that was substantially less than that observed in patients receiving desflurane. Within 5 minutes after increasing the anesthetic concentration, the HR had remained above awake (A) and baseline values at 0.55 MAC (B), reflecting the greater depth of anesthesia present at this time. (From Weiskopf RB, Moore MA, Eger EI, et al. Rapid increase in desflurane concentration is associated with greater transient cardiovascular stimulation than with rapid increase in isoflurane concentration in humans. Anesthesiology 1994;80:1035–45; with permission.)

3. It is speculated that the rapid increase in anesthetic concentration stimulates medullary centers via irritant receptors in the airway, resulting in transient increases in sympathetic nervous system activity.
4. The transient nature of the response may be due to adaptation to the stimulus combined with a direct depressant effect of higher concentrations of the volatile anesthetic.
5. Administration of fentanyl, esmolol, or clonidine 5 minutes before an abrupt increase in anesthetic concentration blunts evidence of cardiovascular stimulation. Fentanyl 1.5 to 4.5 ug·kg^{-1} may be the most clinically useful of these drugs because it blunts the increase in heart rate and blood pressure, has minimal cardiovascular depressant effects, and produces little postanesthetic sedation.

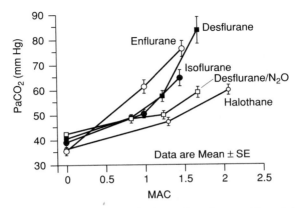

FIGURE 2–11. Volatile anesthetics produce drug-specific and dose-dependent increases in $PaCO_2$ during spontaneous breathing.

V. VENTILATION EFFECTS

A. Pattern of Breathing

1. Inhaled anesthetics produce dose-dependent increases in the frequency of breathing (isoflurane similar to halothane) in association with decreases in tidal volume.

2. The increase in the frequency of breathing is insufficient to offset decreases in total volume, leading to decreases in minute ventilation and increases in $PaCO_2$ (Fig. 2-11).

3. The net effect of these changes is a rapid, regular (in contrast to the awake pattern of intermittent deep breaths separated by varying intervals), and shallow pattern of breathing during general anesthesia.

B. Ventilatory Response to Carbon Dioxide

1. Volatile anesthetics produce dose-dependent depression of ventilation characterized by decreases in the ventilatory response to carbon dioxide and increases in $PaCO_2$ (Fig. 2-11).

   a. Isoflurane is a more profound depressant of ventilation than halothane (volume of ventilation decreases and $PaCO_2$ increases more as a reflection of a greater depression of central neural drive to breathing produced by isoflurane compared to halothane) (Fig. 2-12).

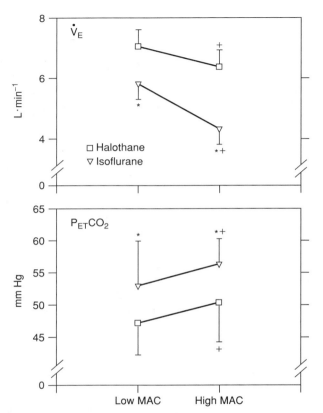

FIGURE 2–12.   Minute ventilation ($\dot{V}_E$) and end-tidal carbon dioxide concentration ($P_{ET}CO_2$), as measured in volunteers breathing halothane or isoflurane in oxygen spontaneously at 1.2 (low) and 2.0 (high) minimum alveolar concentration (MAC). (From Canet J, Sanchis J, Zegri A, Llorente C, Navajas D, Casan P. Effects of halothane and isoflurane on ventilation and occlusion pressure. Anesthesiology 1994;81:563-71; with permission.)

   b. Nitrous oxide does not increase the $PaCO_2$, suggesting that substitution of this anesthetic for a portion of the volatile anesthetic would result in less depression of ventilation.
   c. Surgical stimulation increases minute ventilation about 40% but decreases PCO_2 only about 10%, presumably reflecting increased carbon dioxide production owing to painful stimulation and activation of the sympathetic nervous system.
   d. Duration of administration. After about 5 hours of administration, the increase in $PaCO_2$ produced by volatile anesthetics is less than that present during administration of the same concentration for 1 hour.
  2. The slope of the carbon dioxide response curve is decreased similarly and shifted to the right by anesthetic concentrations of all inhaled anesthetics, including nitrous oxide.
  3. Subanesthetic concentrations (0.1 MAC) of inhaled anesthetics do not alter the ventilatory response to carbon dioxide.
C. Mechanism of Depression
  1. Anesthetic-induced depression of ventilation, as reflected by increases in the $PaCO_2$, most likely reflects direct depressant effects of these drugs on the medullary ventilatory center (central neural drive to breathing).
  2. An additional mechanism may be the ability of halothane and possibly other inhaled anesthetics to interfere selectively with intercostal muscle function, contributing to loss of chest wall stabilization during spontaneous breathing.
D. Management of Depression
  1. The predictable ventilatory depressant effects of volatile anesthetics are most often managed by institution of mechanical ventilation of the lungs.
  2. Assisted ventilation of the lungs is a questionably effective method for counteracting the ventilatory depressant effects of volatile anesthetics, as the apneic threshold (maximal $PaCO_2$ level that does not initiate spontaneous breathing) is only 3 to 5 mmHg lower than the $PaCO_2$ that is present during spontaneous breathing.
E. Ventilatory Response to Hypoxemia
  1. All inhaled anesthetics, including nitrous oxide, pro-

foundly depress (0.1 MAC produces 50% to 70% depression) the ventilatory response to arterial hypoxemia that is normally mediated by the carotid bodies (contrasts with absence of significant depression of the ventilatory response to carbon dioxide in the presence of subanesthetic concentrations).

2. Inhaled anesthetics also attenuate the usual synergistic effect of arterial hypoxemia and hypercapnia on stimulation of ventilation.

F. Airway Resistance

1. In the absence of bronchoconstriction, the bronchodilating effects of volatile anesthetics are difficult to demonstrate because normal bronchomotor tone is low and only minimal additional relaxation is possible.

   a. Volatile anesthetics produce dose-dependent and similar decreases in airway resistance in an animal model.

   b. Relaxant effects of halothane and albuterol on airway smooth muscle are additive, suggesting that the anesthetic acts principally by decreasing afferent vagal nerve traffic from the central nervous system.

2. It has not been documented that the bronchodilating effects of volatile anesthetics are an effective method for treating status asthmaticus that is unresponsive to more conventional treatments.

3. **Desflurane** is an airway irritant as reflected by an increased incidence of coughing and laryngospasm when this drug is administered to unmedicated patients for inhalation induction of anesthesia (limits the rate at which this drug can be delivered).

   a. The addition of nitrous oxide and/or an opioid does not seem to greatly improve the acceptability of desflurane for inhalation induction.

   b. Desflurane is unlikely to replace halothane (and possibly sevoflurane) as the drug of choice for inhalation induction.

VI. HEPATIC EFFECTS

A. Hepatic Blood Flow

1. Isoflurane and desflurane may maintain hepatic oxygen delivery at a more optimal level than halothane, based on measurements of portal vein blood flow and hepatic artery blood flow in animals (Fig. 2–13).

2. Hepatic blood flow tends to decrease, especially at

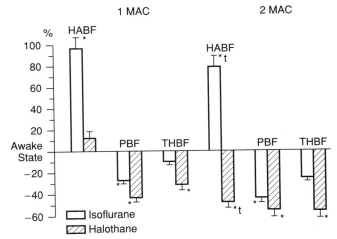

FIGURE 2–13. Changes (%, mean ± SE) in hepatic blood flow during administration of isoflurane or halothane. Decreases in portal vein blood flow (PBF) produced by 1 MAC isoflurane are offset by increases in hepatic artery blood flow (HABF) (autoregulation) such that total hepatic blood flow (THBF) is better maintained during low-dose isoflurane than during low-dose halothane anesthesia. Autoregulation of THBF via changes in HABF is attenuated or absent during 2 MAC isoflurane or halothane anesthesia. (From Gelman S, Fowler KC, Smith LR. Liver circulation and function during isoflurane and halothane anesthesia. Anesthesiology 1984;61:726–30; with permission.)

                deep levels, as a consequence of a decrease in portal venous (but not hepatic arterial) blood flow.

3. During exposure to an inhaled anesthetic, maintenance of hepatic oxygen delivery relative to demand may be important as hepatocyte hypoxia is a significant mechanism in the multifactorial etiology of postoperative hepatic dysfunction.

B. Drug Clearance. Volatile anesthetics may interfere with clearance of drugs (lidocaine, propranolol) from the plasma as a result of decreases in hepatic blood flow or inhibition of drug-metabolizing enzymes.

C. Liver Function Tests. Changes in liver function tests evoked by inhaled anesthetics are not usually clinically important.

Table 2–5
Halothane Hepatotoxicity

Mild Self-Limited Postoperative Hepatotoxicity

Transient increases in plasma transaminase enzyme concentrations

A nonspecific drug effect owing to changes in hepatic blood flow that impair hepatocyte oxygenation

Halothane Hepatitis

Rare (1 in 10,000 to 30,000 patients) and life-threatening

Likely an immune-mediated hepatotoxicity
   Prior exposure to halothane
   Fever
   Arthralgia
   Presence of antibodies
   Genetic susceptibility

D. Hepatotoxicity

1. It is likely that **inadequate hepatocyte oxygenation** (oxygen supply relative to oxygen demand) is the principal mechanism responsible for the mild and transient hepatic dysfunction that frequently follows anesthesia and surgery.

   a. Any anesthetic that decreases alveolar ventilation and/or decreases hepatic blood flow could interfere with hepatocyte oxygenation.

   b. Preexisting liver disease (cirrhosis) may be associated with marginal hepatocyte oxygenation, which would be jeopardized further by the depressant effects of anesthetics on arterial oxygenation and/or hepatic blood flow.

2. **Halothane** is speculated to produce two types of hepatotoxicity (Table 2–5).

   a. In those rare, genetically susceptible patients who develop halothane hepatitis, a reactive oxidative trifluoroacetyl halide metabolite of halothane (not a reductive metabolite) is presumed to acetylate liver proteins which, in effect, changes these proteins from self to nonself (neoantigens).

   b. Antibodies formed against neoantigens result in liver injury.

   c. Antibodies are detectable in the plasma of about 70% of patients who develop halothane hepatitis.

   d. Fatal halothane hepatitis is estimated to occur in 1 in every 110,000 anesthetics.

3. **Enflurane and Isoflurane**
   a. Mild, self-limited postoperative hepatic dysfunction that is associated with enflurane or isoflurane most likely reflects anesthetic-induced alterations in hepatic oxygen delivery relative to demand, resulting in inadequate hepatocyte oxygenation.
   b. Rarely, there may be cross-sensitivity between all halogenated anesthetics that produce the oxidative trifluoroacetyl halide metabolite presumed to be responsible for halothane hepatitis (incidence should be less because the magnitude of metabolism compared with halothane is much less).

4. **Desflurane** is unlikely to result in formation of neoantigens from an oxidative trifluoroacetyl halide metabolite because the magnitude of metabolism of this drug is estimated to be one-tenth that of isoflurane.

VII. RENAL EFFECTS

A. Volatile anesthetics produce similar dose-dependent decreases in renal blood flow, glomerular filtration rate, and urine output that most likely reflect drug-induced decreases in cardiac output and blood pressure.
   1. **Preoperative hydration** attenuates or abolishes many of the changes in renal function associated with volatile anesthetics.
   2. Isoflurane-induced controlled hypotension does not further decrease renal blood flow (compensatory decrease in renal vascular resistance) or glomerular filtration rate compared with the decreases produced by induction of anesthesia.

B. **Nephrotoxicity**
   1. **Fluoride-induced nephrotoxicity** may be more related to intrarenal production of inorganic fluoride (greater with enflurane than sevoflurane) than hepatic metabolism (determines plasma inorganic fluoride concentrations).
   2. Prolonged anesthesia (longer than 9 MAC hours) with sevoflurane (mean peak plasma inorganic fluoride concentration of 47 $\mu M \cdot L^{-1}$) or enflurane (mean peak plasma inorganic fluoride concentration of 23 $\mu M \cdot L^{-1}$) does not impair renal concentrating function, as evidenced by the results of desmopressin testing 1 and 5 days postanesthesia (Fig. 2-14).
   3. Metabolism of other volatile anesthetics to inorganic fluoride is insufficient to cause nephrotoxicity.

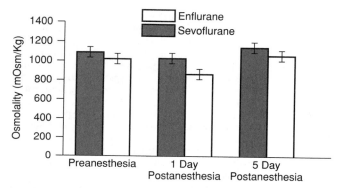

FIGURE 2–14.   Maximal urinary osmolalities (mean ± SEM) in 14 adult male volunteers following administration of desmopressin before and following prolonged administration (more than 9 MAC hours) of enflurane or sevoflurane. (From Frank EJ, Malan TP, Isner RJ, Brown EA, Morgan SE, Brown BR. Renal concentrating function with prolonged sevoflurane or enflurane anesthesia in volunteers. Anesthesiology 1994;80:1019–25; with permission.)

VIII. SKELETAL MUSCLE EFFECTS

    A. Enflurane, isoflurane, desflurane, and sevoflurane produce skeletal muscle relaxation that is about twofold greater than that associated with a comparable dose of halothane.

        1. Nitrous oxide does not relax skeletal muscles and, in combination with opioids, may be associated with skeletal muscle rigidity.

        2. Volatile anesthetics produce dose-dependent enhancement of the effects of neuromuscular blocking drugs, with the effects of enflurane, isoflurane, desflurane, and sevoflurane being similar and greater than those of halothane.

    B. Volatile anesthetics can trigger malignant hyperthermia, but halothane is most potent in this regard. Nitrous oxide, compared with volatile anesthetics, is a weak trigger for malignant hyperthermia.

IX. OBSTETRIC EFFECTS

    A. Volatile anesthetics produce similar and dose-dependent decreases (modest at analgesic concentrations) in uterine smooth muscle contractility and blood flow.

B. Nitrous oxide does not alter uterine contractility in doses used to provide analgesia during vaginal delivery.

C. Uterine relaxation produced by volatile anesthetics may be either desirable (facilitating removal of a retained placenta) or undesirable (increased blood loss).

X. RESISTANCE TO INFECTION

A. Immune changes seen in surgical patients are primarily the result of surgical trauma and endocrine responses (increased catecholamines and corticosteroids) rather than an effect of the anesthetic.

B. Inhaled anesthetics, particularly nitrous oxide, produce dose-dependent inhibition of polymorphonuclear leukocytes and their subsequent migration **(chemotaxis.)**

    1. Chemotaxis is necessary for the inflammatory response to infection.

    2. Decreased resistance to bacterial infection owing to inhaled anesthetics seems unlikely considering the duration of administration and dose of these drugs.

XI. GENETIC EFFECTS

A. In animals, nitrous oxide, but not volatile anesthetics, causes an increased incidence of fetal resorptions.

    1. Nitrous oxide irreversibly oxidizes the cobalt atom of **vitamin B_{12}-dependent enzymes** (methionine synthetase necessary for the formation of myelin and the thymidylate synthetase necessary for the formation of DNA).

    2. Volatile anesthetics do not alter the activity of vitamin B_{12}-dependent enzymes.

B. The speculated but undocumented role of trace concentrations of nitrous oxide in the production of spontaneous abortions has led to the use of scavenging systems designed to remove anesthetic gases, including nitrous oxide, from the operating room.

XII. BONE MARROW FUNCTION

A. Interference with DNA synthesis is responsible for the megaloblastic changes and agranulocytosis that may follow prolonged administration of nitrous oxide.

B. It is presumed that a healthy surgical patient could receive nitrous oxide for 24 hours without harm.

Table 2–6
Anesthetics Absorbed and Recovered as Metabolites

Anesthetic	Metabolites
Nitrous oxide	0.004%
Halothane	15%–20%
Enflurane	2.4%
Isoflurane	0.2%
Desflurane	0.02%
Sevoflurane	3%

XIII. PERIPHERAL NEUROPATHY. Humans who chronically inhale nitrous oxide for nonmedical purposes may develop a sensorimotor polyneuropathy that is often combined with signs of posterior and lateral spinal cord degeneration resembling pernicious anemia.

XIV. TOTAL BODY OXYGEN REQUIREMENTS

    A. Volatile anesthetics decrease total body oxygen requirements in similar amounts, presumably owing to their metabolic depressant effects as well as to the patient's decreased functional needs in the presence of anesthetic-produced depression of organ function.

    B. Oxygen requirements of the heart decrease more than those of other organs, reflecting drug-induced decreases in cardiac work associated with decreases in blood pressure and myocardial contractility.

XV. METABOLISM

    A. Metabolism of inhaled anesthetics may result in organ toxicity (liver, kidneys, reproductive organs) and may influence the rate of decrease in the PA when an anesthetic is discontinued. There is no impact on PA during induction of anesthesia because inhaled anesthetics are administered in great excess of the amount metabolized. (Table 2–6; see Fig. 1–7; see Section VI D1–4).

    B. Determinants of Metabolism (Table 2–7)

    C. Nitrous oxide. An estimated 0.004% of an absorbed dose of nitrous oxide undergoes reductive metabolism to nitrogen in the gastrointestinal tract.

Table 2–7
Determinants of Metabolism of Inhaled Anesthetics

Chemical Structure

Ether bond and carbon-halogen bond are the most likely sites of oxidative metabolism.

Two halogen atoms on a terminal carbon are optimal for dehalogenation.

A terminal carbon with three fluorine atoms is very resistant to metabolism.

Hepatic Enzyme Activity

Blood Concentrations

Subanesthetic concentrations undergo extensive metabolism.

Solubility in Blood and Tissues

Poorly soluble anesthetics tend to be exhaled rather than passed through the liver.

Soluble anesthetics are stored in tissues that act as reservoirs for continued passage through the liver.

Genetic Factors

   D. Halothane
   1. The principal oxidative end metabolites of halothane are trifluoroacetic acid, chloride, and bromide (plasma concentrations of bromide increase 0.5 mEq·L^{-1} for every MAC hour of halothane administration).
   2. A reductive metabolite of halothane is fluoride.
   E. Enflurane undergoes oxidative metabolism to inorganic fluoride and organic fluoride compounds.
   F. Isoflurane undergoes minimal oxidative metabolism to trifluoroacetic and fluoride (peak plasma concentration of less than 5 μM·L^{-1}).
   G. Desflurane undergoes minimal oxidative metabolism (estimated to be one-tenth that of isoflurane) to trifluoroacetic acid.
   H. Sevoflurane metabolism to inorganic fluoride resembles that of enflurane.
   1. Sevoflurane is degraded to fluoromethyl-2, 2-difluoro-1-(trifluoromethyl) vinyl ether (an olefin also known as compound A) in the presence of carbon dioxide absorbent (soda lime and baralyme) and heat (higher than 65°C).

2. Double-bonded breakdown products, such as compound A, can irreversibly bind to tissue macromolecules, potentially resulting in major organ toxicity (no evidence this occurs clinically).
3. In rodents, the lethal concentration of compound A is 400 ppm (using a 750 mL·min^{-1} flow rate, the average concentration of compound A is 8 ppm [soda lime] or 20 ppm [baralyme]).

Chapter

3

Opioid Agonists and Antagonists

Opioid refers to all exogenous substances, natural and synthetic, that bind specifically to any of several subpopulations of opioid receptors and produce at least some agonist (morphine-like) effects (Table 3–1). (Updated and revised from Stoelting RK. Opioid agonists and antagonists. In: Pharmacology and Physiology in Anesthetic Practice. 2nd ed. Philadelphia, JB Lippincott, 1991;70–101.)

I. STRUCTURE ACTIVITY RELATIONSHIPS

A. The alkaloids of opium can be divided into two distinct chemical classes: phenanthrenes and benzylisoquinolines (Figs. 3–1 and 3–2).

B. A close relationship exists between stereochemical structure and potency of opioids, with levorotatory isomers being the most active.

II. MECHANISM OF ACTION

A. Opioids act as agonists at stereospecific opioid receptors present at presynaptic and postsynaptic sites in the central nervous system and peripheral nervous system.

1. Opioid receptors belong to a superfamily of guanine-protein coupled receptors (which also includes muscarinic, adrenergic, and gamma-aminobutyric acid receptors) that constitutes 80% of all known receptors.

a. Opioid receptors have been cloned and their amino acid sequence defined.

b. Based on cloning of opioid receptors, it may be possible to develop opioid agonists and antagonists that react with specific receptor subtypes.

2. Opioid binding sites are categorized as **mu, kappa, and delta receptors** (sigma receptors are not nalox-

      3. Activation of opioid receptors (binding of an exoge-
nous opioid agonist or endogenous ligand) inhibits
the presynaptic release of excitatory neurotransmitters
from terminals of nerves carrying nociceptive activity
(results in hyperpolarization of the neuron due to increased potassium conductance and/or calcium channel inactivation).

  B. Opioids do not alter responsiveness of afferent nerve endings to noxious stimulation, nor do they impair conduction of nerve impulses along peripheral nerves.

III. OPIOID RECEPTORS (Table 3-2)

  A. Endogenous Pain Suppression System

    1. The obvious role of opioid receptors and endogenous
ligands is to function as an endogenous pain-suppres-
sion system.

    2. Opioid receptors are present in areas of the brain
(periaqueductal gray matter of the brain stem) and
spinal cord (substantia gelatinosa) that are involved
with pain perception, integration of pain impulses,
and responses to pain.

  B. Neuraxial Opioids

    1. Placement of opioids in the subarachnoid or epidural
space (diffuse across dura) to manage acute and/or
chronic pain is based on the knowledge that opioid
receptors are present in the substantia gelatinosa of
the spinal cord.

    2. Analgesia produced by neuraxial opioids, in contrast
to intravenous administration of opioids or regional
anesthesia, is not associated with sympathetic nervous
system denervation, skeletal muscle weakness, or loss
of proprioception.

    3. Side effects may accompany the administration of neu-
raxial opioids (Table 3-3).

    4. Clinical signs or symptoms (level of sedation,
breathing rate, pupil size) are unreliable predictors of
ventilatory depression or development of **arterial
hypoxemia** following intrathecal placement of morphine (Fig. 3-3).

      a. Pulse oximetry is useful in detecting inadequate
oxygenation following intrathecal morphine (although it may be associated with false-positive signals and frequent nursing observation is still required).

Table 3–3
Side Effects of Neuraxial Opioids

Pruritus

Urinary retention

Nausea and vomiting

Sedation

Early depression of ventilation (reflects systemic absorption of opioid from its epidural placement site)

Delayed (6 to 24 hours) depression of ventilation (reflects cephalad spread of the opioid in the cerebrospinal fluid; less likely to occur with highly lipid-soluble opioids, such as fentanyl, compared with less lipid-soluble morphine)

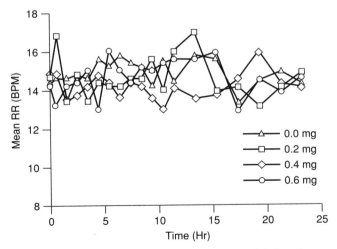

FIGURE 3–3. The respiratory rate (RR) (measured in breaths per minute [BPM]) does not reflect the dose of intrathecal morphine or the presence of depression of ventilation sufficient to result in an increase in $PaCO_2$ or a decrease in PaO_2. (From Bailey PL, Rhondeau S, Schafer PG, et al. Dose-response pharmacology of intrathecal morphine in human volunteers. Anesthesiology 1993;79:49–59; with permission.)

      b. Supplemental oxygen may be an inexpensive and practical approach for minimizing the likelihood of arterial hypoxemia after intrathecal morphine (a continuous infusion of naloxone may interfere with neuraxial analgesia).

      c. Maximum depression of ventilation occurs 3.5 to 7.5 hours after intrathecal administration of morphine (0.2 to 0.6 mg) to volunteers (could be different in surgical patients receiving other anesthetic drugs and presenting with coexisting medical diseases).

      d. Pruritus is usually the first sign and symptom indicative of central opioid action.

IV. OPIOID AGONISTS (Fig. 3-4)

  A. Morphine is the prototype opioid agonist to which all other opioids are compared. Continuous dull pain is relieved by morphine more effectively than is sharp intermittent pain. Analgesia is most prominent when morphine is administered before the painful stimulus occurs **(preemptive analgesia).**

    1. Pharmacokinetics (Table 3-4)

      a. Morphine is well absorbed following intramuscular administration (onset of effect, 15 to 30 minutes; peak effect within 45 to 90 minutes; duration of action, about 4 hours).

      b. Plasma morphine concentrations following rapid intravenous injection do not correlate closely with the opioid's pharmacologic activity (presumably reflecting a delay in penetration of morphine across the blood-brain barrier).

      c. Penetration of morphine into the central nervous system is poor (less than 0.1% of morphine administered intravenously has entered the central nervous system at the time of peak plasma concentrations), partly because of the relatively poor lipid solubility of this opioid.

      d. Morphine, unlike fentanyl, does not undergo significant first-pass uptake into the lungs.

    2. Metabolism of morphine is by conjugation with glucuronic acid in the liver and kidneys to form morphine-3-glucuronide (pharmacologically inactive) and morphine-6-glucuronide (pharmacologically active).

      a. Less than 1% to 2% of a dose of morphine is excreted

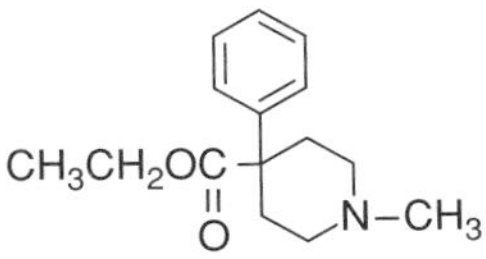

Meperidine

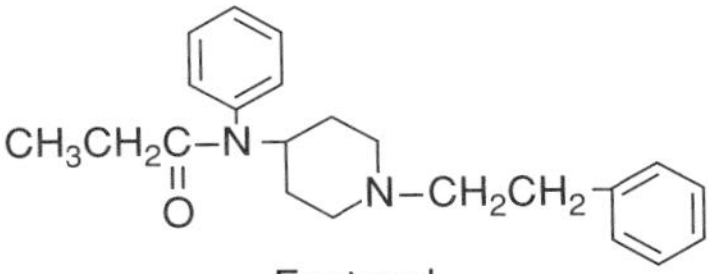

Fentanyl

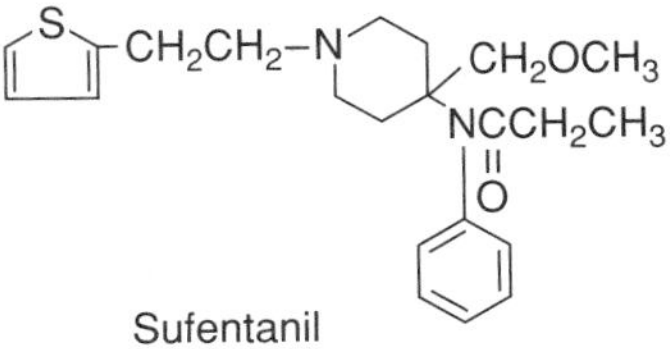

Sufentanil

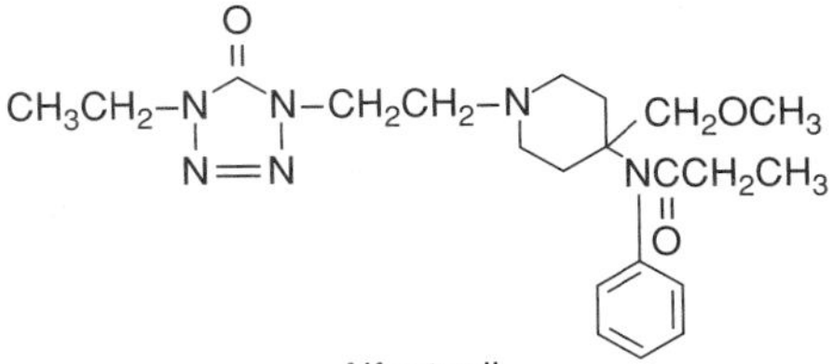

Alfentanil

FIGURE 3–4. Synthetic opioid agonists.

unchanged in the urine (compared to 4% to 6% for fentanyl, 5% to 10% for sufentanil, and less than 1% for alfentanil).

b. An estimated 33% of an administered dose of morphine undergoes nonurinary, nonhepatic metabolism (renal metabolism appears to be significantly involved in the metabolism of morphine).

c. Absence of a decrease in systemic clearance of

Table 3–4
Pharmacokinetics of Opioid Agonists and Antagonists

Opioid	pK	Protein Binding (%)	Volume of Distribution ($L \cdot kg^{-1}$)	Clearance ($mL \cdot kg^{-1} \cdot min^{-1}$)	Elimination Half-Time (min)
Morphine	7.93	26–36	3.2–3.4	15–23	114
Meperidine	8.5	64–82	2.8–4.2	10–17	180–264
Fentanyl	8.43	79–87	3.2–5.9	11–21	185–219
Sufentanil	8.01	92.5	2.86	13	148–164
Alfentanil	6.5	89–92	0.5–1	5–7.9	70–98
Remifentanil					10–21*
Naloxone			1.8	30	60–90

*Data from Westmoreland CL, Hoke JF, Sebel PS, Hug CC, Muir KT. Pharmacokinetics of remifentanil (GI87084B) and its major metabolite (G190291) in patients undergoing elective inpatient surgery. Anesthesiology 1993;79:893–903.)

d. Meperidine (1 mg·kg^{-1} IV) is more effective in treating postoperative shivering (presumably due to kappa receptor stimulation) than are equal analgesic doses of morphine and fentanyl (relatively pure mu receptor agonists).

5. Side Effects (Table 3-5)

a. Orthostatic hypotension occurs more frequently and is more profound after meperidine administration than after comparable doses of morphine.

b. Tachycardia, mydriasis and decreased myocardial contractility are characteristic responses to high doses of meperidine.

c. Delirium and seizures, when they occur, presumably reflect an accumulation of normeperidine, which has stimulating effects on the central nervous system.

d. Meperidine produces less depression of ventilation in the neonate than does morphine.

e. After equal analgesic doses, biliary tract spasm is less after meperidine injection than after morphine injection.

C. Fentanyl is a synthetic opioid agonist that is 75 to 125 times more potent than morphine.

1. Pharmacokinetics (Table 3-4)

a. The more rapid onset and shorter duration of action of fentanyl compared with morphine reflects the former's greater lipid solubility (facilitates entry into the central nervous system followed by prompt redistribution to inactive tissue sites) of fentanyl.

b. Inactive tissue sites for redistribution of fentanyl include skeletal muscles, fat, and the lungs. It is estimated that 75% of the initial fentanyl dose undergoes first-pass pulmonary uptake.

c. Multiple doses or continuous intravenous infusion of fentanyl may result in saturation of inactive tissue sites such that redistribution no longer lowers the plasma opioid concentration. In this situation, fentanyl becomes a long-acting opioid, similar to morphine.

d. There is substantial hepatic first-pass clearance of fentanyl and sufentanil and, to a lesser extent, of alfentanil; this tends to minimize the effect of enterosystemic circulation on plasma drug levels (secondary peaks).

2. Metabolism

a. Fentanyl is metabolized by N-demethylation to norfentanyl, which has decreased analgesic potency and is dependent on renal excretion.

    b. Accumulation of norfentanyl (structurally similar to normeperidine), as occurs in patients with renal failure, has been associated with poor pain control and development of acute toxic delirium.

3. Elimination Half-Time

    a. Despite the clinical impression that fentanyl has a short duration of action, its elimination half-time is longer than that of morphine (Table 3-4).

    b. This longer elimination half-time reflects a larger volume of distribution of fentanyl owing to its higher lipid solubility (reuptake from inactive tissue sites maintains the plasma concentration).

    c. Its prolonged elimination half-time in elderly patients is due to decreased clearance of fentanyl.

4. Clinical Uses. Fentanyl is administered clinically in a wide range of doses.

    a. Low doses of fentanyl (1 to 2 $\mu g \cdot kg^{-1}$ IV) are administered before surgical stimulation to provide preemptive analgesia, to blunt circulatory responses to direct laryngoscopy or sudden changes in the intensity of surgical stimulation, and to provide postoperative analgesia.

    b. Large doses of fentanyl (50 to 150 $\mu g \cdot kg^{-1}$ IV) may be used to produce surgical anesthesia in critically ill patients, providing the advantages of lack of myocardial depressant effects and absence of histamine release. Disadvantages of using fentanyl as the sole anesthetic include failure to reliably prevent sympathetic nervous system responses to surgical stimulation and possible patient awareness. Moreover, lingering postoperative depression of ventilation is predictable when large doses of any opioid are administered during anesthesia.

    c. **Transmucosal** administration (including transnasal delivery) of fentanyl is effective in decreasing anxiety in the preoperative period and facilitating induction of anesthesia, especially in children (associated with significant decreases in breathing rate and arterial hemoglobin saturation with oxygen [as measured by pulse oximetry] and a high incidence of postoperative nausea and vomiting [not prevented by prophylactic droperidol]). Bioavailability of fentanyl administered transmucosally is greater than that following oral administration owing to avoidance of the hepatic first-pass effect.

d. Transdermal fentanyl preparations result in sustained plasma concentrations of the opioid. Fever can increase transdermal absorption.

5. **Side Effects** (Table 3–5)

a. Recurrent depression of ventilation after apparent establishment of acceptable ventilation has been described in the early postoperative period in patients who have received fentanyl (also sufentanil). The cause of this secondary peak of fentanyl is undetermined, but may reflect washout of the opioid from inactive storage sites in the lungs (see Section IV C1d).

b. In comparison with morphine, fentanyl, even in large doses (50 $\mu g \cdot kg^{-1}$ IV), does not evoke the release of histamine (Fig. 3–5).

c. Bradycardia is more prominent with fentanyl than morphine.

d. Seizure activity has been described following rapid intravenous administration of large doses of fentanyl (most likely myoclonus, as the electroencephalogram [EEG] remains normal).

e. In patients with severe head trauma, the administration of fentanyl (3 $\mu g \cdot kg^{-1}$ IV) or sufentanil (0.6 $\mu g \cdot kg^{-1}$ IV) is associated with a modest increase (6 to 8 mmHg) in intracranial pressure that returns to baseline within 15 to 30 minutes. Based on these observations, caution is recommended when administering intravenous fentanyl or sufentanil rapidly to patients with decreased intracranial compliance (Fig. 3–6).

f. Cerebral blood flow velocity is increased by fentanyl and sufentanil.

g. Tonic muscle rigidity and clonic muscle activity (myoclonus) may accompany rapid administration of opioids, especially the high doses used for induction of anesthesia. Myoclonus has also been described on emergence from anesthesia. The underlying mechanism is presumed to be activation of opioid receptors in the brain stem and basal ganglia (naloxone terminates opioid-induced skeletal muscle rigidity).

D. Sufentanil is an analogue of fentanyl. The analgesic potency of sufentanil is about 12 times that of fentanyl (based

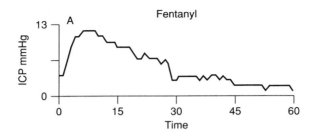

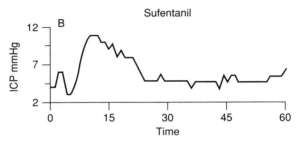

FIGURE 3–6. The time course (minutes) of changes in intracranial pressure (ICP) in a single patient following the administration (at 0 min) of fentanyl (*A*), 3 µg·kg⁻¹ IV, or sufentanil (*B*) 0.6 µg·kg⁻¹ IV, over a 1-minute period. (From Sperry RJ, Bailey PL, Reichman MV, Peterson JC, Peterson PB, Pace NL. Fentanyl and sufentanil increase intracranial pressure in head trauma patients. Anesthesiology 1992;77:416–20; with permission.)

on the plasma concentration of opioid required to produce a similar degree of slowing on the EEG). This parallels the greater affinity of sufentanil for opioid receptors compared with that of fentanyl.

1. **Pharmacokinetics** (Table 3–4)
    a. A high tissue affinity is consistent with the lipophilic nature of sufentanil, which permits rapid penetrance of the blood–brain barrier and onset of central nervous system effects.
    b. A rapid redistribution to inactive tissue sites terminates the effect of small doses, but a cumulative drug effect can accompany large or repeated doses of sufentanil.
    c. Extensive protein binding (principally alpha-1 acid

glycoprotein) of sufentanil compared with fentanyl contributes to the smaller volume of distribution characteristic of sufentanil.

  d. An increased free fraction of sufentanil due to lower concentrations of alpha-1 acid glycoprotein is consistent with the enhanced effect of this opioid in neonates.

  e. The high lipid solubility of sufentanil probably explains the altered pharmacokinetics (increased volume of distribution and prolonged elimination halftime) of this opioid in obese patients.

  f. Sufentanil (also fentanyl), but not alfentanil and morphine, undergo significant first-pass uptake into the lungs following intravenous administration.

  2. Metabolism of sufentanil to pharmacologically inactive or only weakly active metabolites is extensive, with less than 1% of an administered dose appearing unchanged in the urine.

  3. Clinical uses of sufentanil (low dose, 0.1 to 0.4 $\mu g \cdot kg^{-1}$ IV; high dose, 10 to 30 $\mu g \cdot kg^{-1}$ IV) are similar to those described for fentanyl.

E. Alfentanil is an analogue of fentanyl that is less potent (one-fifth to one-tenth) and has one-third the duration of action of fentanyl.

  1. Pharmacokinetics (Table 3-4)

  a. The smaller volume of distribution of alfentanil compared with fentanyl reflects the lower lipid solubility and higher protein binding of alfentanil.

  b. The rapid onset of action of alfentanil (which has a blood–brain equilibration time of 1.5 minutes, resulting in a three- to four-fold more rapid peak analgesic effect than fentanyl or sufentanil) is a result of the lower pK of this drug such that nearly 90% exists in the nonionized form (it readily crosses the blood–brain barrier) at physiologic pH.

  c. The brief duration of action of alfentanil is a result of redistribution to inactive tissue sites (similar to fentanyl) and hepatic metabolism. Unlike fentanyl, continuous intravenous infusion of alfentanil does not result in a significant cumulative drug effect.

  2. Metabolism of alfentanil to inactive metabolites by the liver is extensive (less than 0.5% of an administered dose is excreted unchanged in the urine) and efficient (96% of alfentanil is cleared from the plasma within 60 minutes following injection).

  a. Interindividual variability in the pharmacokinetics

of alfentanil may be attributable to individual differences in metabolism (N-dealkylation) and protein binding.

   b. Hepatic dysfunction (cirrhosis of the liver) causes greater alterations in the clearance of alfentanil than fentanyl or sufentanil.

3. Elimination Half-Time (Table 3-4)

4. Alfentanil is neither a cerebral vasodilator nor a vasoconstrictor and has not been associated with significant increases in intracranial pressure.

5. Clinical Uses

   a. Alfentanil, 150 to 300 $\mu g \cdot kg^{-1}$ IV, produces unconsciousness in about 45 seconds.

   b. Maintenance of anesthesia can be provided by a continuous infusion of alfentanil, 25 to 150 $\mu g \cdot kg^{-1} \cdot h^{-1}$ IV, combined with an inhaled drug (cumulative drug effects are unlikely, even with prolonged infusions of alfentanil).

   c. Alfentanil (because of its rapid blood–brain equilibration) may be useful for attenuating the catecholamine and cardiovascular responses to brief but intense noxious stimuli, such as tracheal intubation (Fig. 3-7).

F. Methadone

   1. Methadone is a synthetic opioid agonist that produces prolonged analgesia (elimination half-time of 35 hours) and is highly effective by the oral route (used to suppress withdrawal symptoms in addicts).

   2. Depression of ventilation by methadone resembles that of morphine, although its sedative and euphoric actions seem to be less.

G. Remifentanil is a synthetic opioid agonist that is structurally related to fentanyl, but unique among opioids because of its ester linkage (Fig. 3-8).

   1. The ester structure renders this opioid susceptible to rapid hydrolysis to inactive metabolites by blood and tissue nonspecific esterases.

   2. Remifentanil, 1 to 8 $\mu g \cdot kg^{-1} \cdot min^{-1}$ IV, is the first true ultra–short-acting opioid for use as a supplement to general anesthesia (elimination half-time of 10 to 20 minutes).

V. OPIOID AGONIST-ANTAGONISTS (Fig. 3-9)

   A. Opioid agonist-antagonists bind to mu receptors (and occasionally, kappa and delta receptors) where they produce

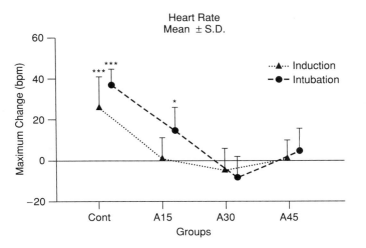

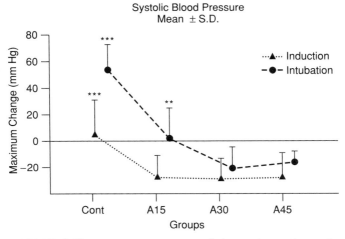

FIGURE 3–7. Dose-response curves of the maximum (percent) changes in heart rate and systolic blood pressure in response to induction of anesthesia and tracheal intubation. *CONT,* control; *A15,* 15 μg·kg^{-1} of alfentanil; *A30,* 30 μg·kg^{-1} of alfentanil; *A45,* 45 μg·kg^{-1} of alfentanil. (From Miller DR, Martineau RJ, O'Brien H, Hull KA, Oliveras L, Hindmarsh T, Greenway D. Effect of alfentanil on the hemodynamic and catecholamine response to tracheal intubation. Anesth Analg 1993;76:1040-6; with permission.)

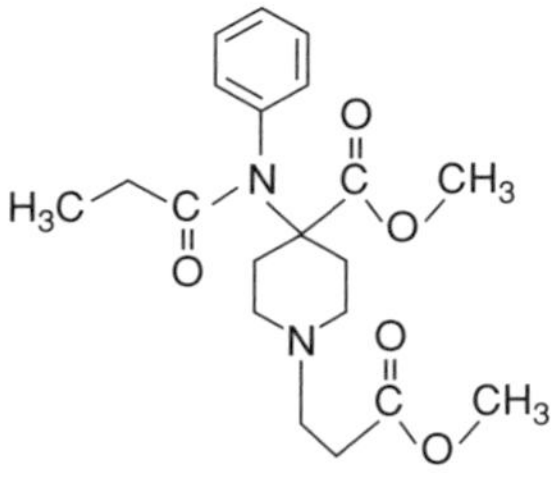

FIGURE 3–8.   Remifentanil.

limited responses (partial agonists) or no effect (competitive antagonists which can attenuate the efficacy of subsequently administered opioids).

1. Advantages of opioid agonist-antagonists include the ability to produce analgesia with limited depression of ventilation and a low potential to produce physical dependence.
2. Analgesic and ventilatory depressant responses are characterized by a ceiling effect beyond which additional doses fail to produce further pharmacologic responses.
3. Side effects of opioid agonist-antagonists are similar to those of opioid agonists; in addition, these drugs may cause dysphoric reactions.

B. Pentazocine

1. **Clinical Uses.** Pentazocine, 10 to 30 mg IV or 50 mg orally (equivalent to 60 mg of codeine), is used most often for the relief of moderate pain. An intramuscular dose of 20 to 30 mg produces analgesia, sedation, and depression of ventilation similar to that produced by 10 mg of morphine (increasing the dose above 30 mg does not increase these effects).

2. **Side Effects**

   a. Sedation, dizziness, and dysphoria (especially with high doses, thus limiting its abuse potential) may accompany the administration of pentazocine.
   b. Nausea and vomiting and increases in common bile duct pressure are less common with pentazocine than with morphine, and miosis does not occur.
   c. Pentazocine increases the plasma concentrations of catecholamines, which may account for the increases in heart rate, systemic blood pressure, and

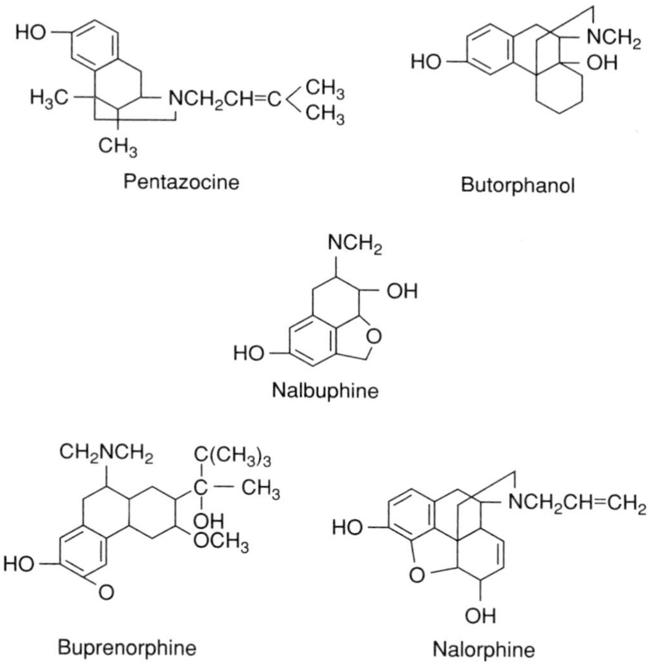

FIGURE 3–9. Opioid agonist-antagonists.

pulmonary artery blood pressure that occasionally accompany administration of this drug.

C. Butorphanol

1. In postoperative patients, butorphanol, 2 to 3 mg IV, produces analgesia and depression of ventilation similar to that provided by 10 mg of morphine.

   a. Because this drug is available only in parenteral form, it is better suited for the relief of acute pain than chronic pain.

   b. Butorphanol, as a kappa receptor agonist-antagonist, stops shivering better than does fentanyl.

2. **Side effects** resemble pentazocine with the exception of dysphoria, which is infrequent following the administration of butorphanol.

D. **Nalbuphine**
1. Nalbuphine, 10 mg IM, produces analgesia similar to morphine. When administered intravenously, it reverses the postoperative depression of ventilation caused by fentanyl but maintains analgesia. Evidence of recurrent hypoventilation may occur 2 to 3 hours following administration of nalbuphine to antagonize the effects of fentanyl.
2. Unlike pentazocine or butorphanol, nalbuphine does not alter systemic or pulmonary arterial pressure. For this reason, nalbuphine may be useful in providing sedation and analgesia during cardiac catheterization.
3. Sedation is the most common side effect; dysphoria is infrequent.

E. **Buprenorphine**
1. Analgesia following buprenorphine, 0.3 mg IM, is equivalent to that afforded by 10 mg of morphine (affinity for mu receptors is 50 times greater than that of morphine).
2. Antagonist effects of buprenorphine reflect its ability to displace opioid agonists from mu receptors.
3. Side effects of buprenorphine include drowsiness, nausea, vomiting, and depression of ventilation; these are similar in magnitude to the side effects of morphine, but may be prolonged and resistant to antagonism with naloxone. Dysphoria is unlikely to occur in association with administration of this drug.

F. **Dezocine**
1. Dezocine is a synthetic opioid with partial agonist characteristics (analgesic potency similar to morphine), reflecting binding to mu-1 opioid receptors.
2. Unlike nalbuphine, dezocine has not been shown to have significant antagonist characteristics.
3. Unlike morphine, but like nalbuphine, dezocine has a ceiling effect on depression of ventilation.

VI. OPIOID ANTAGONISTS

A. Naloxone and naltrexone are pure opioid antagonists with a high affinity for mu receptors and, to a lesser extent, for delta and kappa receptors.
1. Administration of naloxone or naltrexone results in displacement of opioid agonists from opioid receptors.
2. Following this displacement, the binding of naloxone or naltrexone does not activate opioid receptors, and antagonism occurs.

Table 3–6
Side Effects of Naloxone

Reversal of analgesia

Nausea and vomiting

Cardiovascular stimulation
  Tachycardia
  Hypertension
  Pulmonary edema
  Cardiac dysrhythmias (ventricular fibrillation)

Acute withdrawal in newborn with an opioid-dependent mother

    3. In contrast to naloxone, naltrexone is effective orally, producing sustained antagonism of the effects of opioid agonists for as long as 24 hours.

  B. Naloxone
    1. Naloxone, 1 to 4 $\mu g \cdot kg^{-1}$ IV, promptly reverses opioid-induced analgesia and depression of ventilation.
      a. The short duration of action of naloxone (30 to 45 minutes) emphasizes the likely need for supplemental doses.
      b. A continuous infusion of naloxone, 5 $\mu g \cdot kg^{-1} \cdot h^{-1}$ IV, prevents depression of ventilation without altering the analgesia produced by neuraxial opioids.
    2. Side Effects (Table 3-6)
      a. Titration of the dose of naloxone to antagonize depression of ventilation partially but acceptably is a strategy that also preserves partial analgesia.
      b. Sudden antagonism of opioid-induced analgesia (especially with rapid intravenous administration of high doses of naloxone) can activate the sympathetic nervous system, resulting in cardiovascular stimulation.
  C. Nalmefene is a pure opioid antagonist that is equally potent to naloxone but, because of its slower clearance, has a prolonged duration of action.

VII. ANESTHETIC REQUIREMENTS

  A. Even large doses of opioid agonists do not produce the equivalent of 1 MAC as determined for volatile anesthetics (maximum decrease in MAC is about 65%).
  B. Opioid agonists-antagonists decrease MAC for a volatile anesthetic by 20% or less.

Chapter

4

Barbiturates

Barbiturates produce detectable effects for several hours, even following administration of "ultrashort-acting" drugs for induction of anesthesia. (Updated and revised from Stoelting RK. Barbiturates. In: Pharmacology and Physiology in Anesthetic Practice. 2nd ed. Philadelphia, JB Lippincott, 1991;102–17.)

I. COMMERCIAL PREPARATIONS

A. Barbiturates are prepared commercially as sodium salts that are readily soluble in water or saline to form highly alkaline solutions (pH of a 2.5% solution of thiopental is 10.5).

1. These highly alkaline solutions will form a precipitate if mixed in the same syringe with drugs that are acid in solution (opioids, neuromuscular blocking drugs, catecholamines).

2. Bacteriostatic properties of commercial solutions of barbiturates are due to their highly alkaline pH.

B. Recommended concentrations of thiopental and thiamylal are 2.5%, whereas methohexital is used most often as a 1% solution.

II. STRUCTURE ACTIVITY RELATIONSHIPS

A. Barbiturates are defined as any drug derived from barbituric acid (Fig. 4–1).

B. Barbiturates that retain an oxygen atom on the number 2 carbon of the barbituric acid ring are designated **oxybarbiturates,** whereas those with a sulfur atom on the number 2 carbon atom are designated **thiobarbiturates** (Fig. 4–2).

1. Sulfuration increases lipid solubility and is associated with greater hypnotic potency and a more rapid onset but shorter duration of action (thiopental has a more rapid onset and shorter duration of action than its oxybarbiturate analogue, pentobarbital).

2. Addition of a methyl group to the nitrogen atom of

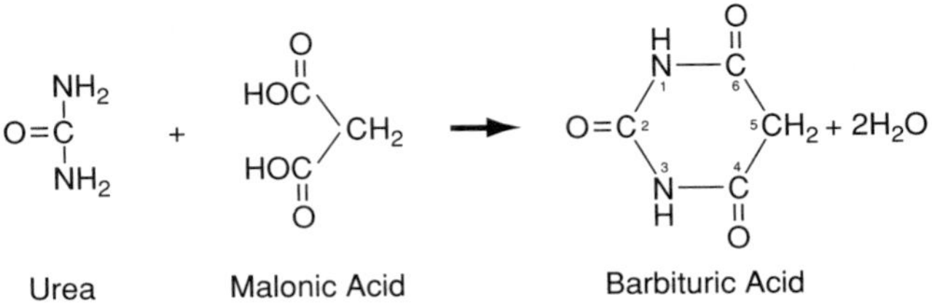

FIGURE 4–1. Barbituric acid is formed by the combination of urea and malonic acid.

the barbituric acid ring, as with methohexital, results in a compound with a short duration of action and also confers convulsive activity manifested as involuntary skeletal muscle movement (seizures may follow administration of methohexital to patients with a history of epilepsy).

III. MECHANISM OF ACTION

A. Barbiturates seem to be uniquely capable of depressing the reticular activating system which is presumed to be important in the maintenance of wakefulness.
   1. This response may reflect the ability of barbiturates to decrease the rate of dissociation of the inhibitory neurotransmitter gamma-aminobutyric acid from its receptors.

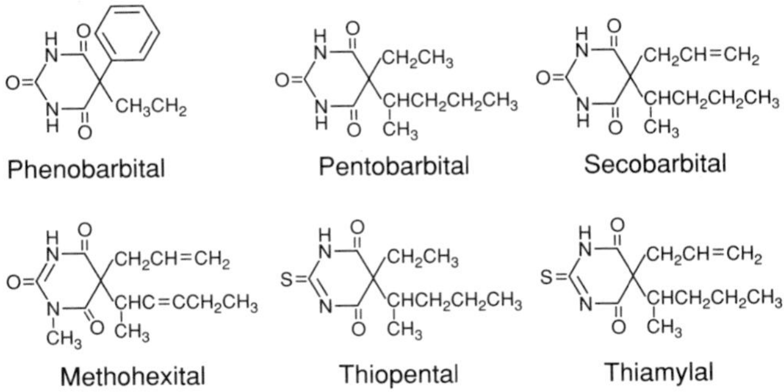

Phenobarbital   Pentobarbital   Secobarbital

Methohexital   Thiopental   Thiamylal

FIGURE 4–2. Barbiturates with sedative-hypnotic properties result from substitutions at the number 2 and 5 carbon atoms of barbituric acid (Fig. 4–1).

2. Gamma-aminobutyric acid causes an increase in chloride conductance through ion channels, resulting in hyperpolarization and, consequently, inhibition of postsynaptic neurons (see Chapter 1, Section VI 4B; Table 1-10; and Fig. 1-13).

B. Barbiturates selectively depress transmission in the sympathetic ganglia, which may contribute to drug-associated decreases in blood pressure.

IV. PHARMACOKINETICS

A. Prompt awakening following intravenous administration of thiopental, thiamylal, and methohexital reflects redistribution of these drugs from the brain to inactive tissue sites (Fig. 4-3). Ultimately, however, elimination from the body depends almost entirely on metabolism, as less than 1% of these drugs is recovered unchanged in the urine.

B. Protein binding of barbiturates parallels lipid solubility (thiopental is the most avidly bound to plasma proteins).
   1. Decreased protein binding of thiopental may explain, in part, the increased drug sensitivity demonstrated by patients with uremia or cirrhosis of the liver.
   2. Protein binding of thiopental in neonates is about half that in adults, suggesting a possible increased sensitivity to this drug in neonates.

C. Distribution of barbiturates in the body is determined principally by their lipid solubility and tissue blood flow (Fig. 4-3).
   1. Brain
      a. Thiopental, thiamylal, and methohexital undergo maximal brain uptake (about 10% of the administered dose) within 30 seconds (rapid onset), followed by a decrease over the next 5 minutes to one-half the initial peak concentration, owing to redistribution of the drug to inactive tissue sites (short duration of action).
      b. Redistribution occurs promptly because the initial high uptake of a lipid-soluble drug into the brain and other highly perfused tissues causes the plasma concentration of barbiturate to decrease, resulting in reversal of the concentration gradient for movement of drug between blood and tissues.
   2. Skeletal muscles are the principal sites for initial redistribution (decline in the plasma concentration) of thiopental.

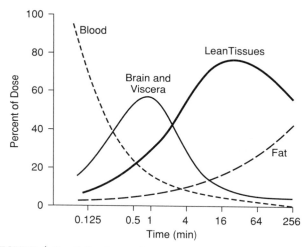

FIGURE 4–3. Following an intravenous bolus, the percentage of thiopental remaining in the blood rapidly decreases as the drug moves from blood to tissues. Time to achievement of peak thiopental levels is a direct function of tissue capacity (solubility) for the barbiturate relative to blood flow. Initially, most thiopental is taken up by the vessel-rich group (VRG) of tissues because of their high blood flow. Subsequently, the drug is redistributed to the skeletal muscles and, to a lesser extent, to fat. The rate of metabolism equals the early rate of removal by fat, and the sum of these two events is similar to uptake of drug by skeletal muscles. (From Saidman LJ. Uptake, distribution, and elimination of barbiturates. In: Eger EI, ed. Anesthetic Uptake and Action. Baltimore, Williams and Wilkins, 1974; with permission.)

> 3. **Fat** is the only compartment in which thiopental continues to accumulate 30 minutes after injection.
>   a. Low fat blood flow limits delivery of barbiturate to this tissue; redistribution to fat will not significantly affect early awakening from a single intravenous dose of barbiturate.
>   b. Large or repeated doses of the lipid soluble barbiturates produce a cumulative drug effect because of the storage capacity of fat.
> 4. **Ionization** influences the distribution of thiopental from blood to tissues (acidosis favors the nonionized fraction, which has greater access to the central nervous system because of its higher lipid solubility).

D. Metabolism

1. Side chain oxidation at the number 5 carbon atom of the benzene ring of the barbiturate to yield carboxylic acid is the most important initial step in terminating pharmacologic activity of barbiturates by metabolism.

2. The reserve capacity of the liver to carry out oxidation of barbiturates is great, and hepatic dysfunction must be extreme before a prolonged duration of action of barbiturates secondary to decreased metabolism occurs.

3. **Thiopental** metabolism is almost complete (99%) and, along with redistribution to inactive tissue sites, is important for awakening following intravenous injection of the drug.

   a. It is unlikely that a single dose of thiopental will produce prolonged effects in patients with cirrhosis of the liver as clearance of thiopental from the plasma is not different from that in normal patients.

   b. Enzyme induction from chronic exposure to environmental pollution is presumed to be the explanation for increased thiopental dose requirements in patients from urban areas compared to those from rural areas.

4. **Methohexital** is less lipid-soluble than thiopental, which means that more of this drug remains in the plasma to be available for prompt metabolism (overall hepatic clearance of methohexital is three to four times that of thiopental) (Fig. 4–4).

   a. Despite this greater hepatic clearance, early awakening from a single dose of methohexital depends primarily on its redistribution to inactive tissue sites.

   b. Recovery (including psychomotor recovery) from methohexital is predictably more rapid than that from thiopental, especially when repeated doses of the drug are administered. This reflects the increased role of metabolism in the clearance of methohexital from the plasma.

E. Renal Excretion

1. All barbiturates are filtered by the renal glomeruli, but the high degree of protein binding limits the magnitude of filtration, whereas high lipid solubility favors reabsorption of any filtered drug back into the circulation.

2. Less than 1% of thiopental, thiamylal, and methohexital is excreted unchanged in the urine.

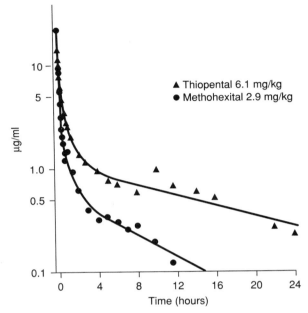

FIGURE 4–4. The rate of decline of the plasma concentration, and thus the elimination half-time, is shorter following the intravenous administration of methohexital than following thiopental administration. (From Hudson RJ, Stanski DR, Burch PG. Pharmacokinetics of methohexital and thiopental in surgical patients. Anesthesiology 1983;59: 215–9; with permission.)

F. **Elimination Half-Time** (Table 4–1)
   1. The shorter elimination half-time of methohexital compared with that of thiopental results entirely from the greater hepatic clearance of methohexital.
   2. Increasing age is associated with slowed passage of thiopental from the central compartment to the peripheral compartment (intercompartmental clearance), resulting in an increased plasma concentration (greater anesthetic effect) in elderly patients (Fig. 4–5). This greater anesthetic effect in elderly patients reflects a pharmacokinetic, not a pharmacodynamic, mechanism.

Table 4–1
Comparative Pharmacokinetics of Barbiturates

	Thiopental	*Methohexital*
Rapid distribution half-time (min)	8.5	5.6
Slow distribution half-time (min)	62.7	58.3
Elimination half-time (h)	11.6	3.9*
Clearance (mL·kg^{-1}·min^{-1})	3.4	10.9*
Volume of distribution (L·kg^{-1})	2.5	2.2

*Significantly different from thiopental.
(Data from Hudson RJ, Stanski DR, Burch PG. Pharmacokinetics of methohexital and thiopental in surgical patients. Anesthesiology 1983; 59:215–9.)

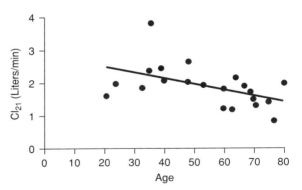

FIGURE 4–5. The rate of intercompartmental clearance of thiopental from the central compartment (V_1) to the peripheral compartment (V_2) slows with increasing age. (From Avram MJ, Krejcie TC, Henthorn TK. The relationship of age to the pharmacokinetics of early drug distribution: The concurrent disposition of thiopental and indocyanine green. Anesthesiology 1990;72:403–11; with permission.)

V. CLINICAL USES

A. Induction of Anesthesia

1. The supremacy of barbiturates for intravenous induction of anesthesia has remained virtually unchallenged since the introduction of thiopental in 1934.
   a. The relative potency of barbiturates used for intravenous induction of anesthesia is: thiopental, 1; thiamylal, 1.1; and methohexital, 2.5.
   b. The usual induction dose of thiopental and thiamylal is 3 to 5 mg·kg^{-1} IV; for methohexital, the induction dose is 1 to 1.5 mg·kg^{-1} IV.
   c. The central nervous system is exquisitely sensitive to intravenous doses of these barbiturates (unconsciousness in less than 30 seconds).
   d. Despite a contrary clinical impression, thiopental dose requirements may not be different for nonalcoholics and alcoholics (Fig. 4–6).
2. Rectal administration of barbiturates (methohexital, 20–30 mg·kg^{-1}) has been used to induce anesthesia in uncooperative or young patients.
   a. Upper airway obstruction may accompany sedation produced by rectal methohexital.
   b. Constant nursing observation and use of pulse oximetry are recommended when methohexital is administered rectally.

B. Treatment of Increased Intracranial Pressure

1. Barbiturates are administered to decrease intracranial pressure which remains persistently high despite deliberate hyperventilation of the lungs and drug-induced diuresis.
2. Barbiturates decrease intracranial pressure by decreasing cerebral blood volume through drug-induced cerebrovascular vasoconstriction and an associated decrease in cerebral blood flow.
   a. An isoelectric electroencephalogram (EEG) confirms the presence of maximal barbiturate-induced depression (about 50%) of cerebral metabolic oxygen requirements.
   b. A hazard of high-dose barbiturate therapy, as used to lower intracranial pressure, is hypotension, which can jeopardize the maintenance of an adequate cerebral perfusion pressure.

C. Cerebral Protection

1. It is unlikely that barbiturate therapy can improve brain survival following global cerebral ischemia owing to

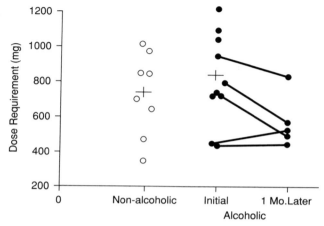

FIGURE 4–6. The dose of thiopental needed to achieve burst suppression with 3 seconds of isoelectric electroencephalogram is similar in nonalcoholics and alcoholic patients with abstinence of 9 to 17 days (initial) and 1 month later. (From Swerdlow BN, Holley FO, Maitre PO, Stanski DR. Chronic alcohol intake does not change thiopental anesthetic requirements, pharmacokinetics, or pharmacodynamics. Anesthesiology 1990;72:455–61; with permission.)

cardiac arrest, as these drugs are effective only when the EEG remains active and metabolic suppression is possible (EEG becomes flat in 20 to 30 seconds following a cardiac arrest).

2. In contrast to global cerebral ischemia, the use of barbiturates in the presence of incomplete (focal) cerebral ischemia results in improved outcome (based on animal studies).

VI. SIDE EFFECTS

A. Cardiovascular System

1. **Hemodynamic effects** of equivalent doses of barbiturates, as administered for the intravenous induction of anesthesia, are similar.

   a. In **normovolemic** subjects, thiopental, 5 mg·kg^{-1} IV, produces a transient 10- to 20-mmHg decrease in blood pressure (similar with rapid or slow intravenous injection) that is offset by a compensatory 15- to 20-beat·min^{-1} increase in heart rate (a carotid-sinus–mediated increase in peripheral sympathetic nervous system activity).

    b. The mild and transient decrease in blood pressure (greatly enhanced in hypovolemic patients) that accompanies induction of anesthesia with barbiturates is principally due to peripheral vasodilation, reflecting decreased sympathetic nervous system outflow from the central nervous system (**direct myocardial depression** is less with barbiturates than with equivalent doses of volatile anesthetics).

  2. Cardiac dysrhythmias following induction of anesthesia with barbiturates are unlikely in the presence of adequate ventilation and oxygenation.

  3. Histamine release is rarely of clinical significance, even following the rapid intravenous injection of thiopental.

B. Ventilation

  1. Barbiturates, as administered for the intravenous induction of anesthesia, produce dose-dependent depression of ventilation (enhanced in presence of other sedative drugs) which often results in transient apnea.

  2. Stimulation of the upper airway, as by laryngoscopy or secretions, in the presence of inadequate depression of laryngeal reflexes by barbiturates may result in **laryngospasm.**

C. Electroencephalogram

  1. The frequency of electrical activity on the EEG decreases as the dose of barbiturate is increased.

  2. Electrical silence (isoelectric EEG) reflects maximal barbiturate-induced decreases (about 50%) in cerebral metabolic oxygen requirements (reflecting a decrease in neuronal, but not metabolic, needs for oxygen).

D. Somatosensory Evoked Responses. Thiopental is an acceptable drug to administer when the ability to monitor evoked potentials is desired.

E. Liver

  1. Induction doses of barbiturates do not alter postoperative liver function test results and produce only modest decreases in hepatic blood flow.

  2. Enzyme induction (increase in liver microsomal protein content) is produced by sustained (2 to 7 days) administration of barbiturates.

  3. Barbiturates stimulate activity of the enzyme (d-aminolevulinic acid) necessary for the production of heme (**acute intermittent porphyria** may be exacerbated in susceptible patients who receive barbiturates).

F. Kidneys. Renal effects of thiopental may include modest decreases in renal blood flow and glomerular filtration rate.

G. Placental Transfer
  1. Barbiturates used for intravenous induction of anesthesia readily cross the placenta, but fetal plasma concentrations are lower than maternal concentrations.
  2. Clearance by the fetal liver and dilution by blood from viscera and extremities result in exposure of the fetal brain to lower barbiturate concentrations than are measured in the umbilical vein.

H. Tolerance and Physical Dependence
  1. Acute tolerance to barbiturates occurs sooner than does barbiturate-induced induction of microsomal enzymes.
  2. Tolerance to the sedative effects and depressant effects of barbiturates on cerebral metabolic oxygen requirements occur in parallel.

I. Intraarterial Injection (Table 4-2)

J. Venous Thrombosis
  1. Venous thrombosis presumably reflects a deposition of barbiturate crystals in the veins (less hazardous than

Table 4–2
Intraarterial Injection of Thiopental

Signs and Symptoms

Excruciating pain
Intense vasoconstriction (obscuring the distal pulses)
Gangrene

Mechanism of Vascular Occlusion (Unproven)

Formation of thiopental crystals (pH becomes too low for the drug to remain in solution; not due to drug's alkalinity)
Hemolysis of erythrocytes and aggregation of platelets
Local release of norepinephrine
Toxic to vascular endothelium

Treatment

Dilution of drug (by injection of saline)
Vasodilation (lidocaine)
Sympathectomy (stellate ganglion block)

arterial deposition because of the ever-increasing diameter of the veins).

2. A dilute solution of barbiturate (2.5% thiopental or thiamylal, or 1% methohexital) decreases the incidence of venous thrombosis.

K. Allergic Reactions

1. Allergic reactions following intravenous administration of barbiturates for induction of anesthesia are infrequent (estimated to occur in 1 in 30,000 patients), but they are often life-threatening (requiring aggressive treatment with epinephrine and intravascular fluid replacement).

2. Most allergic reactions secondary to thiopental administration occur in patients who have received the drug previously without adverse responses.

5

Benzodiazepines

The favorable pharmacologic characteristics of benzodiazepines are the reasons these drugs may be selected in preference to barbiturates (Table 5-1). (Updated and revised from Stoelting RK. Benzodiazepines. In: Pharmacology and Physiology of Anesthetic Practice. 2nd ed. Philadelphia, JB Lippincott, 1991;118-33.)

I. STRUCTURE ACTIVITY RELATIONSHIPS

A. Benzodiazepines are structurally similar and share many active metabolites (Fig. 5-1).

B. The term benzodiazepine refers to the portion of the structure composed of a benzene ring fused to a diazepine ring.

II. MECHANISMS OF ACTION

A. Benzodiazepine receptors are located on the alpha subunits of gamma-aminobutyric acid (GABA) receptors (Fig. 5-2).

    1. Actions of GABA in the central nervous system may be reflected by alterations in sleep, neuronal excitability (prevention of seizures), anxiety, memory, and hypnosis (consistent with the known pharmacologic effects of benzodiazepines).

    2. Benzodiazepines enhance the **chloride-gating function** of GABA by facilitating the binding of this inhibitory neurotransmitter to its receptors (see Chapter 1, Section VI 4B; Table 1-10; and Fig. 1-13).

    3. The resulting enhanced opening of chloride channels leads to hyperpolarization of cell membranes, making them more resistant to excitation.

    4. The anatomic distribution of GABA receptors (almost exclusively in the central nervous system, with the highest density in the cerebral cortex) is consistent with the minimal effects of benzodiazepines outside the central nervous system (minimal circulatory effects).

Table 5–1
Favorable Pharmacologic Characteristics of Benzodiazepines

Selective impairment (affecting encoding of new information [anterograde amnesia], but not stored information [retrograde amnesia])

Minimal depression of ventilation or the cardiovascular system

Specific site of action as anticonvulsants

Relative safety if taken in overdose

Low abuse and physical dependence potential

Availability of a specific pharmacologic antagonist

    B. Benzodiazepines produce dose-dependent suppression of the hypothalamic-pituitary-adrenal axis manifested by decreased plasma concentrations of adrenocorticotropic hormone and cortisol.

    C. Electroencephalographic effects of benzodiazepines resemble those associated with the administration of barbiturates.

    D. Antagonism of the central nervous system effects of benzodiazepines is promptly and selectively achieved following the administration of flumazenil (physostigmine and aminophylline are nonspecific antagonists).

III. DIAZEPAM is the standard with which all benzodiazepines are compared.

    A. Pharmacokinetics (Table 5-2)

        1. High lipid solubility of diazepam facilitates its efficient absorption after oral administration, its rapid entry into the central nervous system (or across the placenta), and its redistribution to inactive tissue sites, especially fat.

        2. Protein binding of diazepam to albumin is extensive and parallels the high lipid solubility of this drug (protein binding limits the efficacy of hemodialysis in removing the drug after an overdose).

        3. Metabolism of diazepam in the liver results in active metabolites (desmethyldiazepam is only slightly less potent than diazepam and is likely to contribute to the return of drowsiness 6 to 8 hours after the administration of diazepam) (Fig. 5-3).

        4. Elimination Half-Time

            a. Cirrhosis of the liver is associated with a prolonged

Table 5–2
Comparative Pharmacology of Benzodiazepines

	Equivalent Dose ($mg \cdot kg^{-1}$)	Volume of Distribution ($L \cdot kg^{-1}$)	Protein Binding (percent)	Clearance ($ml \cdot kg^{-1} \cdot min^{-1}$)	Elimination Half-Time (h)
Diazepam	0.3–0.5	1–1.5	96–98	0.2–0.5	21–37
Midazolam	0.15–0.3	1–1.5	96–98	6–8	1–4
Lorazepam	0.05	0.8–1.3	96–98	0.7–1	10–20

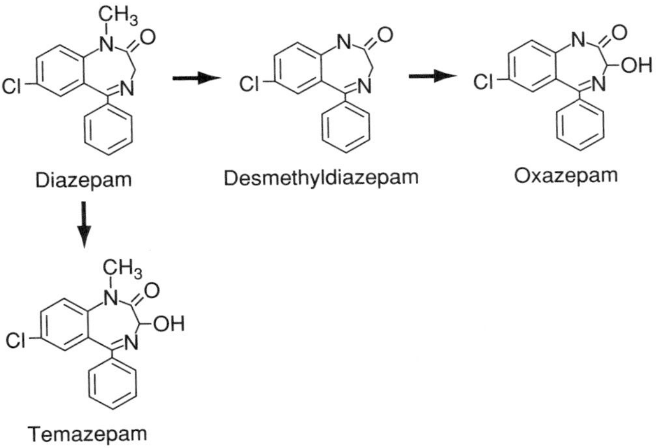

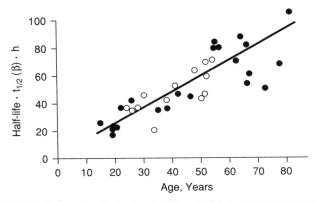

FIGURE 5–3. The principal metabolites of diazepam are desmethyldiazepam and oxazepam. A lesser amount of diazepam is metabolized to temazepam.

FIGURE 5–4. The elimination half-time of diazepam increases progressively with increasing age. (From Koltz U, Avant GR, Hoyumpa A, Schender S, Wilkinson GR. The effects of age and liver disease on the disposition and elimination of diazepam in adult man. J Clin Invest 1975;55:347-59; with permission.)

tering of this drug to patients with chronic obstructive airway disease may result in exaggerated or prolonged depression of ventilation.

2. Cardiovascular System

   a. Diazepam, administered in a dose of 0.5 mg·kg^{-1} IV for induction of anesthesia, typically produces decreases in blood pressure, cardiac output, and systemic vascular resistance that are similar in magnitude to those changes observed during natural sleep (10% to 20% reduction).

   b. Diazepam appears to have no direct action on the sympathetic nervous system, and it does not cause orthostatic hypotension.

   c. Nitrous oxide does not enhance the cardiovascular effects of diazepam (which contrasts with the direct myocardial depression and decreases in blood pressure that occur when nitrous oxide is administered in the presence of opioids).

3. Skeletal Muscle

   a. Skeletal muscle relaxant effects reflect the actions of diazepam on spinal internuncial neurons and not actions at the neuromuscular junction.

   b. Benzodiazepines do not produce adequate relaxation for surgical procedures, nor does their use influence the dose requirements for neuromuscular blocking drugs.

4. Overdose with a benzodiazepine is unlikely to lead to serious sequelae if cardiac and pulmonary function are maintained and other drugs, such as alcohol, are not present.

5. Hepatic and renal function are not noticeably depressed by benzodiazepines.

6. Nausea and vomiting are not increased by benzodiazepines.

C. Drug Interactions

   1. Alcohol may greatly enhance the depressant effects of benzodiazepines, perhaps reflecting a common site of action at GABA receptors (enhancing ion flux through chloride channels). This common site of action is consistent with the effectiveness of diazepam in treating alcohol withdrawal syndrome (delirium tremens).

   2. Cimetidine delays the hepatic clearance of diazepam and desmethyldiazepam and may be associated with enhanced sedation.

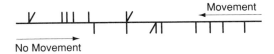

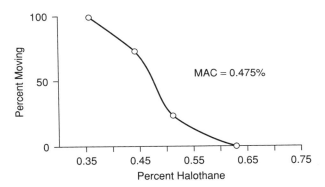

FIGURE 5-5. Diazepam, 0.2 mg·kg^{-1} IV, decreases anesthetic requirements (MAC) for halothane in adult patients from 0.73% to 0.475%. (From Perisho JA, Buechel DR, Miller RD. The effect of diazepam [Valium] on minimum alveolar anesthetic requirements [MAC] in man. Can Anaesth Soc J 1971;18:536-40; with permission.)

    3. Anesthetics
       a. Diazepam decreases the dose of thiopental needed for the induction of anesthesia.
       b. The minimum alveolar concentration (MAC) for volatile anesthetics is decreased by diazepam, with a ceiling effect being reached at about 0.2 mg·kg^{-1} IV (Fig. 5-5).
  D. Abuse and Dependence Liability
    1. The abuse and dependence liability of benzodiazepines is modest in comparison to that of opioids.
    2. Withdrawal symptoms may be accompanied by restlessness and insomnia, but only rarely by seizures.
  E. Benzodiazepines as a class are the most commonly prescribed anxiolytic drugs in the United States (trials comparing different benzodiazepines have failed to demonstrate consistent differences in efficacy) (Table 5-3).
  F. Clinical Uses (Table 5-4)

Table 5-3
Benzodiazepines Used for Anxiolytic Effects

Generic (Trade) Name	Range of Daily Doses (mg)*	Elimination Half-Time	Active Metabolites
Chlordiazepoxide (Librium)	15–100	Long	Dexmethylchlordiazepoxide
Diazepam (Valium)	4–40	Long	Desmethyldiazepam Oxazepam Temazepam
Clorazepate (Tranxene)	15–60	Long	Desmethyldiazepam
Prazepam (Centrax)	20–60	Long	Desmethyldiazepam
Halazepam (Paxipam)	60–160	Long	Desmethyldiazepam
Clonazepam (Klonopin)	0.5–4	Intermediate to long	None
Alprazolam (Xanax)	0.75–4 (anxiety) 1.5–10 (panic disorder)	Short to intermediate	None
Lorazepam (Ativan)	2–6	Short to intermediate	None
Oxazepam (Serax)	30–120	Short	None

*The adult doses given should be decreased for elderly or debilitated patients.
(Modified from Shader RI, Greenblatt DJ. Use of benzodiazepines in anxiety disorders. N Engl J Med 1993;1398–1405; with permission.)

2. **Ventilation**
   a. Midazolam, 0.15 mg·kg^{-1} IV, depresses ventilation similar to diazepam, 0.3 mg·kg^{-1} IV.
   b. Transient apnea may occur following rapid injection of midazolam, especially in the presence of opioids.
3. **Cardiovascular System**
   a. Midazolam-induced hemodynamic changes during induction of anesthesia (0.2 mg·kg^{-1} IV) may resemble those changes produced by thiopental.
   b. Cardiac output is not altered.
   c. In the presence of hypovolemia, administration of midazolam results in enhanced blood pressure-lowering effects similar in magnitude to those produced by other intravenous induction drugs.

E. **Clinical uses** of midazolam are similar to those for diazepam (Table 5-4).
   1. **Preoperative Medication**
      a. Intramuscular administration (0.05-0.1 mg·kg^{-1}) is followed by prompt onset of anxiolysis, amnesia, and hypnotic effects.
      b. In children, oral administration of midazolam, 0.5 mg·kg^{-1}, is an effective preoperative medication.
   2. **Intravenous Sedation.** Midazolam, in doses of 1 to 2.5 mg IV, is effective for sedation in adults during regional anesthesia as well as for brief therapeutic procedures.
      a. Onset is more rapid than with diazepam, and pain on injection is less likely.
      b. Prolonged sedation (4 days or longer) of infants with midazolam has been associated with a withdrawal syndrome (agitation, seizures) when the drug is abruptly discontinued.
   3. **Induction of anesthesia** can be produced by administration of midazolam, 0.1 to 0.2 mg·kg^{-1} IV (thiopental produces induction of anesthesia 50% to 100% faster) (Fig. 5-7).
      a. Elderly patients require less midazolam for the intravenous induction of anesthesia than do young adults.
      b. Onset of unconsciousness is facilitated when a small dose of opioid (fentanyl, 50 to 100 µg IV) precedes the injection of midazolam by 1 to 3 minutes.

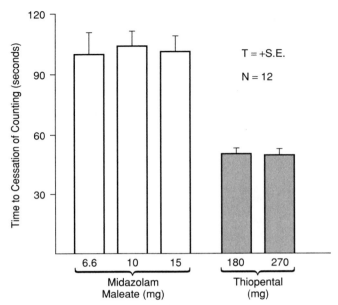

FIGURE 5–7. Induction of anesthesia (as determined by time of cessation of counting) occurs in about 110 seconds following intraveous administration of midazolam compared with about 50 seconds following injection of thiopental. (From Sarnquist FH, Mathers WD, Brock-Utne J, Carr B, Canup C, Brown CR. A bioassay of a water-soluble benzodiazepine against sodium thiopental. Anesthesiology 1980;52:149–53; with permission.)

4. Maintenance of Anesthesia
a. Midazolam may be administered to supplement opioids or inhaled anesthetics during maintenance of anesthesia.
b. Anesthetic requirements (MAC) for volatile anesthetics are decreased in a dose-related manner by midazolam (Fig. 5–8).

V. LORAZEPAM is a more potent amnesic than diazepam.

A. Pharmacokinetics (Table 5–2)
1. Lorazepam is conjugated with glucuronic acid to form

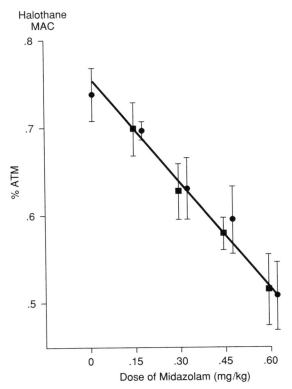

FIGURE 5–8. Midazolam produces dose-dependent decreases in halothane anesthetic requirements (MAC) in patients. Mean ± SE. (From Melvin MA, Johnson BH, Quasha AL, Eger EI. Induction of anesthesia with midazolam decreases halothane MAC in humans. Anesthesiology 1982;57:238–41; with permission.)

      pharmacologically inactive metabolites (in contrast to diazepam).

  2. The elimination half-time of lorazepam is not prolonged in elderly patients or in those treated with cimetidine.

B. Clinical Uses

  1. Preoperative Medication

Table 5–5
Benzodiazepines Used for the Treatment of Insomnia

Oxazepam—most effective in treating insomnia associated with nightly awakenings or shortened sleep times

Flurazepam (15 to 30 mg orally) produces a hypnotic effect in 15 to 30 minutes which lasts 7 to 8 hours

Temazepam (15 to 30 mg orally) is unlikely to be followed by residual drowsiness the next morning)

Triazolam (0.125 to 0.25 mg) has been known to cause marked anterograde amnesia

    a. Lorazepam undergoes reliable absorption after oral and intramuscular injection (recommended oral dose is 50 $\mu g \cdot kg^{-1}$, not to exceed about 4 mg, which produces maximal anterograde amnesia).

    b. The prolonged duration of action of lorazepam limits its usefulness for preoperative medication when rapid awakening at the end of surgery is desirable.

  2. Other Uses. A slow onset of effects limits the usefulness of lorazepam for intravenous induction of anesthesia, intravenous sedation during regional anesthesia, or anticonvulsant therapy.

VI. TREATMENT OF INSOMNIA (Table 5–5)

  A. Potential disadvantages of benzodiazepines used to treat insomnia include rebound insomnia when discontinued, memory loss (especially with triazolam), and residual daytime effects (which should be minimal with triazolam because of its short elimination half-time).

  B. The dosage of benzodiazepines (especially triazolam) should be decreased by about 50% in elderly patients to compensate for decreased clearance and resultant high plasma concentrations of drugs in these patients.

VII. FLUMAZENIL

  A. Flumazenil (8 to 15 $\mu g \cdot kg^{-1}$ IV) is a specific benzodiazepine antagonist that reverses the central nervous system (sedative, memory) effects of benzodiazepines within about 2 minutes (Fig. 5–9).

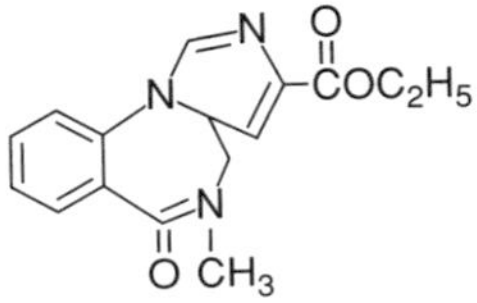

FIGURE 5–9. Flumazenil.

B. This drug has a high affinity for benzodiazepine receptors, where it exerts minimal agonist activity.

   1. This weak agonist activity most likely attenuates evidence of abrupt reversal of agonist effects (acute anxiety, hypertension) and may also be the reason flumazenil does not precipitate withdrawal seizures when administered to patients being treated for seizure disorders.

   2. Flumazenil does not alter anesthetic requirements (MAC) for volatile anesthetics.

   3. Flumazenil is useful in the differential diagnosis of coma when a self-administered drug overdose is suspected.

C. The **duration of antagonism** provided by flumazenil is relatively brief, and return of benzodiazepine agonist effects may require repeated doses of the antagonist.

Chapter

6

Nonbarbiturate Induction Drugs

Nonbarbiturate induction drugs include ketamine, etomidate, and propofol. (Updated and revised from Stoelting RK. Nonbarbiturate induction drugs. In: Pharmacology and Physiology in Anesthetic Practice. 2nd ed. Philadelphia, JB Lippincott, 1991;134–147.)

I. **KETAMINE** is a phencyclidine derivative that produces amnesia, analgesia, and dissociative anesthesia (cataleptic state) (Fig. 6–1).
   A. **Structure Activity Relationships**
      1. Only the racemic mixture, containing equal amounts of the two ketamine isomers, is available for clinical use (*d*-ketamine produces more intense analgesia, more rapid recovery, and a lower incidence of emergence reactions) (see Chapter 1, Section IC).
      2. Both isomers of ketamine appear to be able to inhibit uptake of catecholamines back into postganglionic sympathetic nerve endings (a cocaine-like effect).
   B. **Mechanism of Action.** Ketamine binds to the phenyl-cyclohexyl piperidine (PCP) receptor (may be the same as the sigma receptors previously classified as opioid receptors but now recognized to be nonopioid, as they are not responsive to naloxone).
      1. PCP receptor appears to be coupled to the N-methyl D-aspartate-L-glutamate receptor complex.
      2. Ketamine antagonizes the excitatory transmission mediated by glutamate.
   C. **Pharmacokinetics**
      1. The pharmacokinetics of ketamine resembles that of thiopental (rapid onset of action, relatively short duration of action, high lipid solubility) (Table 6–1).
         a. Initially, ketamine is distributed to highly perfused tissues, such as the brain, where the peak concentration may be four to five times that present in plasma (reflecting its lipid solubility [10 times that

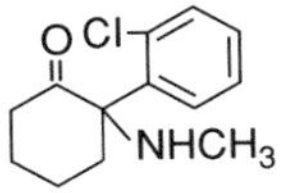

FIGURE 6–1.   Ketamine.

of thiopental] and a drug-induced increase in cerebral blood flow).

   b. Failure of impaired renal function or enzyme induction to alter the duration of action of a single dose of ketamine suggests that redistribution of the drug from the brain to inactive tissue sites is primarily responsible for termination of unconsciousness.

   2. Ketamine stored in tissues may contribute to cumulative drug effects with repeated or continuous administration of the drug.

D. Metabolism

   1. Ketamine is metabolized extensively (like thiopental, important for ultimate clearance) by hepatic microsomal enzymes (norketamine is an active metabolite with one fifth to one third the activity of the parent compound, which may contribute to the prolonged effects of the drug).

   2. Less than 4% of a dose of ketamine is recovered unchanged in the urine.

   3. Accelerated metabolism of ketamine as a result of enzyme induction could explain, in part, the tolerance to the analgesic effects of ketamine that has been observed in patients receiving repeated doses of this drug at short intervals (burn patients).

E. Clinical Uses

   1. Analgesia. Intense analgesia can be achieved for vaginal delivery with subanesthetic doses of ketamine (0.2 to 0.5 $mg \cdot kg^{-1}$ IV) without associated depression of the neonate.

   2. Induction of Anesthesia

   a. Induction of anesthesia is produced by administration of ketamine, 1 to 2 $mg \cdot kg^{-1}$ IV (causing loss of consciousness in 30 to 60 seconds) or 5 to 10 $mg \cdot kg^{-1}$ IM (causing loss of consciousness in 2 to 4 minutes; the high dose requirement reflects a significant first-pass hepatic effect for ketamine).

   b. Administration of an antisialagogue is often recommended (glycopyrrolate may be preferred) to decrease ketamine-induced salivary secretions.

Table 6-1
Comparative Characteristics of Nonbarbiturate Induction Drugs

	Elimination Half-Time (b)	Volume of Distribution (L·kg⁻¹)	Clearance (ml·kg⁻¹·min⁻¹)	Blood Pressure	Heart Rate
Ketamine	1-2	2.5-3.5	16-18	Increased	Increased
Etomidate	2-5	2.2-4.5	10-20	No change	No change
Propofol	0.5-1.5	3.5-4.5	30-60	Decreased	Decreased

    c. Unconsciousness is associated with maintenance of normal or only slightly depressed pharyngeal and laryngeal reflexes.

    d. Return of consciousness usually occurs in 10 to 15 minutes following an intravenous induction dose of ketamine, but complete recovery is often delayed.

    e. Because of its rapid onset of action, ketamine has been used as an intramuscular induction drug in children and difficult-to-manage mentally retarded patients, regardless of age.

    f. Analgesia and the patient's ability to maintain spontaneous ventilation are reasons to select this drug for burn dressing changes.

    g. Induction of anesthesia in **acutely hypovolemic** patients (also those with cardiac tamponade or constrictive pericarditis) is often accomplished with ketamine, taking advantage of the drug's cardiovascular stimulating effects.

    h. Beneficial effects of ketamine on airway resistance (bronchodilation) make this a potentially useful drug for rapid intravenous induction of anesthesia in patients with **asthma.**

  F. Side Effects (Table 6-2)

    1. Central Nervous System

      a. The ability of ketamine to increase cerebral blood flow and thus intracranial pressure (may not occur if the $PaCO_2$ is maintained at normal levels) is blunted by the prior administration of other drugs (thiopental, midazolam).

      b. Ketamine does not alter the seizure threshold in epileptic patients.

      c. Nystagmus produced by ketamine may be undesirable in patients undergoing eye muscle surgery.

Table 6–2
Side Effects of Ketamine

Increased intracranial pressure

Sympathetic nervous system stimulation
  Increased systemic and pulmonary artery blood pressure
  Increased heart rate
  Increased cardiac output

Salivary and tracheobronchial secretions

Emergence delirium

2. Cardiovascular System

   a. A unique feature of ketamine that distinguishes it from other intravenous induction drugs is its ability to stimulate the cardiovascular system.

   b. The cardiovascular stimulating effects of ketamine (systolic blood pressure increases 20 to 40 mmHg during the first 3 to 5 minutes following intravenous injection of ketamine, decreasing thereafter to predrug levels over the next 10 to 20 minutes) are blunted by the prior administration of a benzodiazepine (most effective) or concomitant administration of inhaled anesthetics, including nitrous oxide.

   c. The administration of ketamine to patients with coronary artery disease or pulmonary hypertension has been questioned because of increased myocardial oxygen requirements that may accompany this drug's sympathomimetic effects on the heart.

   d. **Critically ill patients** occasionally respond to ketamine with unexpected decreases in blood pressure and cardiac output, which may reflect depletion of catecholamine stores and exhaustion of sympathetic nervous system compensating mechanisms (no evidence that alternative drugs, such as etomidate, produce less hypotension in these patients).

   e. **Mechanisms of Cardiovascular Effects.** The mechanisms for ketamine-induced cardiovascular effects are complex, but direct stimulation of the central nervous system leading to increased sympathetic nervous system outflow is the most likely explanation.

3. Ventilation and Airway

   a. Despite maintaining upper airway skeletal muscle tone, ketamine anesthesia does not negate the need for protection of the lungs against aspiration by placement of a cuffed tube in the trachea.

   b. Ketamine is an effective bronchodilator.

4. Emergence Delirium

   a. **Mechanism.** Emergence delirium probably occurs secondary to ketamine-induced changes in the central nervous system that lead to a misinterpretation of auditory and visual stimuli.

   b. **Incidence.** The incidence of emergence delirium following ketamine administration ranges from 5% to 30%.

   c. **Prevention.** Benzodiazepines (midazolam, admin-

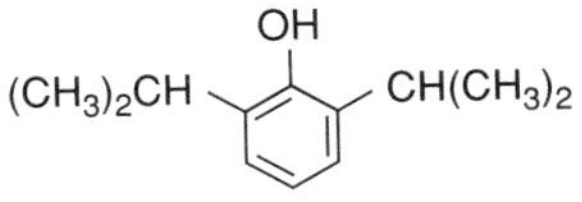

FIGURE 6–3. Propofol.

   b. This enzyme inhibition lasts 4 to 8 hours following an induction dose of etomidate.

  7. Nausea and vomiting is more common after the induction of anesthesia with etomidate than after thiopental.

III. PROPOFOL

  A. Propofol is a substituted isopropylphenol that is administered intravenously as a 1% solution (Fig. 6–3).

   1. Propofol inhibits activity at both supraspinal and spinal synapses by interacting with the gamma-aminobutyric acid (GABA) receptor complex to potentiate effects mediated by this receptor.

   2. It seems that propofol exerts its actions at the chloride ion channel without binding directly to GABA receptors (see Chapter 1, Section VI, 4B, Table 1–10, and Fig. 1–13).

   3. Propofol, unlike other hypnotics, possesses strong (preferential) depressant subcortical actions (antiemetic, antipruritic, anxiolytic) that outlast its cortico-hypnotic effects.

  B. Pharmacokinetics (Table 6–1)

   1. Clearance of propofol from the plasma exceeds hepatic blood flow, emphasizing that tissue uptake as well as metabolism is important in removing this drug from the plasma.

    a. Less than 0.3% of a dose is excreted unchanged in the urine along with pharmacologically inactive metabolites.

    b. Despite the rapid clearance of propofol by metabolism, there is no evidence of impaired elimination in patients with **cirrhosis.**

    c. Renal dysfunction does not influence the clearance of propofol.

    d. Patients older than 60 years of age exhibit a decreased rate of plasma clearance of propofol compared with younger adults.

   2. Rapid clearance of propofol from the plasma is the

Table 6–3
Hypnotic and Nonhypnotic Therapeutic Applications of Propofol

Hypnotic Applications
Induction of anesthesia
Maintenance of anesthesia
Monitored anesthesia care
Sedation during regional anesthesia

Nonhypnotic Applications
Antiemetic
Antipruritic
Proconvulsant (?)
Anticonvulsant
Anxiolysis

reason this drug may be administered as a continuous infusion without an excessive cumulative effect.
3. Propofol readily crosses the placenta.
C. **Clinical Uses** (Table 6-3)
  1. **Induction of Anesthesia**
     a. Administration of propofol, 2 to 2.5 mg·kg^{-1} IV (equivalent to 3 to 5 mg·kg^{-1} IV of thiopental), produces unconsciousness within about 30 seconds.
     b. Awakening is more rapid and complete than that following intravenous induction of anesthesia with thiopental or methohexital. This is the most important advantage of propofol over other drugs used to produce intravenous induction of anesthesia, especially for outpatient surgery.
  2. **Maintenance of anesthesia** may be provided by a continuous infusion of propofol, often in combination with nitrous oxide (75-300 mg·kg^{-1}·min^{-1}).
  3. **Monitored anesthesia care** may be provided by a continuous intravenous infusion of propofol (25-100 mg·kg^{-1}·min^{-1}).
D. **Nonhypnotic Applications of Propofol** (Table 6-3)
  1. **Antiemetic Effect**
     a. The mechanisms mediating the antiemetic action of propofol are unknown but likely include direct effects on the chemoreceptor trigger zone and/or vomiting center (Fig. 6-4).
     b. Subhypnotic doses of propofol (10 to 15 mg IV)

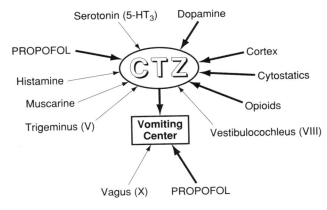

FIGURE 6–4. The antiemetic effects of propofol may be due to effects at the chemoreceptor trigger zone (CTZ) and/or vomiting center. (From Borgeat A, Wilder Smith OHG, Suter PM. The nonhypnotic therapeutic applications of propofol. Anesthesiology 1994;80:642–56; with permission.)

may be used in the Postanesthesia Care Unit to treat postoperative nausea and vomiting.

2. **Antipruritic effects** are useful in patients treated with neuraxial opioids (propofol, 10 mg IV or 0.5 to 1 mg·kg^{-1}·h^{-1}).

3. **Proconvulsant properties** are controversial, being based on case reports of postpropofol "seizures" or opisthotonus.

 a. Propofol has not been proven to cause cortical seizure activity, based on electroencephalographic (EEG) findings, in the absence of a preexisting seizure disorder (conversely, there is evidence that use of propofol in patients with epilepsy is safe, but the drug may interfere with the recording of spikes on the EEG).

 b. Reported excitatory phenomena may reflect the ability of low doses of propofol to depress inhibitory but not excitatory subcortical centers (also occurs with other hypnotic agents).

Table 6–4
Side Effects of Propofol

Delayed seizures (?)

Decreased blood pressure

Bradycardia and/or heart block

Apnea

Allergic reactions

Fever (bacterial contamination of drug)

---

      c. Proexcitatory effects of propofol can be circumvented by using an adequate dosage regimen.

      d. It is presumed that propofol-induced "seizures" during induction or emergence from anesthesia are due to spontaneous excitatory movements of subcortical origin.

    4. Anticonvulsant properties of propofol are well documented (controls status epilepticus, shortens duration of electrically induced seizure activity, and masks seizure foci during temporal lobe mapping).

    5. Anxiolysis may accompany subhypnotic doses of propofol.

    6. Dreaming (amorous behavior or hallucinations) has been described in patients recovering from propofol anesthesia.

  E. Side Effects (Table 6-4)

    1. Central Nervous System

      a. Propofol has a vasoconstrictive effect on cerebral vasculature.

      b. Propofol is likely to be followed by decreased cerebral blood flow and a corresponding decrease in intracranial pressure.

    2. Cardiovascular System

      a. Propofol decreases blood pressure, cardiac output, and systemic vascular resistance to a greater extent than comparable doses of thiopental (Fig. 6-5).

      b. Blood pressure effects of propofol may be exaggerated in hypovolemic patients, elderly patients, and those with compromised left ventricular function.

      c. Despite decreases in blood pressure, heart rate often remains unchanged. This is in contrast to the modest heart rate increases that typically accom-

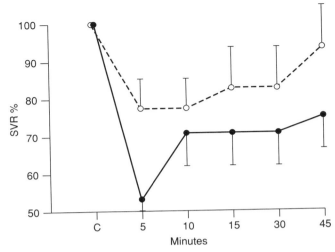

FIGURE 6–5. Comparative changes (expressed in percent changes [mean ± SD]) from control values (C) in systemic vascular resistance (SVR) in the 45 minutes following the administration of thiopental, 5 mg·kg⁻¹ IV (open circles) or propofol, 2.5 mg·kg⁻¹ IV (solid circles). (From Rouby J-J, Andreev A, Leger P, et al. Peripheral vascular effects of thiopental and propofol in humans with artificial hearts. Anesthesiology 1991;75:32–42; with permission.)

      pany rapid intravenous injection of thiopental (possibly reflecting a sympatholytic or vagotonic effect of propofol).

    d. Bradycardia and/or heart block has been observed following induction of anesthesia with propofol (sympathetic nervous system activity being decreased more than parasympathetic nervous system activity), resulting in the occasional recommendation that an anticholinergic drug be given when vagal stimulation is likely to occur in association with use of this drug.

  3. Ventilation. Propofol is a profound depressant of ventilation (transient apnea likely following rapid intravenous injection), and this effect is enhanced by opioids.

  4. Allergic reactions to propofol may reflect prior sensitization to drugs that contain a common antigenic component (phenyl nucleus, isopropyl side chain). Patients known to be allergic to muscle relaxants may be at increased risk for an allergic reaction to propofol.

5. Miscellaneous Effects

   a. Intraarterial administration of propofol does not damage vascular endothelium.

   b. The vehicle for propofol does not contain antibacterial preservatives, emphasizing the importance of maintaining strict asepsis when handling the drug and the need to discard any unused drug at the conclusion of single patient use.

   c. Free radical scavenging properties of propofol resemble those of vitamin E (free radicals may contribute to repefusion injury and acute inflammatory processes, such as acute lung injury, sepsis, and multisystem organ failure).

IV. ELTANOLONE

A. Eltanolone is a naturally occurring metabolite of progesterone that possesses sedative effects but lacks significant endocrine activity.

B. Low water solubility of eltanolone is circumvented by its formulation in an oil-and-water emulsion, currently in use as the solvent for propofol.

C. Intravenous administration of eltanolone produces a rapid onset of unconsciousness that is of short duration.

   1. Blood pressure decreases are modest following injection of eltanolone.

   2. Cerebral blood flow and cerebral oxygen consumption are decreased by eltanolone.

7

Local Anesthetics

Local anesthetics are drugs that produce reversible conduction blockade of impulses (autonomic, sensory, somatic motor) along central and peripheral nerve pathways following regional anesthesia. (Updated and revised from Stoelting RK. Local anesthetics. In: Pharmacology and Physiology in Anesthetic Practice. 2nd ed. Philadelphia, JB Lippincott, 1991;148–71.) Lidocaine is the standard to which all other local anesthetics are compared.

I. COMMERCIAL PREPARATIONS

   A. Local anesthetics are poorly soluble in water and, therefore, are marketed most often as water-soluble hydrochloride salts (the acidic pH contributes to the stability of the local anesthetic).
   B. An acidic pH of the local anesthetic solution is important if epinephrine is present, as this catecholamine is unstable at an alkaline pH.

II. STRUCTURE ACTIVITY RELATIONSHIPS

   A. Local anesthetics consist of a lipophilic (essential for anesthetic activity) and a hydrophilic portion, separated by a connecting hydrocarbon chain (Fig. 7–1).
   1. In almost all instances, an ester (—CO—) or an amide (—NHC—) bond links the hydrocarbon chain to the lipophilic aromatic ring (basis for the classification of local anesthetics as esters or amides).
   2. The important differences between ester and amide local anesthetics relate to the site of metabolism and the potential for producing allergic reactions.
   B. Modifying the chemical structure of a local anesthetic alters its pharmacologic effects (lengthening the connecting hydrocarbon chain or increasing the number of carbon atoms on the tertiary amine or aromatic ring often results in a drug with different lipid solubility,

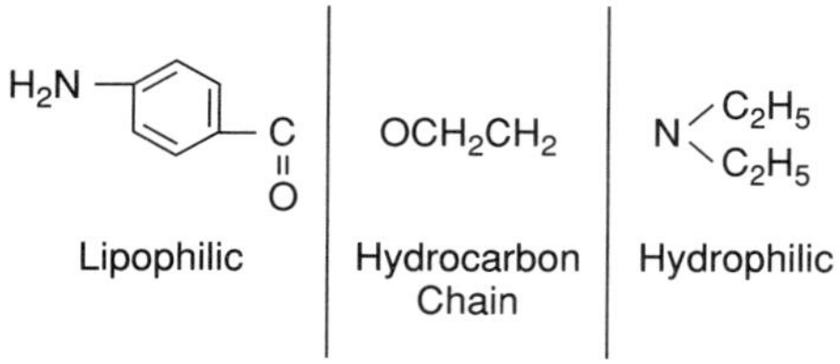

FIGURE 7–1. Local anesthetics consist of a lipophilic and hydrophilic portion separated by a connecting hydrocarbon chain.

potency, rate of metabolism, and duration of action) (Fig. 7–2 and Table 7–1).

III. PHARMACOKINETICS

    A. Local anesthetics are weak bases that have pH values somewhat above physiologic pH (as a result, less than 50% of the local anesthetic exists in a lipid-soluble nonionized form at physiologic pH) (Table 7–1).

        1. Acidosis in the environment into which the local anesthetic solution is injected (infection) further increases the ionized fraction (poor quality of local anesthesia).

        2. Local anesthetics with pKs nearest to physiologic pH have the most rapid onset of action, reflecting the presence of an optimal ratio of ionized to nonionized drug fraction.

        3. Intrinsic vasodilator activity (which is greater for lidocaine than for mepivacaine) will influence potency and duration of action (greater vascular absorption and shorter duration of action of lidocaine).

    B. Absorption and Distribution

        1. Absorption of a local anesthetic from its site of injection into the systemic circulation is influenced by the site of injection and dosage, use of epinephrine, and pharmacologic characteristics of the drug (Fig. 7–3).

        2. The ultimate plasma concentration of a local anesthetic is determined by the rate of tissue distribution and the rate of clearance (metabolism and excretion) of the drug (Fig. 7–4).

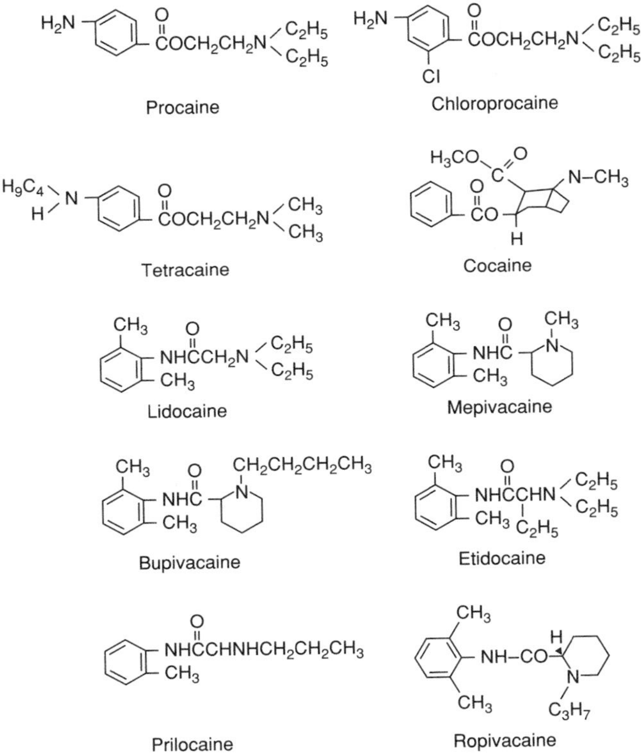

FIGURE 7–2. Ester and amide local anesthetics.

- **a.** After distribution to highly perfused tissues, the local anesthetic is redistributed to less well-perfused tissues, including skeletal muscles and fat.
- **b.** Lipid solubility of the local anesthetic is important in redistribution, as well as being a primary determinant of intrinsic local anesthetic activity.
3. **Protein binding** of local anesthetics parallels lipid solubility and is inversely related to the plasma concentration of drug.

(text continues on page 128)

Table 7-1
Comparative Pharmacology of Local Anesthetics

Classification	Potency	Onset	Duration After Infiltration (min)	Maximum Single Dose for Infiltration (adult, mg)*
Esters				
Procaine	1	Slow	45–60	500
Chloroprocaine	4	Rapid	30–45	600
Tetracaine	16	Slow	60–180	100 (topical)
Amides				
Lidocaine	1	Rapid	60–120	300
Mepivacaine	1	Slow	90–180	300
Bupivacaine	4	Slow	240–480	175
Etidocaine	4	Slow	240–480	300
Prilocaine	1	Slow	60–120	400
Ropivacaine[†]				

Classification	Toxic Plasma Concentration ($\mu g \cdot mL^{-1}$)	pK	Fraction Nonionized (percent) pH 7.2	pH 7.4	pH 7.6	Protein Binding (percent)
Esters						
Procaine		8.9	2	3	5	6
Chloroprocaine		8.7	3	5	7	
Tetracaine		8.5	5	7	11	76

Amides

						Elimination Half-Times (min)
Lidocaine	>5	7.9	17	25	33	70
Mepivacaine	>5	7.6	28	39	50	77
Bupivacaine	~1.5	8.1	11	15	24	95
Etidocaine	~2	7.7	24	33	44	94
Prilocaine	>5	7.9	17	24	33	55
Ropivacaine[†]	>4	8.1			94	

Classification	Lipid Solubility	Volume of Distribution (L)	Clearance (L·min⁻¹)	Elimination Half-Times (min)
Esters				
Procaine	0.6			
Chloroprocaine				
Tetracaine	80			
Amides				
Lidocaine	2.9	91	0.95	96
Mepivacaine	1.0	84	9.78	114
Bupivacaine	28	73	0.47	210
Etidocaine	141	133	1.22	156
Prilocaine	0.9			
Ropivacaine[†]				

*Use only as guideline; dose may be increased if solution contains epinephrine.

[†]Resembles bupivacaine.

(Reprinted from Covino BG, Vassallo, HL. Local anesthetics: Mechanisms of Action and Clinical Use. New York, Grune and Stratton, 1976, p. 73; with permission.)

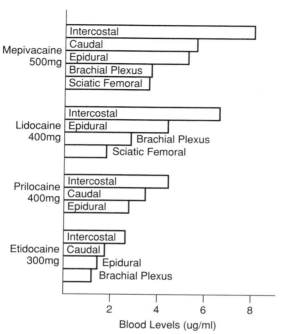

FIGURE 7–3. Peak plasma concentrations of local anesthetic are influenced by the site of injection for accomplishment of regional anesthesia. (From Covino BG, Vassallo HL. Local anesthetics: Mechanisms of Action and Clinical Use. New York, Grune and Stratton, 1976; with permission.)

    C. Lung Extraction. Passage of local anesthetics into the lungs will limit the concentration of drug that reaches the systemic circulation for distribution to the coronary and cerebral circulations.

    D. Placental Transfer

        1. Plasma protein binding influences the rate and degree of diffusion of local anesthetics across the placenta (more lidocaine than bupivacaine crosses the placenta).

        2. Acidosis in the fetus, which may occur during prolonged labor, can result in accumulation of local anesthetic in the fetus **(ion trapping)** (Fig. 7-5).

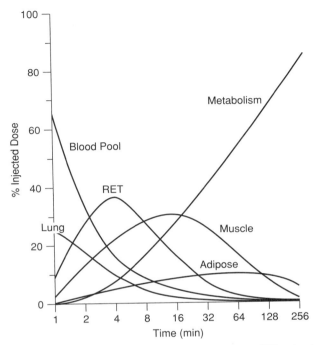

FIGURE 7–4. Perfusion model for the distribution of lidocaine in various tissues and its elimination after an intravenous infusion for 1 minute. *RET*, rapidly equilibrating (highly perfused) tissues. (From Benowitz N, Forsyth RP, Melmon KL, et al. Lidocaine disposition kinetics in monkey and man. I. Prediction by a perfusion model. Clin Pharmacol Ther 1974;16:87–92; with permission.)

       3. Ester local anesthetics, because of their rapid hydrolysis, are not available to cross the placenta in significant amounts.

    E. Clearance. Clearance values and elimination half-times for amide local anesthetics (rapid hydrolysis of ester local anesthetics limits measurement of these values) probably represent mainly hepatic metabolism, since renal excretion of unchanged drug is minimal.

    F. Metabolism of Amide Local Anesthetics

      1. Amide local anesthetics undergo varying rates of me-

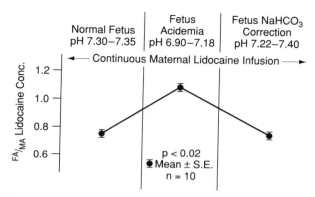

FIGURE 7–5. Fetal-maternal arterial (FA/MA) lidocaine ratios are greater during fetal acidemia compared with a normal pH. Mean ± SE. (From Biehl D, Shnider SM, Levinson G, Callender K. Placental transfer of lidocaine: Effects of fetal acidosis. Anesthesiology 1978;48:409–12; with permission.)

tabolism by microsomal enzymes located primarily in the liver (prilocaine > lidocaine and mepivacaine > bupivacaine and etidocaine).

   a. Slower metabolism of amide compared with ester local anesthetics means that sustained increases in the plasma concentrations of amide local anesthetics (and thus systemic toxicity) are more likely than with ester local anesthetics.

   b. Cumulative drug effects of amide local anesthetics are more likely than with ester local anesthetics.

2. Lidocaine

   a. The principal metabolic pathway of lidocaine is oxidative dealkylation in the liver to monoethylglycinexylidide (somewhat less potent than lidocaine in protecting against cardiac dysrhythmias), which is followed by its hydrolysis to xylidide (Fig. 7–6).

   b. Hepatic disease or decreases in hepatic blood flow, as can occur during anesthesia, can decrease the rate of metabolism of lidocaine (a reason to consider decreasing the rate of intravenous infusion of lidocaine being administered to treat cardiac dysrhythmias when an awake patient is rendered unconscious by general anesthesia).

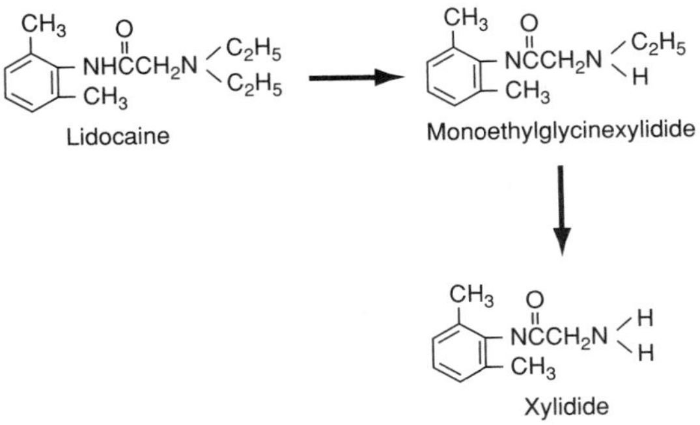

FIGURE 7–6. Metabolism of lidocaine.

3. **Mepivacaine**
   a. Clearance of mepivacaine is decreased in neonates, leading to a prolonged elimination half-time.
   b. Mepivacaine lacks vasodilator activity (in contrast to lidocaine) and so is an alternative when addition of epinephrine to the local anesthetic solution is not recommended.
4. **Bupivacaine** metabolism has not been fully elucidated in humans.
5. **Prilocaine**
   a. **Ortho-toludine,** the principal metabolite of prilocaine, is capable of converting hemoglobin to methemoglobin.
   b. The unique ability of prilocaine to cause dose-related **methemoglobinemia** (more likely when the prilocaine dose exceeds 600 mg) limits the clinical usefulness of this local anesthetic, except when used for intravenous regional anesthesia.
   c. **Treatment** of significant methemoglobinemia (decreased oxygen-carrying capacity and cyanosis) is with methylene blue, 1 to 2 mg·kg^{-1} IV over 5 minutes.
G. **Metabolism of Ester Local Anesthetics**
   1. Ester local anesthetics undergo varying rates of hydrolysis (chloroprocaine > procaine > tetracaine) by cholinesterase enzyme, principally in the plasma. The resulting metabolites are pharmacologically inactive, although **para-aminobenzoic acid** may be

an antigen responsible for subsequent **allergic reactions.**

   a. **Systemic toxicity** is inversely proportional to the rate of hydrolysis.
   b. Cerebrospinal fluid contains little or no cholinesterase enzyme, and anesthesia produced by subarachnoid placement of tetracaine will persist until the drug has been absorbed into the circulation.
   c. Patients with **atypical plasma cholinesterase** may be at increased risk for developing excess systemic concentrations of an ester local anesthetic owing to absent or limited plasma hydrolysis.
   d. Plasma cholinesterase activity may be decreased in parturients and in patients being treated with certain chemotherapeutic drugs.

   2. Cocaine
   a. The exception to hydrolysis of ester local anesthetics in the plasma is cocaine, which undergoes significant metabolism in the liver.
   b. Water-soluble metabolites of cocaine in the urine may be present for 24 to 36 hours (a useful marker of cocaine use or abstention).

H. Renal Elimination
   1. Poor water solubility of local anesthetics usually limits renal excretion of unchanged drug to less than 5% of the injected dose (except in the case of cocaine, 10% to 12% of which can be recovered unchanged in the urine).
   2. Water-soluble metabolites of local anesthetics, such as para-aminobenzoic acid resulting from metabolism of ester local anesthetics, are readily excreted in the urine.

I. Use of Vasoconstrictors
   1. Epinephrine (1:200,000) may be added to local anesthetic solutions to produce vasoconstriction, which limits systemic absorption and maintains the drug concentration in the vicinity of the nerve fibers to be anesthetized.
   a. Addition of epinephrine to a lidocaine solution prolongs the duration of conduction blockade by about 50%.
   b. The impact of epinephrine in prolonging the duration of conduction blockade and decreasing systemic absorption of bupivacaine (greater lipid sol-

ubility causes avid binding to tissues) is less than that observed with lidocaine.

    c. Alpha-agonist effects of epinephrine may also contribute to sensory anesthesia.

    d. Decreased systemic absorption of local anesthetic due to vasoconstriction produced by epinephrine increases the likelihood that the rate of metabolism will match that of absorption, thus decreasing the possibility of systemic toxicity.

  2. Whenever local anesthetic solutions containing epinephrine are administered in the presence of inhaled anesthetics, the possibility of enhanced cardiac irritability should be considered.

  3. Systemic absorption of epinephrine may accentuate hypertension in vulnerable patients.

J. Combinations of Local Anesthetics

  1. Local anesthetics may be combined in an effort to produce a rapid onset (chloroprocaine) and prolonged duration (bupivacaine) of action.

  2. Local anesthetic toxicity of combinations of drugs is additive rather than synergistic.

IV. MECHANISM OF ACTION

A. Local anesthetics prevent transmission of nerve impulses (conduction blockade) by inhibiting passage of sodium ions (Na^+) through ion-selective Na^+ channels in nerve membranes.

  1. The Na^+ channel is a specific receptor for local anesthetics.

  2. Failure of ion channel permeability to Na^+ to increase slows the rate of depolarization such that threshold potential is not reached and, thus, an action potential is not propagated (Fig. 7-7).

B. Sodium Channels

  1. Na^+ channels exist in activated-open, inactivated-closed, and rested-closed states during various phases of the action potential.

  2. It is speculated that local anesthetics stabilize Na^+ channels in inactivated-closed states such that changes in Na^+ permeability cannot occur. As a result, conduction of nerve impulses in the form of propagated action potentials cannot occur.

C. Frequency-Dependent Blockade

  1. Local anesthetic molecules can gain access to recep-

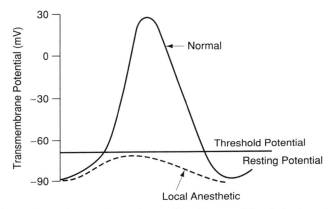

FIGURE 7–7. Local anesthetics slow the rate of depolarization of the nerve action potential such that threshold potential is not reached. As a result, an action potential cannot be propagated in the presence of local anesthetic, and conduction blockade results.

tors only when Na^+ channels are in activated-open states.

2. For this reason, selective conduction blockade of nerve fibers by local anesthetics may be related to the nerve's characteristic frequencies of activity, as well as to its anatomical properties, such as its diameter.

V. MINIMUM CONCENTRATION

A. The minimum concentration of local anesthetic necessary to produce conduction blockade of nerve impulses is termed the **Cm** (analogous to MAC for inhaled anesthetics).

1. The Cm is unique for each local anesthetic (differing potencies for each drug).

2. The Cm is influenced by the nerve diameter (with larger-diameter fibers requiring a higher Cm) and the presence or absence of myelin (necessary to expose at least two nodes of Ranvier to an adequate concentration).

B. **Differential Conduction Blockade.** This phenomenon is illustrated by selective blockade of nerve fibers based on their diameter and myelination (preganglionic sympathetic nervous system B fibers are blocked with lower concentrations than C and A fibers).

C. **Changes During Pregnancy.** Increased sensitivity (more rapid onset of conduction blockade) may be present during pregnancy.

VI. SIDE EFFECTS

A. Allergic Reactions

1. Allergic reactions to local anesthetics (or their preservatives) are rare (accounting for less than 1% of all adverse reactions to local anesthetics) despite the frequent use of these drugs.

   a. Ester local anesthetics that produce metabolites related to para-aminobenzoic acid are more likely than amide local anesthetics (not metabolized to para-aminobenzoic acid) to evoke an allergic reaction.

   b. **Preservatives,** such as methylparaben, are structurally similar to para-aminobenzoic acid. These preservatives are present in commercial preparations of both ester and amide local anesthetics.

2. **Cross-Sensitivity**

   a. A common metabolite, para-aminobenzoic acid, is the reason for cross-sensitivity between ester local anesthetics.

   b. A similar cross-sensitivity does not exist between classes of local anesthetics (a patient who is allergic to an ester local anesthetic can receive a preservative-free amide local anesthetic without adverse effect).

3. **Documentation of Allergy** (Table 7–2)

B. Systemic Toxicity

1. Systemic toxicity from a local anesthetic is due to an excess plasma concentration of the drug.

   a. Most adverse responses that are often attributed to allergic reactions are, instead, manifestations of excess plasma concentrations of the local anesthetic.

   b. Accidental direct intravascular injection of local anesthetic solutions during performance of peripheral nerve block anesthesia or epidural anesthesia is the most common mechanism for production of excess plasma concentrations of local anesthetics.

blockade of cardiac Na⁺ channels by bupivacaine, further contributing to its selective cardiac toxicity.

C. **Neurotoxicity**
  1. Intrathecal placement of hyperbaric lidocaine 5%, despite extensive use to produce spinal anesthesia, has been associated with lumbosacral root irritation (usually transient).
      a. Pooling of the hyperbaric lidocaine solution on the sacral side of the lordotic curve, especially when the solution is injected through a small-caliber continuous spinal catheter, may increase the risk of neurotoxicity.
      b. Stretching of nerves created by the lithotomy position may increase the risk of neurotoxicity from hyperbaric lidocaine.
      c. Neurotoxicity seems less likely when 5% lidocaine is administered in saline rather than in 7.5% dextrose.
  2. Chloroprocaine is not recommended for spinal anesthesia because of reports of cauda equina syndrome following intrathecal placement (possibly reflecting the neurotoxic effects of the preservative).

VII. **USES OF LOCAL ANESTHETICS** (Table 7–5)

  A. **Regional Anesthesia**
   1. **Topical anesthesia** is established by contact of the local anesthetic solution with mucous membranes (mouth, tracheobronchial tree, esophagus, genitourinary tract).
       a. Lidocaine, tetracaine, and cocaine are the local anesthetics selected most often for topical anesthesia.
       b. Cocaine's usefulness for topical anesthesia reflects its ability to produce localized vasoconstriction, thereby decreasing blood loss and improving surgical visualization.
       c. Procaine and chloroprocaine penetrate mucous membranes poorly and are ineffective for topical anesthesia.
       d. Topical anesthesia applied to the tracheobronchial tree inhibits ciliary activity, which may impair removal of secretions.
       e. Local anesthetics are absorbed into the systemic

Table 7–7
Physiologic Effects of Spinal Anesthesia

Arteriolar dilatation (blood pressure does not decrease proportionally because of compensatory vasoconstriction in areas with intact sympathetic nervous system innervation)

Decreased systemic vascular resistance

Venous dilatation (decreases venous return leading to decreases in cardiac output, especially in the presence of hypovolemia; is treated with head-down position and prompt administration of drugs with alpha agonist activity)

Heart rate slowing (blockade of preganglionic cardiac accelerator fibers)

Apnea (ischemic paralysis of medullary ventilatory centers due to a profound hypotension)

the accompanying level of **sympathetic nervous system blockade** (Table 7-7).

B. Analgesia
1. Continuous low-dose intravenous infusion of lidocaine to maintain a plasma concentration of 1 to 2 $\mu g \cdot ml^{-1}$ decreases the severity of postoperative pain without producing systemic toxicity.
2. Lidocaine may be administered intravenously in the perioperative period as a cough suppressant (intubation and extubation of the trachea).

C. Prevention or Treatment of Increases in Intracranial Pressure
1. Lidocaine, $1.5 \ mg \cdot kg^{-1}$ IV, is as effective as thiopental in preventing increases in intracranial pressure (as well as increases in blood pressure) as may be evoked by intubation of the trachea.
2. An advantage of using lidocaine rather than barbiturates is a lesser likelihood of drug-induced hypotension.

VIII. COCAINE TOXICITY (Table 7-8)

IX. ROPIVACAINE

A. Ropivacaine is a long-acting amide local anesthetic that resembles bupivacaine in its chemical structure, pK, protein binding, and clinical uses (Table 7-1; Fig. 7-1).

Table 7–8
Manifestations of Cocaine Toxicity

Hypertension

Tachycardia (treated with esmolol)

Coronary artery vasoconstriction (myocardial ischemia, myocardial infarction, cardiac dysrhythmias)

Cerebrovascular accidents

Decreased uterine blood flow (fetal hypoxemia)

Hyperpyrexia

Seizures

    B. This drug is unique among local anesthetics because it is prepared as the S-isomer rather than as a racemic mixture.

        1. Cardiac toxicity of the S-isomer may be less than that of racemic preparations.

        2. Ropivacaine's lipid solubility and depressant effect on cardiac excitation and conduction are intermediate between those of lidocaine and bupivacaine.

    C. Ropivacaine produces less motor blockade than bupivacaine, which may be an advantage for obstetric patients in labor and for those experiencing acute and chronic pain.

    D. Ropivacaine 0.5% and bupivacaine 0.5% are comparable when used for brachial plexus block and epidural anesthesia.

8

Neuromuscular Blocking Drugs

The principal pharmacologic effect of neuromuscular blocking drugs is to interrupt transmission of nerve impulses at the neuromuscular junction. (Updated and revised from Stoelting RK. Neuromuscular blocking drugs. In: Pharmacology and Physiology in Anesthetic Practice. 2nd ed. Philadelphia, JB Lippincott, 1991;172–225.)

I. INTRODUCTION

A. On the basis of distinct electrophysiologic differences in their mechanisms of action and duration of action, neuromuscular blocking drugs can be classified as either **depolarizing** or **nondepolarizing** (Table 8–1).

B. Clinically, the most common method for determining the type and degree of neuromuscular blockade present is to observe or record the skeletal muscle response (most often, contraction of the adductor pollicis muscle innervated by the ulnar nerve) that is evoked by a supramaximal electrical stimulus delivered from a peripheral nerve stimulator (diaphragm is more resistant to neuromuscular blocking drugs than are peripheral muscles).

1. **A single twitch** response evoked using a peripheral nerve stimulator reflects events at the **postjunctional membrane**.

2. The response to **continuous stimulation (tetanus)** reflects events at the **presynaptic membrane**.

3. The **electromyogram** (EMG) serves the same purpose as the peripheral nerve stimulator.

II. CLINICAL USES

A. The principal uses of neuromuscular blocking drugs are to provide **skeletal muscle relaxation** to facilitate tracheal intubation and to provide optimal surgical working conditions.

Table 8–1
Classification of Neuromuscular Blocking Drugs

Depolarizers
  Succinylcholine

Nondepolarizers
  Long-acting
    d-Tubocurarine
    Metocurine
    Gallamine
    Pancuronium
    Doxacurium
    Pipecuronium

  Intermediate-acting
    Atracurium
    Vecuronium
    Rocuronium

  Short-acting
    Mivacurium

---

1. These drugs lack central nervous system depressant effects and cannot substitute for anesthetic drugs.
2. Ventilation of the lungs must be provided mechanically whenever substantial neuromuscular blockade is present.

B. Drug Selection. The choice between depolarizing and nondepolarizing neuromuscular blocking drugs is influenced by their speed of onset, duration of action, and capacity for producing side effects (circulatory side effects reflect the actions of these drugs at sites other than the neuromuscular junction).

C. Sequence of Onset of Neuromuscular Blockade
1. Neuromuscular blocking drugs affect small, rapidly moving muscles (eyes, digits) before those of the abdomen (diaphragm).
   a. The onset of neuromuscular blockade following the administration of nondepolarizing neuromuscular blocking drugs is more rapid but less intense at the laryngeal muscles than at the peripheral muscles (reflects differential rates of equilibration between plasma and various skeletal muscles) (Fig. 8–1).
   b. Recovery of laryngeal muscles is more rapid than that of the adductor pollicis muscle (Fig. 8–1).
2. The maximum effect of neuromuscular blocking drugs

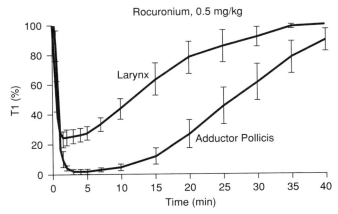

FIGURE 8–1. The effects of rocuronium (in terms of maximum depression of twitch) were less intense and duration of action was less at the adductor muscles of the larynx than at the adductor pollicis. (From Plaud B, Donati F. Rocuronium [ORG 9426] neuromuscular blockade at the adductor muscles of the larynx and adductor pollicis in humans. Can J Anaesth 1992;39:665–9; with permission.)

at the laryngeal muscles may not correspond to the initial onset of twitch depression as monitored at the adductor pollicis (see Section VIII B).

   a. With short- and intermediate-acting neuromuscular blocking drugs, the period of laryngeal paralysis is brief and may be dissipating before a maximum effect is reached at the thumb (adductor pollicis) (Fig. 8–1).

   b. The orbicularis oculi (facial nerve) is a better monitor of the onset of neuromuscular blockade for drugs such as mivacurium at the vocal cords (recurrent laryngeal nerve) than is the adductor pollicis (ulnar nerve) (Fig. 8–2) (see Section VIII B).

III. STRUCTURE ACTIVITY RELATIONSHIPS

   A. Neuromuscular blocking drugs are structurally similar to the endogenous neurotransmitter acetylcholine (Fig. 8–3).

   1. Succinylcholine is two molecules of acetylcholine linked through acetate methyl groups.

   2. Bulky and rigid molecules that are characteristic of

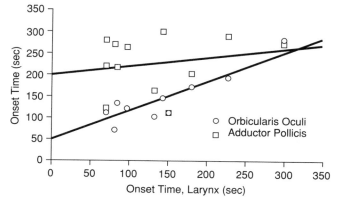

FIGURE 8–2.   Onset time to loss of visible detectable response in the orbicularis oculi and adductor pollicis, versus measured onset time to 100% depression of response in laryngeal muscles. No correlation was found between adductor pollicis and laryngeal muscle onset time. Onset time in the orbicularis oculi correlated significantly with that of the laryngeal muscles ($P < 0.001$). (From Unureanu D, Meistelman C, Frossard J. Donati F. The orbicularis oculi and the adductor pollicis muscles as monitors of atracurium block of laryngeal muscles. Anesth Analg 1993;77:775–9; with permission.)

        nondepolarizing neuromuscular blocking drugs contain portions similar to acetylcholine.

B. Acetylcholine has a positively charged quaternary ammonium group (four carbon atoms attached to one nitrogen atom) that attaches to the negatively charged cholinergic receptor (neuromuscular junction).

    1. The electrostatic attraction of the negatively charged nicotinic cholinergic receptor for the positively charged quaternary ammonium group of acetylcholine also occurs at cholinergic sites other than the neuromuscular junction (lack of specificity), including cardiac muscarinic receptors and nicotinic autonomic ganglia receptors.

    2. Circulatory effects of neuromuscular blocking drugs may reflect drug-induced **histamine release** or attachment of these drugs to receptors at sites other than the neuromuscular junction (especially with high doses).

    3. All neuromuscular blocking drugs contain at least one

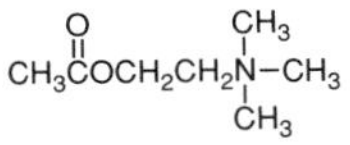

Acetylcholine

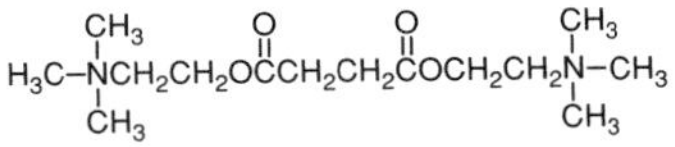

Succinylcholine

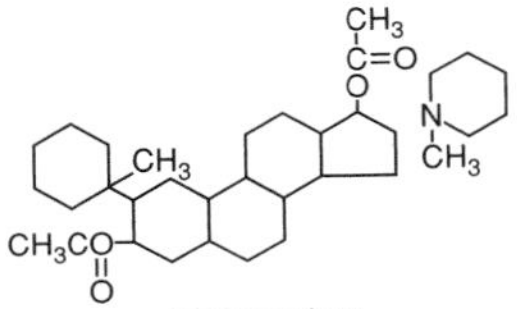

Pancuronium

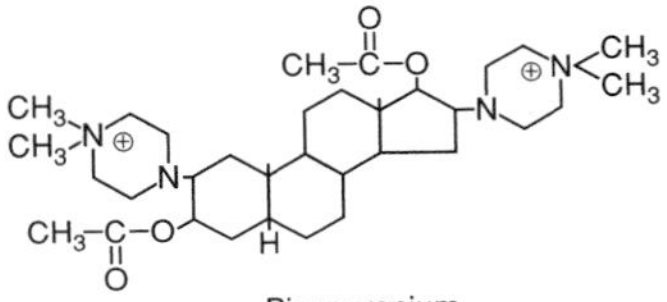

Pipecuronium

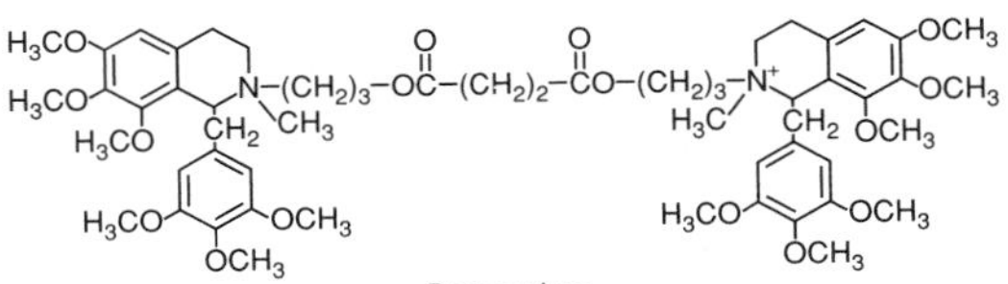

Doxacurium

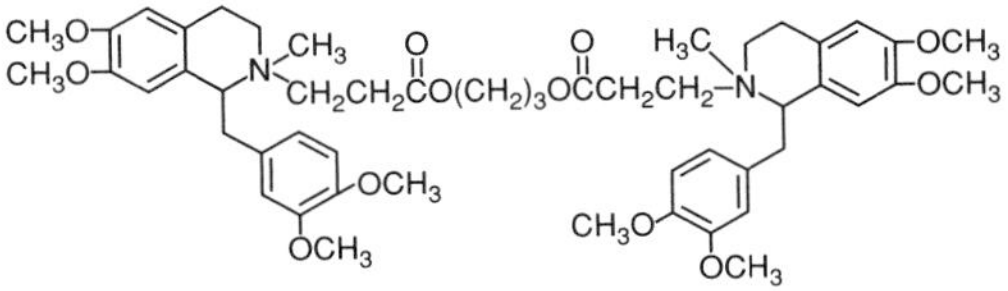

Atracurium

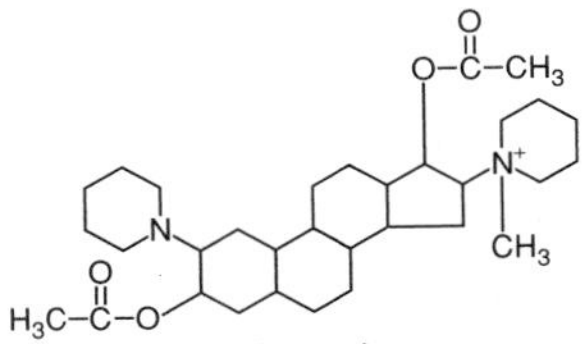

Vecuronium

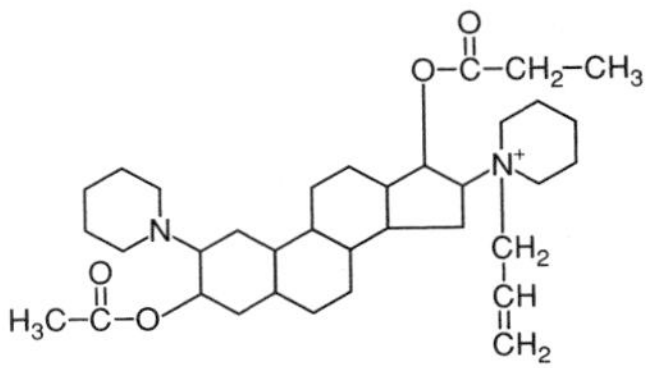

Rocuronium

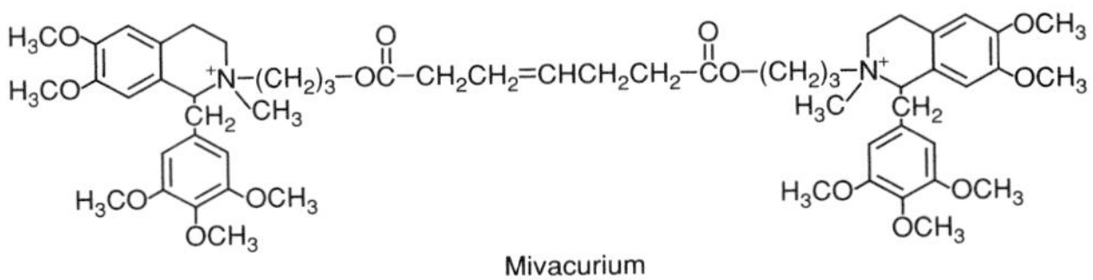

Mivacurium

FIGURE 8–3. Acetylcholine and neuromuscular blocking drugs.

quaternary ammonium group (allergic cross-sensitivity between all neuromuscular blocking drugs reflects the antigenic effects of the quaternary ammonium group).

4. Aminosteroid muscle relaxants (pancuronium, vecuronium, rocuronium) lack hormonal activity.

IV. NEUROMUSCULAR JUNCTION

A. The neuromuscular junction consists of a prejunctional motor nerve ending separated from a highly folded postjunctional membrane of the skeletal muscle fiber by a synaptic cleft (Fig. 8–4).

1. The resting transmembrane potential of approximately -90 mV across nerve and skeletal muscle membranes is maintained by the unequal distribution of potassium (K^+) and sodium (Na^+) ions across the membrane.

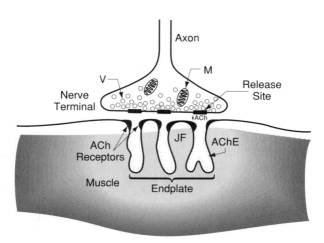

FIGURE 8–4.   Schematic depiction of the neuromuscular junction. Acetylcholine (ACh) is present in vesicles (V) of the axon for release in response to nerve impulses. The neurotransmitter diffuses across the synaptic cleft to attach to receptors that are concentrated on the junctional folds (JF) of the skeletal muscle endplate. Acetylcholinesterase (AChE) is present in the JF to facilitate rapid hydrolysis of ACh. (From Drachman DA. Myasthenia gravis. N Engl J Med 1978;298:136–42; with permission.)

      2. Nicotinic cholinergic receptors are situated on both the presynaptic and postsynaptic membranes.

B. Acetylcholine

    1. Acetylcholine is synthesized and stored in the motor nerve ending for release as a neurotransmitter in response to arrival of a nerve impulse.

    2. Acetylcholine traverses the synaptic cleft and attaches to nicotinic cholinergic receptors on postsynaptic membranes, causing a change in membrane permeability to ions.

      a. This change in permeability causes a decrease in the transmembrane potential from approximately -90 mV to -45 mV (threshold potential), at which point a propagated **action potential** (depolarization) spreads over the surface of the skeletal muscle (contraction).

      b. Acetylcholinesterase (true cholinesterase) situated in close proximity to cholinergic receptors is responsible for rapid hydrolysis (less than 15 ms) of acetylcholine, leading to a restoration (repolarization) of membrane permeability.

C. Postjunctional Nicotinic Receptors

    1. Nicotinic cholinergic receptors are present in large numbers on postjunctional membranes, forming a channel that allows the flow of ions (Fig. 8–5).

      a. These ion channels are open (in the active state) and allow the flow of ions only when an acetylcholine molecule occupies each of the subunits.

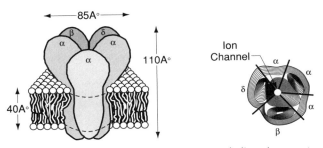

FIGURE 8–5. The postjunctional nicotinic cholinergic receptor consists of five subunits designated alpha (two subunits), beta, gamma, and delta. (From Taylor P. Are neuromuscular blocking agents more efficacious in pairs? Anesthesiology 1985;63:1–3; with permission.)

    b. This flow of ions is the basis for normal neuromuscular transmission.

    c. Alpha subunits, in addition to being the binding sites for acetylcholine, are the sites occupied by neuromuscular blocking drugs.

    d. Occupation of one or both alpha subunits by a nondepolarizing neuromuscular blocking drug causes the channel to remain closed (ions cannot flow so depolarization does not occur; hence the term nondepolarizing neuromuscular blocking drugs).

      e. A nondepolarizing neuromuscular blocking drug may show a preference for one of the two alpha subunits, resulting in synergism if two drugs with different preferences for each alpha subunit are administered simultaneously.

      f. Succinylcholine, by binding to each subunit, causes the channel to remain open (mimics acetylcholine), resulting in sustained depolarization (in contrast to acetylcholine) that prevents propagation of an action potential (hence the term depolarizer).

2. Extrajunctional Cholinergic Receptors

    a. Neural activity suppresses synthesis of these receptors.

    b. Whenever motor nerves are less active (denervation or trauma to skeletal muscle), extrajunctional cholinergic receptors proliferate, providing additional sites for ion flow (hyperkalemia following succinylcholine, resistance to the effects of nondepolarizing neuromuscular blocking drugs).

    c. Varying numbers of extrajunctional cholinergic receptors may account for differences in response to neuromuscular blocking drugs among individuals and in the presence of various disease states.

D. Prejunctional Nicotinic Receptors. These receptors influence the release of neurotransmitters and provide an additional site for attachment of neuromuscular blocking drugs.

V. DEPOLARIZING NEUROMUSCULAR BLOCKING DRUGS

A. Succinylcholine is the only nondepolarizing neuromuscular blocking drug that is used clinically, most often to facilitate tracheal intubation.

1. Administered in a dose of 0.5 to 1 mg·kg^{-1} IV, the onset of action of succinylcholine is prompt (30 to 60 seconds) and the duration of its action is brief (3 to 5 minutes).
2. The ED$_{90}$ for succinylcholine is 0.27 mg·kg^{-1}.
3. A small dose of succinylcholine (0.1 mg·kg^{-1} IV) has been found to be reliable in the treatment of laryngospasm.

B. Mechanism of Action

1. Succinylcholine attaches to each of the alpha subunits of the nicotinic cholinergic receptor and mimics the action of acetylcholine, thus depolarizing the postjunctional membrane.
   a. Compared with acetylcholine, the hydrolysis of succinylcholine is slow, resulting in sustained depolarization (opening) of the receptor ion channels.
   b. Neuromuscular blockade develops because a depolarized postjunctional membrane cannot respond to a subsequent release of acetylcholine (depolarizing neuromuscular blockade, or phase I blockade).
2. Sustained opening of receptor ion channels (and the resulting depolarization of postjunctional membranes) produced by succinylcholine is associated with leakage of K$^+$ from the interior of cells sufficient to produce an average 0.5 mEq·L^{-1} increase in serum K$^+$ concentrations.
3. A single large dose (more than 2 mg·kg^{-1} IV), repeated doses, or a continuous infusion of succinylcholine may result in postjunctional membranes that do not respond normally to acetylcholine, even when postjunctional membranes have become repolarized (desensitization neuromuscular blockade, or phase II blockade).
4. Characteristics of phase I blockade (Table 8–2)
5. Characteristics of phase II blockade (Table 8–2)

C. Duration of Action

1. The brief duration of action of succinylcholine (3 to 5 minutes) is principally due to its hydrolysis by plasma cholinesterase (pseudocholinesterase) enzyme (Fig. 8–6).
   a. **Succinylcholine** is 1/20 to 1/80 as potent as a neuromuscular blocker.
   b. Rapid hydrolysis makes it difficult to obtain pharmacokinetic data for succinylcholine.

Table 8–2
Characteristics of Succinylcholine

Phase I Blockade
  Decreased single twitch
  Decreased but sustained response to continuous stimulation
  Train-of-four ratio more than 0.7
  Augmentation of neuromuscular blockade by anticholinesterase
    drugs

Phase II Blockade (resembles nondepolarizing neuromuscular
  blockade)
  Decreased single twitch
  Fade during continuous stimulation
  Train-of-four ratio lower than 0.7
  Antagonism of neuromuscular blockade by anticholinesterase
    drugs (confirmed with a small dose of edrophonium [0.1 to 0.2
    $mg \cdot kg^{-1}$ IV])
  Onset manifests as tachyphylaxis to succinylcholine (usually after
    a total dose of 2 to 4 $mg \cdot kg^{-1}$ IV)

  c. Plasma cholinesterase has an enormous capacity
     to hydrolyze succinylcholine such that only a
     small fraction of the original intravenous dose of
     drug actually reaches the neuromuscular junction
     (influences the duration of action of succinylcho-
     line by controlling the amount of neuromuscular
     blocking drug that is hydrolyzed before reaching
     the neuromuscular junction).
2. **Plasma Cholinesterase Activity**
  a. **Liver disease** must be severe before decreases
     in plasma cholinesterase production sufficient to
     prolong succinylcholine-induced neuromuscular
     blockade occur.
  b. Potent anticholinesterase drugs (insecticides,
     agents used to treat glaucoma or myasthenia gra-
     vis) and chemotherapeutic drugs (nitrogen mus-
     tard, cyclophosphamide) may decrease plasma
     cholinesterase activity so that prolonged neuro-
     muscular blockade follows administration of suc-
     cinylcholine.
3. **Atypical Plasma Cholinesterase**
  a. The presence of atypical plasma cholinesterase
     (several genetically related variants) is often rec-

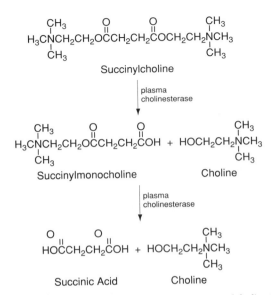

FIGURE 8–6. The brief duration of action of succinylcholine is principally due to its rapid hydrolysis in the plasma by cholinesterase enzyme to inactive metabolites.

ognized only after an otherwise healthy patient experiences prolonged neuromuscular blockade (1 to 3 hours) following a conventional dose of succinylcholine (Table 8–3).

b. Dibucaine inhibits the activity of normal plasma cholinesterase by approximately 80% (dibucaine number 80) compared with only approximately 20% inhibition of the activity of atypical enzyme (dibucaine number 20).

c. A dibucaine number of 20 occurs in approximately 1 in every 3200 patients (homozygous for atypical plasma cholinesterase enzyme).

d. A dibucaine number of 40 to 60 occurs in approximately 1 in every 480 patients (heterozygous for atypical plasma cholinesterase enzyme).

e. The dibucaine number reflects the quality of plasma cholinesterase (ability to metabolize suc-

Table 8–3
Hereditary Variants of Plasma Cholinesterase

Genotype	Dibucaine Number	Fluoride Number	Response to Succinylcholine	Frequency
$E^u E^u$	80	60	Normal	96%
$E^a E^a$	20	20	Greatly prolonged	1 in 3200
$E^u E^a$	60	45	Slightly prolonged	1 in 480
$E^u E^f$	75	50	Slightly prolonged	1 in 200
$E^f E^a$	45	35	Greatly prolonged	1 in 20,000

E^u, normal gene; E^a, atypical enzyme gene; E^f, fluoride-sensitive gene

cinylcholine), not the quantity of the enzyme that is circulating in the plasma (decreased circulating levels due to liver disease do not alter the dibucaine number).

D. Adverse Side Effects (Table 8–4)

1. Intravenous administration of succinylcholine produces modest and transient (usually shorter than 5 minutes) increases in intraocular pressure (occurs even in the absence of extraocular muscle contraction, suggesting that the cycloplegic action of succinylcholine is primarily responsible) (Fig. 8–7).

2. Hyperkalemia, myoglobinuria, and cardiac dysrhythmias may follow the administration of succinylcholine to children with undiagnosed myopathies (Duchenne's muscular dystrophy occurs only in males and is always associated with a preexisting increase in creatinine phosphokinase concentration).

E. Administration of succinylcholine, 1 mg·kg^{-1} IV, to brain-injured patients does not alter cerebral blood flow velocity, intracranial pressure, or the electroencephalogram (Fig. 8–8).

F. Incomplete jaw relaxation (not trismus) after a halothane-succinylcholine sequence is not uncommon in children, and is considered to be a normal response.

VI. LONG-ACTING NONDEPOLARIZING NEUROMUSCULAR BLOCKING DRUGS

A. Long-acting nondepolarizing neuromuscular blocking drugs are characterized by an onset of maximum neuro-

Table 8–4
Adverse Side Effects of Succinylcholine

Cardiac dysrhythmias (bradycardia reflects the ability of succinylcholine to mimic the normal effects of acetylcholine at cardiac muscarinic cholinergic receptors, especially when a second dose is administered about 5 minutes after the first dose)

Increased heart rate and/or blood pressure (reflects the ability of succinylcholine to mimic the normal effects of acetylcholine at autonomic nervous system ganglia)

Hyperkalemia
    Unhealed third-degree burns
    Denervation leading to skeletal muscle atrophy (may develop
      within 96 hours and may persist for 6 months or longer)
    Severe skeletal muscle trauma
    Upper motor neuron lesions
    Muscular dystrophy

Myalgia (particularly prominent in the muscles of the neck, back, abdomen, especially in young patients undergoing elective surgery; neck muscle soreness may be misinterpreted as a sore throat secondary to tracheal intubation)

Myoglobinuria

Increased intragastric pressure (prevent by prior administration of a nonparalyzing dose of nondepolarizing muscle relaxant)

Increased intraocular pressure (transient, lasting only 5 to 10 minutes)

Sustained skeletal muscle contraction (masseter spasm)

Trigger for malignant hyperthermia

muscular blockade in 3 to 5 minutes and a duration of action of 60 to 90 minutes (dose necessary to depress twitch 95% [ED_{95}] is frequently used as an index of equal potency for drug comparisons) (Table 8–5).

B. Mechanism of Action

    1. Nondepolarizing neuromuscular blocking drugs are classically thought to act by combining with postganglionic nicotinic cholinergic receptors (act competitively with acetylcholine at alpha subunits of the receptor) without causing any activation (change in configuration) of these receptors.

    2. Occupation of as many as 70% of the nicotinic cholinergic receptors by a neuromuscular blocking drug does not produce evidence of neuromuscular block-

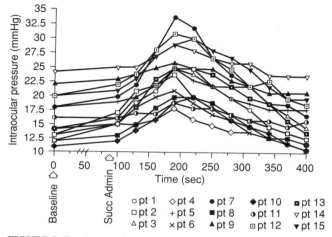

FIGURE 8–7.   Intraocular pressure changes following administration of succinylcholine (Succ Admin), 1.5 mg·kg^{-1} IV, to patients in whom all extraocular muscles had been previously detached. (From Kelly RE, Dinner M, Turner LS, Haik B, Abramson DH, Daines P. Succinylcholine increases intraocular pressure in the human eye with the extraocular muscles detached. Anesthesiology 1993;79:948–52; with permission.)

ade, as reflected by the twitch response to a single stimulus.

C. Characteristics of Nondepolarizing Neuromuscular Blockade (Table 8–6)

D. Pharmacokinetics (Table 8–5)

  1. Nondepolarizing neuromuscular blocking drugs, because of their quaternary ammonium groups, are highly ionized at physiologic pH and possess limited lipid solubility.

    a. The volume of distribution is small, being limited principally to extracellular fluid.

    b. These drugs cannot easily cross lipid barriers (blood–brain barrier, renal tubular epithelium, gastrointestinal epithelium, placenta).

  2. Size of the Initial Dose

    a. The magnitude of neuromuscular blockade, as characterized by twitch response, is proportional to the plasma concentration of the neuromuscular blocking drug.

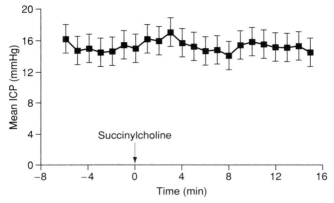

FIGURE 8–8. Succinylcholine (1 mg·kg⁻¹ IV), when administered to patients with neurologic injury (median Glasgow coma scale score of 6), did not change the mean intracranial pressure (ICP). (From Kovarik WD, Mayberg TS, Lam AM, Mathisen TL, Winn HR. Succinylcholine does not change intracranial pressure, cerebral blood flow velocity, or the electroencephalogram in patients with neurologic injury. Anesth Analg 1994;78:469-73; with permission.)

    b. The size of the initial dose or a supplemental dose of nondepolarizing neuromuscular blocking drug determines the resulting plasma concentration of drug.

  3. The response to nondepolarizing neuromuscular blocking drugs is influenced by pharmacokinetic factors (relative impact varies among the neuromuscular blocking drugs) that probably explain variable patient responses to these drugs (Table 8-7).

  4. The absence of age-related changes in responsiveness of the neuromuscular junction (changes in pharmacodynamics) is confirmed by similar dose-response curves in elderly and young adults receiving nondepolarizing neuromuscular blocking drugs (Fig. 8-9).

  5. Response of Pediatric Patients

    a. Neonates and infants are more sensitive to nondepolarizing neuromuscular blocking drugs.

    b. Nevertheless, the initial dose administered to achieve the same plasma concentration of nondepolarizing neuromuscular blocking drug is similar

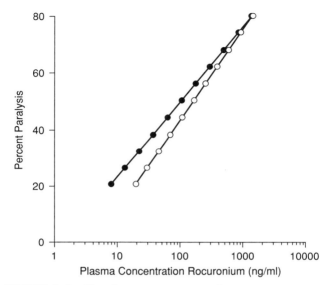

FIGURE 8–9.   The plasma concentration of rocuronium necessary to produce a specific degree of paralysis is not different in elderly (*solid circles*) and young adults (*open circles*). (From Matteo RS, Ornstein E, Schwartz AE, Ostapkovich N, Stone JG. Pharmacokinetics and pharmacodynamics of rocuronium [ORG 9426] in elderly surgical patients. Anesth Analg 1993;77:1193–7; with permission.)

    b. A sympathomimetic effect of pancuronium apparently plays a minor role in heart rate responses (beta blockade does not predictably prevent heart rate responses to pancuronium).

    c. The magnitude of heart rate increase evoked by pancuronium seems more dependent on the pre-existing heart rate (an inverse relationship) than the dose or rate of drug administration.

    d. Marked increases in heart rate seem more likely to occur in patients with altered atrioventricular conduction of cardiac impulses such as occur in atrial fibrillation.

    e. Cardiac stimulating effects of pancuronium may also increase the incidence of myocardial ischemia in patients with coronary artery disease.

Table 8-8
Mechanisms of Neuromuscular Blocking Drug-Induced Cardiovascular Effects

ED_{95} Dose	Histamine Release	Cardiac Muscarinic Receptors	Nicotinic Receptors at Autonomic Ganglia
Succinylcholine	Slight	Modest stimulation	Modest stimulation
Pancuronium	None	Modest blockade	None
Pipecuronium	None	None	None
Doxacurium	None	None	None
Atracurium	Slight	None	None
Vecuronium	None	None	None
Rocuronium	None	None(?)	None
Mivacurium	Slight	None	None

3. Doxacurium

a. Doxacurium is devoid of histamine-releasing or cardiovascular side effects.

b. Pharmacokinetics of doxacurium resemble pancuronium (dependence on renal clearance mechanisms) (Table 8–5).

c. Intensity of neuromuscular blockade produced by doxacurium is similar in young and elderly adults (ED_{95} similar in both), although a longer duration of action (T10–25) can be expected in the elderly.

d. Reversal of doxacurium-induced residual neuromuscular blockade with neostigmine may take longer than 10 minutes, and may be incomplete.

4. Pipecuronium

a. This steroidal nondepolarizing neuromuscular blocking drug is devoid of histamine-releasing or cardiovascular side effects.

b. Pharmacokinetics of pipecuronium resemble pancuronium (dependence on renal clearance mechanisms) (Table 8–5).

c. Hepatic cirrhosis does not alter the pharmacokinetics or pharmacodynamics of pipecuronium.

d. The pharmacologic actions of pipecuronium in otherwise healthy patients do not differ between young and elderly adults.

5.
Only small hemodynamic differences between pancuronium, doxacurium, and pipecuronium were observed following administration of $2 \times ED_{95}$ doses of these drugs (Figs. 8–10 and 8–11).

F. Causes of Altered Responses (Table 8–9)

1. Volatile anesthetics
most likely enhance the effects of nondepolarizing neuromuscular blocking drugs by virtue of anesthetic-induced depression of the central nervous system (decreases the tone of skeletal muscles) and, possibly, decreased sensitivity of postjunctional membranes to depolarization.

a. Plasma concentrations of nondepolarizing neuromuscular blocking drug necessary to decrease the twitch response 90% are lower during administration of a volatile anesthetic than of nitrous oxide-opioid.

b. This difference in plasma concentrations confirms that volatile anesthetic-induced potentiation of neuromuscular blockade represents a

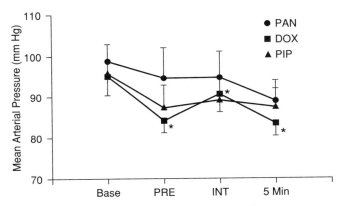

FIGURE 8–10. Mean arterial pressure awake (BASE) was measured in awake patients and then 5 minutes after anesthetic induction (PRE) with fentanyl, 50 µg·kg^{-1} IV, plus 2 × ED$_{95}$ of pancuronium (PAN), doxacurium (DOX), or pipecuronium (PIP) immediately after tracheal intubation (INT), and 5 minutes after tracheal intubation (5 MIN). There were no differences between treatment groups at any time. *P < .05 compared with baseline. (From Rathmell JP, Brooker RF, Prielipp RC, Butterworth JF, Gravlee GP. Hemodynamic and pharmacodynamic comparison of doxacurium and pipecuronium with pancuronium during induction of cardiac anesthesia: Does the benefit justify the cost? Anesth Analg 1993;513–9; with permission.)

change in pharmacodynamics, rather than pharmacokinetics.

2. **Calcium** produces unpredictable effects in antagonizing antibiotic-induced enhancement of neuromuscular blockade produced by nondepolarizing neuromuscular blocking drugs.

3. Possible enhancement of neuromuscular blockade should be considered when administering cardiac antidysrhythmic doses of **lidocaine** intravenously to patients recovering from general anesthesia that included use of a nondepolarizing neuromuscular blocking drug.

4. Monitoring neuromuscular blockade with a peripheral nerve stimulator attached to a paretic or paralyzed extremity may **underestimate** the degree of **neuromuscular blockade** and **overestimate** the

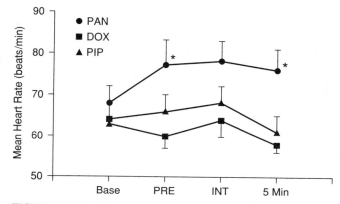

FIGURE 8–11.   Heart rate at various times following induction of anesthesia and administration of $2 \times ED_{95}$ of pancuronium, doxacurium, and pipecuronium. *$P < .05$ compared to baseline. (See legend for Figure 8-10 for a description of labels.) (From Rathmell JP, Brooker RF, Prielipp RC, Butterworth JF, Gravlee GP. Hemodynamic and pharmacodynamic comparison of doxacurium and pipecuronium with pancuronium during induction of cardiac anesthesia: Does the benefit justify the cost? Anesth Analg 1993;76:513–9; with permission.)

degree of **recovery** from neuromuscular blockade present at muscles utilized for breathing.

5. **Succinylcholine Followed by a Nondepolarizing Neuromuscular Blocking Drug.** Following administration of a dose of succinylcholine for intubation of the trachea the subsequent onset of nondepolarizing neuromuscular blockade is faster and recovery is delayed (unexpected since these two classes of drugs should be antagonistic).

6. **Combination of Neuromuscular Blocking Drugs**

   a. The combination of pancuronium and metocurine (also vecuronium and metocurine) produces neuromuscular blockade that is synergistic rather than additive, presumably reflecting the differing sites of action (prejunctional versus postjunctional) of these two drugs.

   b. The combination of nondepolarizing neuromuscular blocking drugs permits achievement of the

Table 8–9
Causes of Altered Responses to Nondepolarizing
Neuromuscular Blocking Drugs

Drugs that Enhance Neuromuscular Blockade

Volatile anesthetics (dose-dependent enhancement of magnitude and duration; greater enhancement with desflurane and isoflurane than with halothane)

Aminoglycoside antibiotics (excepting penicillins and cephalosporins)

Local anesthetics

Cardiac antidysrhythmic drugs (lidocaine, quinidine)

Loop diuretics (osmotic diuretics that do not alter glomerular filtration rate are exceptions)

Magnesium

Lithium

Phenytoin

Cyclosporine

Changes Unrelated to Concurrent Drug Therapy

Hypothermia (slows renal and hepatic clearance mechanisms)

Acid-base changes (respiratory acidosis enhances; other changes are unpredictable)

Serum potassium concentration (acute decreases enhance whereas increases oppose the action of nondepolarizing neuromuscular blocking drugs)

Thermal (burn) injury (resistance to the effects of nondepolarizing neuromuscular blocking drugs)

Allergic reaction (the cross-sensitivity between all neuromuscular blocking drugs reflects the antigenic effect of quaternary ammonium groups)

---

same degree of neuromuscular blockade with a smaller dose of each drug (fewer dose-related cardiovascular effects).

VII. INTERMEDIATE-ACTING NONDEPOLARIZING NEUROMUSCULAR BLOCKING DRUGS (Table 8-10)

A. Atracurium, vecuronium, and rocuronium are intermediate-acting nondepolarizing neuromuscular blocking drugs with efficient clearance mechanisms (reason for

Table 8–10

Characteristics of Intermediate-Acting Nondepolarizing Neuromuscular Blocking Drugs (Compared with Long-Acting Drugs)

Similar onset rate of maximum neuromuscular blockade (the exception being rocuronium, the onset of which approximates that of succinylcholine)

Duration of action is approximately one third that of long-acting drugs

Rate of recovery is 30% to 50% more rapid than with long-acting drugs

Minimal to absent cardiovascular effects (especially vecuronium and rocuronium)

Useful for short operations (outpatients)

Less likely to be associated with residual weakness postoperatively, even when administered for prolonged operations

intermediate duration of action) that minimize the likelihood of significant cumulative effects with repeated injections or continuous infusions of these drugs (Table 8–6).

B. Chemical Structure

    1. Atracurium is a bisquaternary ammonium nondepolarizing neuromuscular blocking drug that is adjusted to a pH of 3.25 to 3.65 in the commercial solution to minimize the likelihood of spontaneous *in vitro* degradation.

        a. In view of its *in vitro* acid pH, atracurium probably should not be mixed with alkaline drugs (barbiturates) or exposed to alkaline solutions as may be used for intravenous infusions.

        b. The **potency** of atracurium stored at room temperature decreases approximately 5% every 30 days.

    2. Vecuronium is a monoquaternary steroidal analogue of pancuronium that is supplied as a lyophilized powder that must be dissolved in sterile water prior to its use.

        a. Absence of a quaternary methyl group decreases the vagolytic property of vecuronium compared with pancuronium.

        b. The monoquaternary structure of vecuronium increases its lipid solubility (less dependent on renal excretion) compared with pancuronium.

   3. **Rocuronium** is a steroidal neuromuscular blocking
      drug that is structurally related to vecuronium.
C. **Metabolism** (Table 8-5)
   1. **Atracurium** was designed to undergo spontaneous
      pH- and temperature-dependent *in vivo* chemode-
      gradation (**Hofmann elimination**) as well as bio-
      degradation by ester hydrolysis (nonspecific ester-
      ases that are unrelated to plasma cholinesterase).
      a. Ester hydrolysis is the principal mechanism for
         metabolism of atracurium, whereas Hofmann
         elimination provides a unique alternative route
         of spontaneous degradation that may be impor-
         tant in patients with severe renal or hepatic failure
         (estimated that two thirds of atracurium is de-
         graded by ester hydrolysis and one third by Hof-
         mann elimination) (Fig. 8-12).
      b. The duration of action of atracurium is indepen-
         dent of hepatic or renal function and is not altered
         in the presence of atypical plasma cholinesterase
         levels.
      c. The rate of Hofmann elimination is slowed by
         acidosis (pH lower than 7.4) or decreases in body
         temperature (lower than 37°C).
      d. In contrast to Hofmann elimination, the rate of
         ester hydrolysis of atracurium is enhanced by de-
         creases in blood pH to lower than 7.4.
      e. Laudanosine is the result of metabolism of atracu-
         rium by ester hydrolysis and Hofmann elimina-
         tion. This inactive metabolite at the neuromuscu-
         lar junction may cross the blood–brain barrier
         and stimulate the central nervous system (un-
         likely after usual doses of atracurium adminis-
         tered during surgery). Administration of atracu-
         rium during liver transplantation is associated
         with clinically insignificant increases in the
         plasma concentration of laudanosine (laudano-
         sine depends upon renal excretion for its clear-
         ance from the plasma).
   2. **Vecuronium,** because of its increased lipid solubil-
      ity compared with pancuronium, has greater access
      to hepatocytes (undergoes deacetylation to metabo-
      lites with modest activity at the neuromuscular junc-
      tion) and undergoes substantial biliary excretion (an
      estimated 50% of the intravenous dose of vecuro-
      nium may be present in the liver 30 minutes after
      injection).

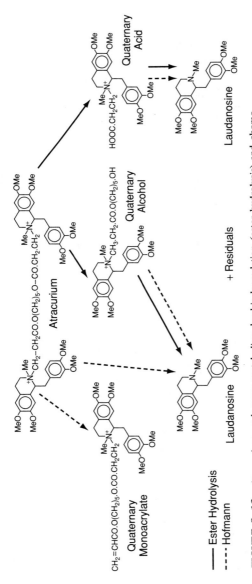

FIGURE 8–12. Atracurium undergoes metabolism by biodegradation (ester hydrolysis) and chemodegradation (Hoffmann elimination). (From Stiller RL, Cook DR, Chakravorti S. In vitro degradation of atracurium in human plasma. Br J Anaesth 1985;57:1085–8; with permission.)

3. **Rocuronium** is not metabolized, but rather is excreted unchanged in the bile and urine.

D. Onset and Duration of Action (Table 8-5)

1. The onset of action of atracurium and vecuronium is similar to the long-acting nondepolarizing neuromuscular blocking drugs, but the duration of action is approximately one third that of the long-acting drugs.

2. The onset of action of rocuronium is more rapid than that of the other intermediate-acting drugs (low potency permits administration of a dose that contains sufficient molecules to produce a rapid pharmacologic effect).

   a. Onset time (injection to maximum twitch depression) is similar for rocuronium (0.9 and 1.2 $mg \cdot kg^{-1}$ IV) and succinylcholine (1 $mg \cdot kg^{-1}$ IV) (Fig. 8-13).

   b. The duration of action of rocuronium resembles atracurium and vecuronium.

   c. The duration of action of rocuronium is prolonged in elderly patients because of decreased clearance of the drug (pharmacodynamics are not altered by aging) (Fig. 8-9).

3. **Priming Principle**

   a. The priming principle is based on the concept that the onset of neuromuscular blockade can be accelerated if spare receptors are initially occupied by a small subparalyzing dose (approximately 10% of the drug's ED_{95}) followed in approximately 4 minutes by the larger dose of the drug (2 to 3 × ED_{95}).

   b. The initial subparalyzing dose is presumed to decrease the safety margin of neuromuscular transmission, allowing a more rapid onset of effect after the second larger dose.

E. Rate of Recovery

1. The rate of recovery from 10% to 25% of control twitch response is more rapid with intermediate-acting than with long-acting nondepolarizing neuromuscular blocking drugs.

   a. Abdominal musculature is adequately relaxed at 10%, but not 25%, of control twitch response.

   b. Typically, neuromuscular blockade can be antagonized 20 to 30 minutes after initial injection of 2 × ED_{95} of an intermediate-acting nondepolarizing neuromuscular blocking drug.

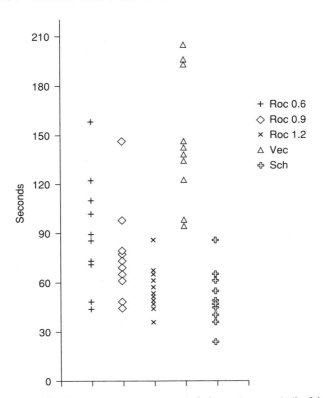

FIGURE 8–13. Onset to maximum twitch depression was similar following the intravenous administration of rocuronium (Roc) at doses of 0.9 mg·kg^{-1} and 1.2 mg·kg^{-1} and succinylcholine (Sch), 1 mg·kg^{-1}. (From Magorian T, Flannery KB, Miller RD. Comparison of rocuronium, succinylcholine, and vecuronium for rapid sequence induction of anesthesia in adult patients. Anesthesiology 1993;79:913–8; with permission.)

    2. Atracurium has an elimination half-time of 22 minutes (about one-third that of long-acting nondepolarizing neuromuscular blocking drugs), which reflects the drug's rapid metabolism.

    3. Vecuronium undergoes rapid hepatic metabolism and biliary excretion, resulting in a duration of action similar to that of atracurium despite a longer elimination half-time.

    4. Rocuronium has a duration of action similar to that of vecuronium.

    5. The rapid clearance of intermediate-acting nondepolarizing neuromuscular blocking drugs makes it difficult to derive valid ED_{95} values from dose-response techniques based on repeated dose regimens.

F. Cumulative Effects

    1. Consistency of onset-to-recovery intervals after repeated supplemental doses of atracurium is a unique characteristic of this drug that reflects the absence of a significant cumulative effect.

        a. Rapid elimination of atracurium from the plasma, independent of hepatic or renal function, is the reason for the lack of significant cumulative drug effects.

        b. Lack of significant drug accumulation minimizes the likelihood of persistent neuromuscular blockade when prolonged surgical procedures require repeated doses or sustained continuous infusion of atracurium.

    2. Repeated supplemental doses of vecuronium produce slight but detectable increases in the duration of neuromuscular blockade (cumulative effect) that is more than that observed with atracurium but much less than that produced by pancuronium.

    3. Whenever supplemental doses of atracurium, vecuronium, or rocuronium exceed the rate of plasma clearance, cumulative drug effects are possible.

G. Pharmacologic and Physiologic Interactions (Table 8-9)

    1. Histamine release sufficient to cause cardiovascular changes (doubling of plasma histamine concentration) does not occur predictably, even with high doses of vecuronium or rocuronium.

    2. Atracurium does not evoke sufficient histamine release to cause cardiovascular changes until about 3 $\times$ ED_{95} dose is administered.

        a. Slowing the rate of intravenous atracurium injection (over 30 to 75 seconds rather than bolus) decreases the likelihood of drug-induced histamine release.

        b. Histamine release evoked by neuromuscular blocking drugs does not occur repeatedly because histamine stores are not replenished for several days (a decrease in blood pressure due to initial drug-induced histamine release is less likely to occur to the same magnitude on repeat dosing).

    c. Bronchospasm due to atracurium-induced histamine release may be more likely in patients with a history of asthma.

H. Renal Dysfunction

1. In contrast to long-acting nondepolarizing neuromuscular blocking drugs, renal failure does not influence the duration of action of even large doses of atracurium.

2. The elimination half-time of vecuronium is prolonged in patients with renal failure, reflecting a decreased clearance of the drug (duration of action is not predictably prolonged).

3. Rocuronium is dependent, to some extent, on renal clearance.

4. Tolerance to the neuromuscular blocking effects of intermediate-acting nondepolarizing neuromuscular blocking drugs may develop in patients with renal failure.

I. Hepatic Dysfunction

1. Hepatic failure does not alter the elimination half-time of atracurium.

2. High doses of vecuronium (0.2 mg·kg^{-1} IV) administered to patients with hepatic cirrhosis are associated with a prolonged elimination half-time and, thus, prolonged duration of action.

3. Dose requirements for pancuronium and vecuronium, but not atracurium, are decreased during liver transplantation.

4. Rocuronium is dependent, to some extent, upon elimination in the bile.

J. Circulatory Effects

1. Atracurium in doses up to $2 \times ED_{95}$, does not predictably evoke sufficient histamine release to cause circulatory effects (Fig. 8–14).

    a. The rapid intravenous injection of $3 \times ED_{95}$ of atracurium decreases mean arterial pressure (average decrease of about 22%).

    b. These circulatory changes are transient, occurring 60 to 90 seconds after administration of atracurium and disappearing within 5 minutes.

    c. Plasma histamine concentrations increase transiently and parallel heart rate and blood pressure

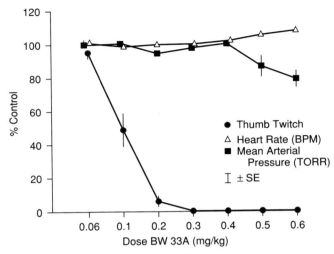

FIGURE 8–14. Heart rate and blood pressure changes do not occur following the rapid intravenous administration of atracurium (BW 33A) up to doses equivalent to $2 \times ED_{95}$ (0.4 mg·kg^{-1} IV). Larger doses of atracurium may produce transient increases in heart rate and decreases in blood pressure. (From Basta SJ, Ali HH, Savarese JJ, et al. Clinical pharmacology of atracurium besylate (BW 33A): A new nondepolarizing muscle relaxant. Anesth Analg 1982;61:723–9; with permission.)

                changes when atracurium (0.6 mg·kg^{-1} IV) is administered rapidly.

    d. Cardiovascular effects of atracurium are attenuated by slow intravenous injection of the drug (over 30 to 75 seconds) or pretreatment with H-1 and H-2 receptor antagonists.

2. Vecuronium is typically devoid of circulatory effects (even with doses that exceed $3 \times ED_{95}$ of the drug), emphasizing the lack of vagolytic or histamine-releasing effects.

    a. Bradycardia attributed to vecuronium may reflect the absence of a vagolytic effect of this drug, especially in the presence of opioids.

    b. Sinus node exit block has been described in association with vecuronium injection.

3. Rocuronium (at doses equivalent to 2, 3, and $4 \times$

ED_{95}) does not cause changes in heart rate, mean arterial pressure, or plasma histamine concentration (Figs. 8–15, 8–16, and 8–17).

K. Obstetric Patients

1. The short duration of action of intermediate-acting nondepolarizing neuromuscular blocking drugs makes these drugs attractive selections for producing skeletal muscle relaxation during general anesthesia for cesarean section (insufficient amounts of these drugs cross the placenta to produce effects in the fetus).

2. Rocuronium may be an alternative to succinylcholine when rapid intubation of the trachea is desirable in these patients.

L. Pediatric Patients

1. Infants appear to be more sensitive than children or adults to the neuromuscular blocking effects of atracurium.

2. In infants, the onset of neuromuscular blockade produced by vecuronium is more rapid (because of high

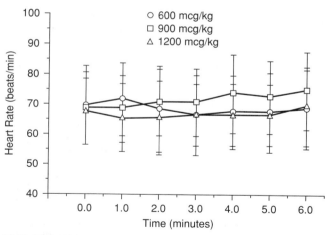

FIGURE 8–15. Changes in heart rate (mean ± SD) after intravenous administration of three different doses of rocuronium to adult patients. (From Levy JH, Davis GK, Duggan J, Szalm F. Determination of the hemodynamics and histamine release of rocuronium [ORG 9426] when administered in increased doses under N_2O/O_2 - sufentanil anesthesia. Anesth Analg 1994;78:318–21; with permission.)

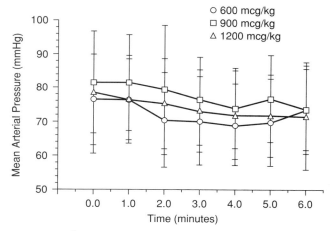

FIGURE 8–16. Changes in mean arterial pressure (mean ± SD) after intravenous administration of three different doses of rocuronium to adult patients. (From Levy JH, Davis GK, Duggan J, Szalm F. Determination of the hemodynamics and histamine release of rocuronium [ORG 9426] when administered in increased doses under N_2O/O_2 - sufentanil anesthesia. Anesth Analg 1994;78:318–21; with permission.)

cardiac output) than in adults, whereas the duration of action is longer (because of immature hepatorenal and/or biliary clearance mechanisms).

M. Elderly Patients

1. Increasing age has no effect on the neuromuscular blocking effects of atracurium, presumably reflecting the independence of atracurium clearance mechanisms from age-related effects on renal and hepatic function.

2. Increasing age may be associated with decreased dose requirements and prolonged rate of recovery from nondepolarizing neuromuscular blocking drugs (other than atracurium), presumably reflecting age-related decreases in hepatic and renal clearance mechanisms.

3. Evidence of unchanging responsiveness of the neuromuscular junction to nondepolarizing neuromuscular blocking drugs despite increasing age can be found in the similarity of the plasma concentration of these drugs that is necessary to depress twitch

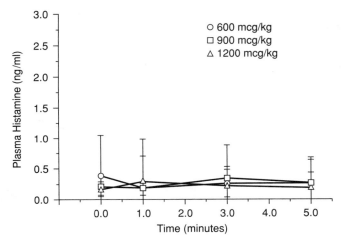

FIGURE 8–17. Changes in plasma histamine concentration (mean ± SD) after intravenous administration of three different doses of rocuronium to adult patients. (From Levy JH, Davis GK, Duggan J, Szalm F. Determination of the hemodynamics and histamine release of rocuronium [ORG 9426] when administered in increased doses under N_2O/O_2 - sufentanil anesthesia. Anesth Analg 1994;78:318–21; with permission.)

response in elderly patients and young adult patients.

N. Obesity may be associated with an increased duration of action of vecuronium.

O. Intracranial pressure is not changed following administration of intermediate-acting nondepolarizing neuromuscular blocking drugs.

P. Intraocular pressure is not changed following administration of intermediate-acting nondepolarizing neuromuscular blocking drugs.

Q. Malignant hyperthermia is not triggered by intermediate-acting nondepolarizing neuromuscular blocking drugs. Prolonged neuromuscular blockade may occur in patients who have been pretreated with **dantrolene.**

R. Critically Ill Patients
  1. Prolonged administration (longer than 6 days) of steroid-based nondepolarizing neuromuscular blocking

drugs to facilitate mechanical ventilation of the lungs in critically ill patients has been associated with generalized skeletal muscle weakness and atrophy **(tetraparesis)** and areflexia **(neurogenic atrophy)** that may persist for weeks or months (electrodiagnostic studies of the neuromuscular junction suggest a presynaptic disorder similar to the Lambert-Eaton syndrome).

   a. The presence of renal failure and accumulation of active metabolites (3-desacetylvecuronium) may contribute to prolonged neuromuscular blockade in patients being treated with vecuronium.

   b. Patients being chronically treated with steroids (as for asthma) may be at increased risk for developing myopathy following prolonged infusions of neuromuscular blocking drugs.

   c. Development of acute quadriparesis in an asthmatic treated with atracurium suggests that the steroid nucleus may not be essential in causing this side effect.

2. Nondepolarizing neuromuscular blocking drugs injected directly into the cerebrospinal fluid of rats cause dose-dependent central nervous system excitation and seizures (reason for concern about possible central nervous system side effects in patients receiving these drugs for prolonged periods).

S. Postoperative Weakness

1. Impaired neuromuscular activity in the Postanesthesia Care Unit (train-of-four ratio less than 0.7) despite prior administration of anticholinesterase drugs is more common in patients receiving a long-acting (pancuronium), rather than an intermediate-acting (atracurium, vecuronium), neuromuscular blocking drug.

2. The lower incidence of residual neuromuscular blockade after administration of short- or intermediate-acting neuromuscular blocking drugs is a consequence of their more rapid spontaneous clearance.

3. Use of short- or intermediate-acting neuromuscular blocking drugs, even for operations lasting longer than 2 hours, may be justified to minimize the risk of residual paresis in the postoperative period (an example of the benefit of a more expensive drug compared to a less expensive [pancuronium] but longer-acting drug).

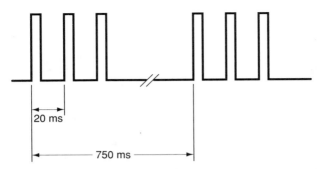

FIGURE 8–18. Stimulation pattern in double-burst suppression is characterized by three impulses at a frequency of 50 Hz separated by 750 ms. (From Bevan DR, Donati F, Kopman AF. Reversal of neuromuscular blockade. Anesthesiology 1992;77:785–805; with permission.)

        a. Train-of-four values greater than 0.7 are usually not associated with evidence of clinical weakness (as tested by eye opening, head lift, and vital capacity).

        b. It is not possible to accurately estimate, either visually or manually, a train-of-four ratio (middle two twitches interfere with comparison of the first and last twitch) with sufficient certainty to exclude residual skeletal muscle weakness in the postoperative period (double-burst suppression [two trains of three stimuli separated by 750 ms] is easier to perceive as two separate twitches and more accurate in discerning the presence of fade) (Fig. 8–18).

        c. The ability to sustain a head lift for 5 seconds indicates sufficient strength to protect the upper airway against obstruction and aspiration of gastric contents.

VIII. MIVACURIUM

    A. Mivacurium is a short-acting nondepolarizing neuromuscular blocking drug that is hydrolyzed by plasma cholinesterase at a rate equivalent to 88% that of succinylcholine (Table 8–5).

    B. Administration of an ED_{95} dose (0.08 mg·kg^{-1}) of mivacurium results in maximum twitch depression (onset) within 3.8 minutes (2.5 minutes with $2 \times ED_{95}$) and spontaneous recovery to 95% twitch height within 24.5 minutes (30.6 minutes with $2 \times ED_{95}$).

1. Increasing the dose of mivacurium administered to facilitate tracheal intubation to 0.2 to 0.25 mg·kg^{-1} shortens the onset by 30 to 60 seconds while prolonging the duration of action by only 2 to 5 minutes.

2. Following administration of $2 \times ED_{95}$ of mivacurium, 95% twitch depression of the orbicularis oculi muscle occurs sooner than that of the adductor pollicis muscle (Fig. 8-19).

   a. Tracheal intubating conditions are acceptable at the time of maximum twitch depression of the

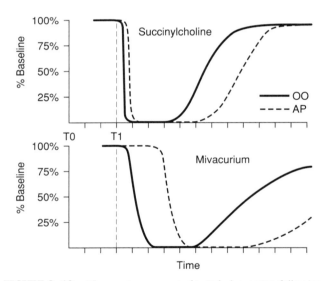

FIGURE 8–19. The maximum onset of twitch depression following administration of mivacurium, 0.15 mg·kg^{-1} IV, was more rapid when twitch response was monitored at the orbicularis oculi (OO) muscle than at the adductor pollicis (AP) muscle. The onset of maximum twitch depression following administration of succinylcholine, 1 mg·kg^{-1} IV, was similar at both muscles. Time is represented as 1 minute per division. (From Sayson SC, Morgan PD. Onset of action of mivacurium chloride. A compression of neuromuscular blockade monitoring at the adductor pollicis and the orbicularis oculi. Anesthesiology 1994;81:35–42; with permission.)

orbicularis oculi (permits earlier tracheal intubation than afforded by waiting for maximum twitch depression of the adductor pollicis).

b. Diaphragmatic activity (cough) may accompany tracheal intubation following the administration of $2 \times ED_{95}$ of mivacurium, regardless of whether the orbicularis oculi or adductor pollicis muscle is monitored.

3. Prolonged neuromuscular blockade following administration of mivacurium may occur in patients with decreased plasma cholinesterase activity (renal failure, cirrhosis of the liver) and atypical cholinesterase enzyme (Fig. 8–20).

4. The effect of anticholinesterase drugs is additive (despite their potential to inhibit plasma cholinesterase)

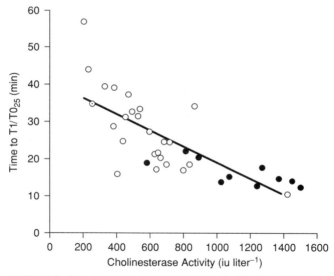

FIGURE 8–20. Recovery from neuromuscular blockade produced by mivacurium is prolonged in patients with decreased cholinesterase activity as may be associated with cirrhosis of the liver (*open circles*). Solid circles represent normal patients, whereas circles with a dot represent heterozygous patients. (From Devlin JC, Head-Rapson AG, Parker CJR, Hunter JM. Pharmacodynamics of mivacurium chloride in patients with hepatic cirrhosis. Br J Anaesth 1993;71:227–31; with permission.)

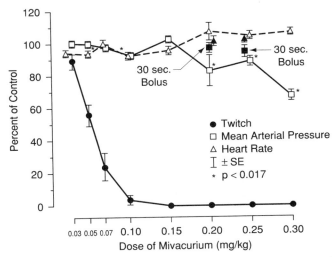

FIGURE 8–21. Neuromuscular and cardiovascular dose response of mivacurium after injection over 10 to 15 seconds (except where indicated as 30 seconds). (From Savarese JJ, Ali HH, Basta SJ, et al. The cardiovascular effects of mivacurium chloride [BW B1090U] in patients receiving nitrous oxide-opiate-barbiturate anesthesia. Anesthesiology 1989;70:386–94; with permission.)

to the rapid rate of spontaneous recovery from miva-curium-induced neuromuscular blockade.

5. The **cardiovascular effects** of mivacurium are minimal at doses of up to $2 \times ED_{95}$ (Fig. 8–21).

C. Mivacurium does not trigger malignant hyperthermia.

9

Anticholinesterase Drugs and Cholinergic Agonists

Anticholinesterase drugs inhibit the enzyme acetylcholinesterase (true cholinesterase), which is normally responsible for the hydrolysis of acetylcholine. One molecule of acetylcholinesterase is capable of hydrolyzing 300,000 molecules of acetylcholine every minute. (Updated and revised from Stoelting RK. Anticholinesterase drugs and cholinergic agonists. In: Pharmacology and Physiology in Anesthetic Practice. 2nd ed. Philadelphia, JB Lippincott, 1991;226–41.)

I. CLASSIFICATION

A. Anticholinesterase drugs are classified according to the mechanism by which they inhibit the activity of acetylcholinesterase (Fig. 9–1).

1. **Reversible Inhibition**

   a. Edrophonium produces reversible inhibition of acetylcholinesterase by electrostatic attachment to the anionic site and hydrogen bonding at the esteratic site of the enzyme, thus preventing acetylcholine (the natural substrate) from approximating correctly with the enzyme (Fig. 9–2).

   b. Because a true chemical (covalent) bond is not formed, acetylcholine can easily compete with edrophonium for access to acetylcholinesterase, making the inhibition truly reversible.

2. **Formation of Carbamyl Esters**

   a. **Physostigmine, neostigmine, and pyridostigmine** produce reversible inhibition of acetylcholinesterase by forming a carbamyl-ester complex at the esteratic site of the enzyme (Fig. 9–3).

   b. Carbamylated acetylcholinesterase cannot hydro-

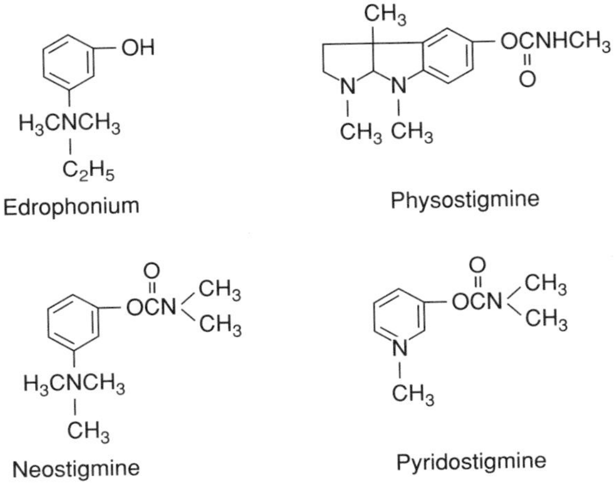

FIGURE 9–1. Anticholinesterase drugs.

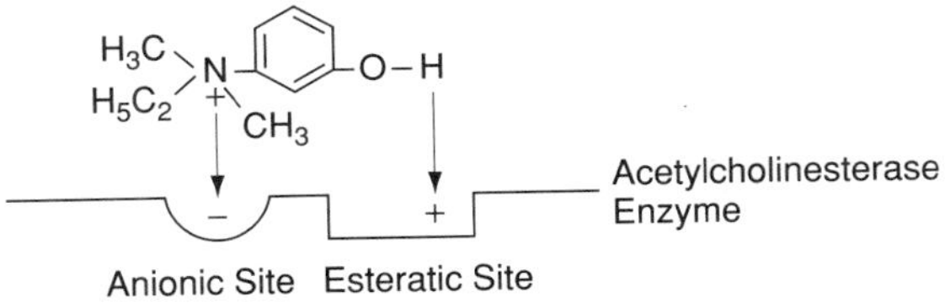

FIGURE 9–2. Edrophonium produces reversible inhibition of acetylcholinesterase by electrostatic attachment to the anionic site and hydrogen bonding at the esteratic site of the enzyme.

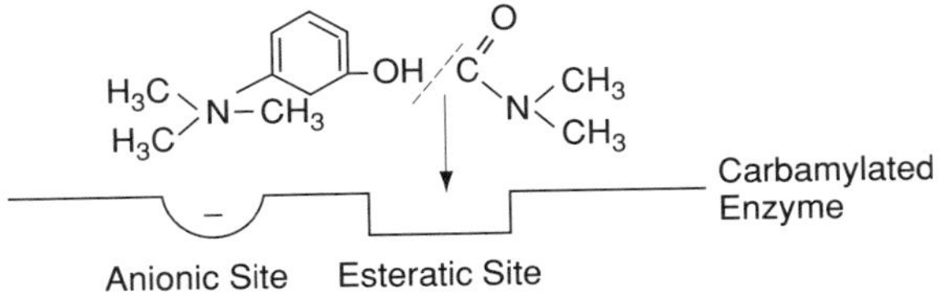

FIGURE 9–3. Certain drugs, such as physostigmine, neostigmine, and pyridostigmine, produce reversible inhibition of acetylcholinesterase by forming a carbamyl-ester complex at the esteratic site of the enzyme.

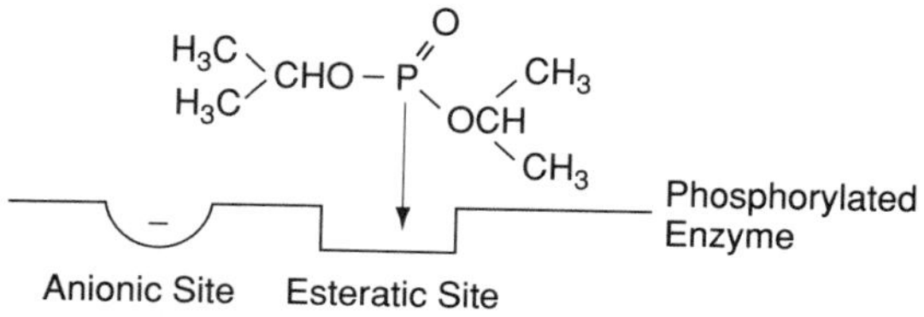

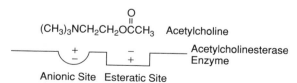

FIGURE 9–4. Organophosphate anticholinesterase drugs produce irreversible inhibition of acetylcholinesterase by forming a phosphorylate complex at the esteratic site of the enzyme.

lyze acetylcholine until the carbamate-enzyme bond dissociates.
  c. Neostigmine also has presynaptic actions, as manifested by an increased rate of repetitive firing following a single impulse.
3. **Irreversible Inactivation**
  a. Organophosphate anticholinesterase drugs (echothiophate, insecticides, nerve gases) combine with acetylcholinesterase at the esteratic site to form a stable inactive complex that does not undergo hydrolysis (Fig. 9–4).
  b. Spontaneous regeneration of acetylcholinesterase requires several hours or does not occur, thus requiring synthesis of new enzyme.

II. STRUCTURE ACTIVITY RELATIONSHIPS   Acetylcholinesterase consists of an anionic and an esteratic site, arranged so that they are complementary to the natural substrate acetylcholine (Fig. 9–5).

FIGURE 9–5.   The anionic and esteratic sites of acetylcholinesterase are arranged so that they are complementary to the quaternary nitrogen and ester linkage of acetylcholine, respectively.

III. PHARMACOKINETICS

A. In patients with normal renal and hepatic function, there are no significant pharmacokinetic differences among the anticholinesterase drugs (differences in potency most likely reflect pharmacodynamic effects) (Table 9-1).

B. The fact that edrophonium dose-response curves are not parallel to those for neostigmine and pyridostigmine suggests that different mechanisms of action may be involved for the different anticholinesterase drugs (Fig. 9-6).

C. **Lipid Solubility**
   1. Anticholinesterase drugs containing a quaternary ammonium group (edrophonium, neostigmine, pyridostigmine) are poorly lipid soluble and thus do not easily penetrate lipid cell barriers, such as the blood-brain barrier (lack central nervous system effects).
   2. Physostigmine is a tertiary amine and, like organophosphates, can easily cross lipid barriers (central nervous system effects are likely).

D. **Volume of Distribution** (Table 9-1)
   1. The large volume of distribution (Vd) of quaternary ammonium anticholinesterase drugs is surprising because these drugs would not be expected to cross lipid membranes easily.
   2. Presumably, this large Vd reflects extensive tissue storage.

E. **Onset of Action** (Fig. 9-7)
   1. The more rapid onset of action of edrophonium may reflect a presynaptic (acetylcholine release) rather than a postsynaptic (acetylcholinesterase inhibition) action.
   2. A postsynaptic action may be predominant for drugs with a slower onset of action, such as neostigmine and pyridostigmine.

F. **Renal Clearance** (Table 9-1)
   1. Dependence on renal clearance means that plasma concentrations of anticholinesterase drugs will be sustained as long, if not longer, than nondepolarizing neuromuscular blocking drugs (especially long-acting drugs), making the occurrence of recurarization unlikely.
   2. In anesthetized patients receiving a functioning renal transplant, the pharmacokinetics of anticholinesterase drugs are similar to those in patients with normal renal function.

Table 9–1

Comparative Characteristics of Anticholinesterase Drugs Administered to Antagonize Nondepolarizing Neuromuscular Blockade

	Elimination Half-Time (min)		Volume of Distribution (L·kg⁻¹)		Clearance (ml·kg⁻¹·min⁻¹)		Renal Contribution to Total Clearance (%)	Speed of Onset	Duration (min)	Principal Site of Action
	Normal	Anephric	Normal	Anephric	Normal	Anephric				
Edrophonium (0.5 mg·kg⁻¹)	110	206	1.1	0.7	9.6	2.7	66	Rapid	60	Presynaptic Presynaptic
Neostigmine (0.043 mg·kg⁻¹)	80	183	0.7	0.8	9.0	3.4	54	Intermediate	60	Postsynaptic
Pyridostigmine (0.35 mg·kg⁻¹)	112	379	1.1	1.0	8.6	2.1	76	Delayed	90	Postsynaptic

(Data from Cronnelly R, Stanski, DR, Miller RD, Sheiner LB, Sohn YJ. Renal function and the pharmacokinetics of neostigmine in anesthetized patients. Anesthesiology 1979; 51:222–6; Cronnelly R, Stanski DR, Miller RD, Sheiner LB. Pyridostigmine kinetics with and without renal function. Clin Pharmacol Ther 1980; 28:78–81; Cronnelly R, Morris RB. Antagonism of neuromuscular blockade. Br J Anaesth 1982; 54:183–93; Morris RB, Cronnelly R, Miller RD, Stanski DR, Fahey MR. Pharmacokinetics of edrophonium and neostigmine when antagonizing d-tubocurarine neuromuscular blockade in man. Anesthesiology 1981; 54:399–402; with permission.)

188

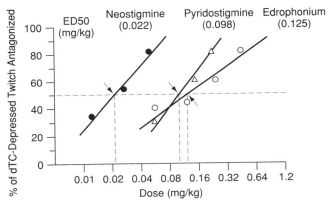

FIGURE 9–6. The dose-response curve for edrophonium is not parallel to the curves for neostigmine and pyridostigmine, suggesting different mechanisms of action for the various anticholinesterase drugs. (From Cronnelly R, Morris RB, Miller RD. Edrophonium: Duration of action and atropine requirements in humans during halothane anesthesia. Anesthesiology 1982;57:261–6; with permission.)

G. Metabolism
  1. In the absence of renal function, hepatic metabolism accounts for 50% of a dose of neostigmine, 30% of edrophonium, and 25% of pyridostigmine.
  2. Metabolites of anticholinesterase drugs are inactive.

H. Influence of Patient Age
  1. The time course of onset and duration of antagonism produced by equipotent doses of neostigmine are similar in infants, children, and adults.
  2. Dose requirements are less for neostigmine, but not for edrophonium (implies different mechanisms for antagonism of neuromuscular blockade) in neonates and children compared with adults.
  3. The duration of maximum response produced by neostigmine and pyridostigmine, but not edrophonium, is more prolonged in elderly adults than in younger adults.

IV. PHARMACOLOGIC EFFECTS

  A. Pharmacologic effects of anticholinesterase drugs are predictable and reflect the accumulation of acetylcholine at

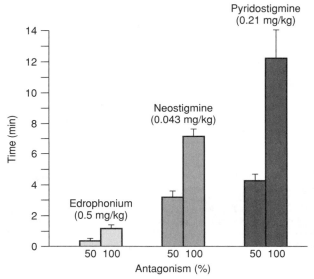

FIGURE 9–7. Comparison of the onset of action of anticholinesterase drugs as reflected by antagonism of drug-induced neuromuscular blockade. Mean ± SE. (From Cronnelly R, Morris RB, Miller RD. Edrophonium: Duration of action and atropine requirements in humans during halothane. Anesthesiology 1982;57:261–6; with permission.)

muscarinic and nicotinic cholinergic receptor sites (Table 9–2).

1. Depending on the reason for administration of anticholinesterase drugs, these effects may be considered therapeutic or undesirable.
2. Muscarinic cholinergic effects are evoked by lower concentrations of acetylcholine than are required for production of nicotinic effects at autonomic ganglia and the neuromuscular junction.
   a. For this reason, drug-assisted antagonism of nondepolarizing neuromuscular blockade with an anticholinesterase drug also includes administration of an anticholinergic drug (Table 9–3).
   b. The anticholinergic drug selectively blocks the effects of acetylcholine at muscarinic cholinergic receptors, and leaves intact the response to acetylcholine at nicotinic cholinergic receptors.

Table 9–2
Pharmacologic Effects of Anticholinesterase Drugs

Muscarinic Cholinergic Effects (Blockade with an Anticholinergic Drug)

Bradycardia
Enhanced gastric fluid secretion
Hyperperistalsis (may increase incidence of nausea and vomiting)
Miosis and inability to focus for near vision
Salivation

Nicotinic Cholinergic Effects

Stimulation of autonomic ganglia
Stimulation at the neuromuscular junction

---

   c. Bradycardia and/or sinus arrest have been described when neostigmine plus an anticholinergic drug are administered to reverse neuromuscular blockade in patients who previously had undergone heart transplants. It is presumed that direct activation by neostigmine of excitatory cholinergic receptors on cardiac ganglion cells results in release of acetylcholine and heart rate slowing in these denervated hearts.

   d. Skeletal muscle weakness may occur in patients with myasthenia gravis who are treated with anticholinesterase drugs but is rare in patients receiving anticholinesterase drugs for drug-assisted antagonism of neuromuscular blockade.

   e. Increased peristalsis produced by anticholinesterase drugs is unlikely to influence the incidence of anastomotic bowel leakage. Avoidance of routine antagonist-assisted reversal of neuromuscular blockade (possible in selected patients receiving intermediate- or short-acting neuromuscular blocking drugs) may decrease the likelihood of postoperative nausea and vomiting.

B. Neostigmine and pyridostigmine, but not edrophonium, produce marked and prolonged inhibition of plasma cholinesterase.

V. CLINICAL USES (Table 9-4)

A. Antagonist-Assisted Reversal of Neuromuscular Blockade

Table 9-3
Choice of Anticholinesterase Drug

Train-of-Four Visible Twitches	Estimated Train-of-Four Fade	Anticholinesterase Drug and Dose ($mg \cdot kg^{-1}$ IV)	Anticholinergic Drug and Dose* ($\mu g \cdot kg^{-1}$ IV)
None[†]			
≤ 2	++++	Neostigmine, 0.07	Glycopyrrolate, 7; atropine, 15
3–4	+++	Neostigmine, 0.04	Glycopyrrolate, 7; atropine, 15
4	++	Edrophonium, 0.5	Atropine, 7–15
4	±	Edrophonium, 0.25	Atropine, 7

*Administered simultaneously with an anticholinesterase drug.
[†]Postpone antagonist-assisted reversal until some evoked response is visible.
(Adapted from Bevan DR, Donati F, Kopman AF. Reversal of neuromuscular blockade. Anesthesiology 1992;77:785–805.)

ticholinergic drug attenuates or prevents undesirable muscarinic cholinergic effects of the anticholinesterase drug).

b. Atropine has a rapid onset of action (about 1 minute) and a duration of 30 to 60 minutes, and it crosses the blood–brain barrier. Glycopyrrolate has a slower onset (2 to 3 minutes) of action, but does not easily cross the blood–brain barrier.

c. The more delayed onset of the cardiac vagolytic effects of glycopyrrolate is appropriately matched for the slower onset of action of neostigmine and pyridostigmine, whereas the more rapid onset of vagolytic activity provided by atropine more closely parallels the onset of activity produced by edrophonium.

d. Late bradycardia is more likely when short-acting atropine, rather than long-acting glycopyrrolate, is combined with neostigmine.

7. Excessive Neuromuscular Blockade. Persistence of neuromuscular blockade despite large doses of anticholinesterase drugs is often an indication to ventilate the patient's lungs mechanically until neuromuscular blockade dissipates with time.

8. Events That Influence Reversal of Neuromuscular Blockade (Table 9–5; Fig. 9–9)

9. 4-Aminopyridine

a. This drug is an effective antagonist of nondepolarizing neuromuscular blockade without associated muscarinic cholinergic effects.

Table 9–5
Factors that Influence Speed of Reversal of Neuromuscular Blockade

Intensity of preexisting neuromuscular blockade (Table 9–3 and Fig. 9–9)

Antagonist selected (edrophonium is less effective than neostigmine in antagonizing deep neuromuscular blockade; Table 9–3)

Dose of anticholinesterase drug

Spontaneous recovery rate

Miscellaneous factors
  Antibiotics
  Hypothermia
  Respiratory acidosis
  Hypothermia

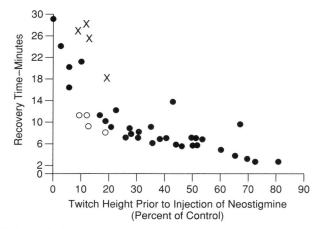

FIGURE 9–9. The rate of antagonism of drug-induced neuromuscular blockade parallels the magnitude of blockade present just before administration of the anticholinesterase drug. (From Katz RL. Clinical neuromuscular pharmacology of pancuronium. Anesthesiology 1971; 34:550–6; with permission.)

    b. The mechanism involved is thought to be a decrease in potassium conductance that prolongs the nerve action potential and produces greater calcium influx.

    c. Central nervous system stimulation (restlessness, excitement, confusion) may accompany administration of this drug.

B. Treatment of Central Nervous System Effects of Certain Drugs. Physostigmine (15 to 60 μg·kg−1 IV) crosses the blood–brain barrier and thus is effective in antagonizing the adverse central nervous system effects of certain drugs (see Chapter 10, Sections V and VI).

C. Treatment of Myasthenia Gravis

    1. The quaternary ammonium structure of neostigmine and pyridostigmine limits the oral absorption of these drugs (oral dose being about 30 times greater than the intravenous dose).

    2. In assessing the anticholinesterase drug therapy of myasthenia gravis, edrophonium, 1 mg IV, is administered every 1 to 2 minutes until a change in symptoms is observed.

Table 9–6
Acute Intoxication by Anticholinesterase Drugs (Insecticides, Nerve Gases)

Symptoms
Muscarinic (miosis, difficulty focusing, salivation, bronchoconstriction, bradycardia, abdominal cramps)
Nicotinic (ranging from skeletal muscle weakness to paralysis)
Central nervous system (confusion, ataxia, seizures, coma)

Treatment
Atropine (35 to 70 $\mu g \cdot kg^{-1}$ IV every 3 to 10 minutes until muscarinic symptoms disappear; no effect at the neuromuscular junction)
Pralidoxime (15 $mg \cdot kg^{-1}$ IV every 20 minutes until skeletal muscle weakness is reversed)
Supportive measures (tracheal intubation, mechanical ventilation of the lungs)
Diazepam (seizures)

    a. Inadequate therapy is indicated if edrophonium results in a decrease in myasthenic symptoms.
    b. Excess anticholinesterase therapy (cholinergic crisis) is indicated if edrophonium results in an increase in myasthenic symptoms.

VI. OVERDOSE OF ANTICHOLINESTERASE DRUGS
(Table 9-6)

VII. SYNTHETIC CHOLINERGIC AGONISTS (Table 9-7)

Table 9–7
Synthetic Cholinergic Agonists

Carbachol (topical treatment of narrow-angle glaucoma)
Bethanechol (treatment of adynamic ileus, urinary retention)
Pilocarpine (topical miotic)

10

Anticholinergic Drugs

Anticholinergic drugs competitively antagonize the effects of the neurotransmitter acetylcholine at cholinergic postganglionic muscarinic receptors (heart, salivary glands, smooth muscle of the gastrointestinal and genitourinary tract). (Updated and revised from Stoelting RK. Anticholinergic drugs. In: Pharmacology and Physiology in Anesthetic Practice. 2nd ed. Philadelphia, JB Lippincott, 1991;242-51.) Acetylcholine is also the neurotransmitter at postganglionic nicotinic receptors (neuromuscular junction, autonomic ganglia), but usual clinical doses of anticholinergic drugs exert little or no effect at nicotinic cholinergic receptors (suggesting that these drugs are selectively antimuscarinic).

I. STRUCTURE ACTIVITY RELATIONSHIPS

A. Naturally occurring anticholinergic drugs (atropine, scopolamine) are esters formed by the combination of tropic acid and an organic base (tropine or scopine) (Fig. 10-1).

1. Structurally, these drugs resemble cocaine.

2. Anticholinergic effect is almost entirely due to the levorotatory form.

B. Glycopyrrolate is a synthetic anticholinergic drug that contains mandelic rather than tropic acid (Fig. 10-1).

C. Like acetylcholine, anticholinergic drugs contain a cationic portion that can fit into the muscarinic cholinergic receptor.

II. MECHANISM OF ACTION

A. Anticholinergic drugs combine reversibly with muscarinic cholinergic receptors and thus prevent access of the neurotransmitter acetylcholine to these sites.

1. As a result, cell membrane changes do not occur despite the continued release of acetylcholine.

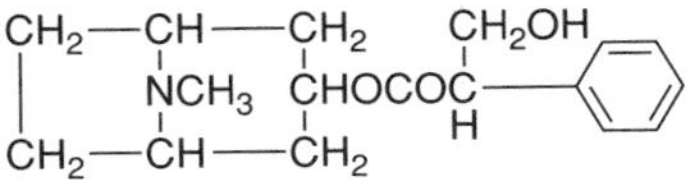

Atropine

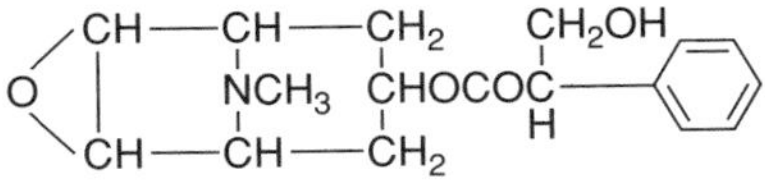

Scopolamine

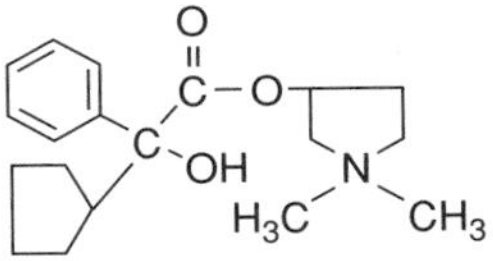

Glycopyrrolate

FIGURE 10–1. Naturally occurring and synthetic anticholinergic drugs.

> 2. The effect of anticholinergic drugs (competitive antagonists) can be overcome by increasing the concentration of acetylcholine in the area of the muscarinic receptors.

B. Evidence for **subclasses** of muscarinic receptors can be found in the variable sensitivity among different cholinergic receptors (muscarinic cholinergic receptors that control salivation are inhibited by lower doses of anticholinergic drugs than are required to inhibit muscarinic receptors at the heart and eyes), as well as in the differences in potency among the anticholinergic drugs (Table 10–1).

C. Small intravenous doses of anticholinergic drugs (including glycopyrrolate, which cannot readily cross the blood-brain barrier) can produce heart rate slowing as a reflection of a weak **peripheral muscarinic cholinergic agonist effect.**

III. PHARMACOKINETICS

A. Oral absorption of anticholinergic drugs is not sufficiently predictable to warrant use of this approach (absorption after intramuscular injection is prompt).

Table 10-1
Comparative Effects of Anticholinergic Drugs

	Sedation	Antisialagogue	Increased Heart Rate	Relaxation of Smooth Muscle	Mydriasis/ Cycloplegia	Prevention of Motion Sickness	Decreased Gastric Hydrogen Ion Secretion	Altered Fetal Heart Rate
Atropine	+	+	+++	++	+	+	±	0
Scopolamine	+++	+++	+	+	+++	+++	±	?
Glycopyrrolate	0	++	++	++	0	0	±	0

0, none; +, mild; ++, moderate; +++, marked

B. Atropine and scopolamine are lipid-soluble tertiary amines (easily penetrating the blood–brain barrier), whereas glycopyrrolate is a poorly lipid-soluble quaternary ammonium compound (minimal ability to cross the blood–brain barrier and produce central nervous system effects).

C. Metabolism of anticholinergic drugs is greatest for scopolamine (less than 1% of a dose being recovered unchanged in the urine).

IV. CLINICAL USES (Table 10-2)

A. Preoperative Medication

1. Sedation

a. Scopolamine is selected when sedation and/or amnesia is the reason for including an anticholinergic drug in the preoperative medication (100 times more potent than atropine in depressing the reticular activating system).

b. Scopolamine greatly enhances the sedative effects of concomitantly administered drugs, especially opioids and benzodiazepines.

c. Central nervous system effects (restlessness, confusion, delayed awakening) are more likely after the administration of scopolamine than after atropine, especially in elderly patients (unlikely following administration of glycopyrrolate).

Table 10–2
Clinical Uses of Anticholinergic Drugs

Preoperative medication
  Sedation
  Antisialagogue effect
Treatment of reflex-mediated bradycardia
Prevention of the cardiovascular effects of anticholinesterase drugs (see Table 9–3)
Bronchodilation
Biliary and ureteral smooth muscle relaxation
Mydriasis and cycloplegia
Antagonism of gastric hydrogen ion secretion
Prevention of motion-induced sickness
Constituents in nonprescription cold remedies

2. Antisialagogue Effect

a. Scopolamine is approximately three times more potent as an antisialagogue than atropine (selected when sedation and an antisialagogue effect are desired).

b. Glycopyrrolate is approximately two times more potent as an antisialagogue than atropine (selected when an antisialagogue effect in the absence of sedation is desired).

B. Treatment of Reflex-Mediated Bradycardia

1. Anticholinergic drugs are the drugs of choice for treating intraoperative bradycardia resulting from increased parasympathetic nervous system activity (most often atropine, 15 to 70 $\mu g \cdot kg^{-1}$ IV).

2. During anesthesia that includes a volatile drug, the dose of atropine required to increase heart rate may be decreased compared with that required in awake patients, perhaps reflecting depression of vagal centers during anesthesia.

3. Atropine and scopolamine cross the placenta but fetal heart rate is not significantly changed.

C. Prevention of Cardiovascular Effects of Anticholinesterase Drugs (see Chapter 9, Section V)

1. Atropine and glycopyrrolate have muscarinic blocking (vagolytic) effects but exert no activity at the nicotinic receptors (neuromuscular junction).

2. Administered intravenously just before or in combination with an anticholinesterase drug (antagonist-assisted reversal of neuromuscular blockade), these drugs attenuate or blunt muscarinic responses (bradycardia, salivation, hyperperistalsis) provoked by the anticholinesterase drug (see Table 9–3).

D. Bronchodilation

1. The effectiveness of anticholinergic drugs as bronchodilators reflects their antagonism of acetylcholine's effects on airway smooth muscle via muscarinic receptors.

a. Relaxation of bronchial smooth muscle lowers airway resistance and increases dead space.

b. Magnitude of decrease in airway resistance depends largely on the degree of preexisting bronchomotor tone.

2. Administration of anticholinergic drugs for preanesthetic medication could result in inspissation of secretions (unlikely with a single dose) rather than bronchodilation.

3. **Ipratropium**
   a. Bronchodilation is more likely to occur when anticholinergic drugs are administered by a metered dose inhaler (ipratropium, 40 to 80 μg, delivered by two to four actuations of the inhaler).
   b. Systemic effects of inhaled ipratropium do not occur, reflecting the minimal systemic absorption (less than 1% of the inhaled dose) of this quaternary ammonium drug.
   c. Although not considered the initial bronchodilator of choice for the treatment of asthma-induced bronchospasm, ipratropium may be used to augment bronchodilation produced by beta agonists.

E. **Biliary and Ureteral Smooth Muscle Relaxation**
   1. Atropine may prevent spasm of the ureter produced by morphine (may be used in the treatment of renal colic).
   2. Atropine is unlikely to overcome opioid-induced spasm of the sphincter of Oddi.

F. **Mydriasis and Cycloplegia**
   1. Anticholinergic drugs placed topically on the cornea block the action of acetylcholine on the circular muscles of the iris (mydriasis) and ciliary muscles (cycloplegia).
      a. These changes could increase intraocular pressure in patients with glaucoma.
      b. An anticholinesterase drug (pilocarpine), when applied topically to the cornea, prevents mydriasis due to atropine.
   2. Doses of intramuscular atropine used for preoperative medication are probably inadequate to increase intraocular pressure, even in susceptible patients, assuming that medications used to treat glaucoma are continued (also true for anticholinergic drugs administered intravenously with anticholinesterase drugs to antagonize nondepolarizing neuromuscular blocking drugs).
   3. Scopolamine is a more potent mydriatic than either atropine or glycopyrrolate.

G. **Antagonism of Gastric Hydrogen Ion Secretion**
   1. The high doses of anticholinergic drugs required to inhibit gastric hydrogen ion secretion are often associated with unacceptable secretory, ocular, and cardiac side effects (H-2 receptor antagonists are more selective).
   2. High doses of anticholinergic drugs, administered in-

travenously, prevent excess peristalsis of the gastrointestinal tract that would otherwise be associated with antagonism of nondepolarizing neuromuscular blocking drugs using anticholinesterase drugs (parasympathetic nervous system provides almost exclusive innervation of the gastrointestinal tract).

H. Prevention of Motion-Induced Sickness

1. Transdermal absorption of scopolamine (postauricular application delivers 5 $\mu g \cdot h^{-1}$) provides sustained therapeutic plasma concentrations that protect against motion-induced nausea without introducing prohibitive side effects, such as sedation, cycloplegia, or drying of secretions.

   a. It is presumed that scopolamine blocks transmission to the medulla of impulses arising from overstimulation of the vestibular apparatus of the inner ear.

   b. Administration of transdermal scopolamine after the onset of symptoms is less effective than prophylactic application at least 4 hours before the noxious stimulus.

2. Anisocoria has been attributed to contamination of the eye following digital manipulation of the transdermal scopolamine.

V. CENTRAL ANTICHOLINERGIC SYNDROME

A. Scopolamine, and to a lesser extent, atropine, can enter the central nervous system and produce symptoms characterized as the central anticholinergic syndrome (restlessness and confusion that may progress to somnolence and unconsciousness).

1. It is presumed that these responses reflect blockade of muscarinic cholinergic receptors in the central nervous system.

2. Physostigmine, a tertiary amine anticholinesterase drug, when administered in doses of 15 to 60 $\mu g \cdot kg^{-1}$ IV, offers specific treatment for the central anticholinergic syndrome.

B. Glycopyrrolate does not easily cross the blood–brain barrier, and thus is not likely to cause a central anticholinergic syndrome.

VI. OVERDOSE

A. Deliberate or accidental overdose with an anticholinergic drug produces a rapid onset of symptoms characteristic

Table 10–3
Symptoms of Anticholinergic Drug Overdose

Dry mouth (making speech difficult)

Blurred vision and photophobia

Tachycardia

Dry and flushed skin

Rash over face, neck, upper chest (blush area; selective dilation of cutaneous vessels)

Increased body temperature (especially in children; reflects inhibition of sweating via sympathetic nervous system nerves that release acetylcholine)

Increased minute ventilation (bronchodilation)

Skeletal muscle weakness (nicotinic cholinergic receptor blockade)

Hypotension

Seizures

Coma

Paralysis of medullary ventilator center

---

of muscarinic cholinergic receptor blockade (Table 10-3).

B. Small children and infants seem particularly vulnerable to developing life-threatening symptoms following an overdose of anticholinergic drug.

C. Physostigmine, 15 to 60 $\mu g \cdot kg^{-1}$ IV, is the specific treatment for an anticholinergic drug overdose (repeated doses of this anticholinesterase drug may be necessary to prevent recurrence of symptoms).

VII. DECREASED BARRIER PRESSURE

A. Intravenous administration of atropine or glycopyrrolate has been shown to decrease lower esophageal sphincter pressure, thereby decreasing barrier pressure (the difference between gastric pressure and lower esophageal sphincter pressure) and inherent resistance to reflux of acidic fluid into the esophagus.

B. The clinical significance, if any, of drug-induced decreases in lower esophageal sphincter pressure remains undocumented.

Chapter

11

Nonopioid and Nonsteroidal Analgesic, Antipyretic, and Antiinflammatory Drugs

Aspirin (acetylsalicylic acid) is the prototype of the nonopioid analgesic, antipyretic, and antiinflammatory drugs (salicylates) (Fig. 11-1). (Updated and revised from Stoelting RK. Nonopioid and nonsteroidal analgesic, antipyretic, and antiinflammatory drugs. In: Pharmacology and Physiology in Anesthetic Practice. 2nd ed. Philadelphia, JB Lippincott, 1991;252–63.) Aspirin and nonsteroidal antiinflammatory drugs (NSAIDs) are among the most commonly prescribed pharmacologic agents, accounting for nearly 4% of all prescriptions filled. Among those patients older than 65 years (in whom there is a high incidence of arthritis and musculoskeletal complaints), it is estimated that 10% to 15% regularly take NSAIDs. In this regard, these drugs generate the greatest number of adverse drug reactions (gastrointestinal irritation, prolonged bleeding, decreased renal function, bronchospasm).

I. MECHANISMS OF ACTION

   A. Aspirin-like drugs produce analgesia through their ability to irreversibly acetylate cyclooxygenase (prostaglandin synthetase) enzyme, leading to a decrease in the synthesis and release of prostaglandins from cells (see Fig. 20–2).

   B. Inhibition of cyclooxygenase decreases the formation of **thromboxane** (a potent vasoconstrictor and stimulant of platelet aggregation) and **prostacyclin** (a potent vasodilator and inhibitor of platelet aggregation).

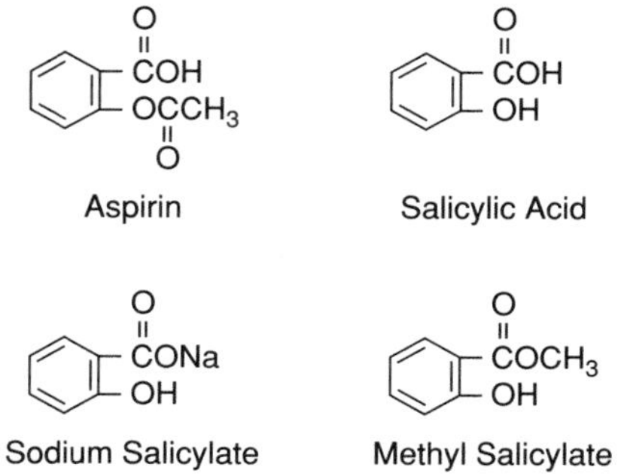

FIGURE 11–1.   Salicylates.

1. A 650-mg dose of aspirin will irreversibly acetylate cyclooxygenase in platelets for the life span of the platelet, which is 8 to 11 days.
   a. The effect of aspirin on platelet function is clinically detectable as prolongation of the **bleeding time.**
   b. Low doses of aspirin (60 to 100 mg daily) may prevent coronary thrombosis.
2. The analgesic action of aspirin is confined to a small dose range, below which there is little effect and above which an increase in dose produces toxic effects with little increase in analgesia.

II. CLINICAL USES (Table 11-1)

III. SALICYLATES

A. Pharmacokinetics

1. Orally administered salicylates are rapidly absorbed from the small intestine, and to a lesser extent, from the stomach.
   a. Buffered effervescent preparations undergo more rapid systemic absorption and cause less gastrointestinal irritation than do the corresponding tablet formulations.
   b. Alkalinization of the urine may increase urinary excretion of salicylates.
2. **Protein binding** of salicylates may result in displacement of other drugs from these binding sites (oral hypoglycemics).

Table 11–1
Clinical Uses of Aspirin and Aspirin-Like Drugs

Analgesia (especially for soft tissue inflammation associated with
  prostaglandin release; not effective for visceral pain)
  Headache
  Musculoskeletal disorders (osteoarthritis, rheumatoid arthritis)
  Postoperative analgesia
  Cancer pain
  Dysmenorrhea

Antipyretic (prevention of pyrogen-induced release of
  prostaglandins)

Inhibition of platelet aggregation (prevention of thrombosis)

Closure of patent ductus arteriosus (indomethacin)

Decreased incidence of pregnancy-induced hypertension

   3. Clearance
       a. Aspirin is rapidly hydrolyzed in the liver to salicylic
             acid (renal excretion is dependent on urine pH).
       b. Salicylic acid is conjugated with glycine to form
             salicyluric acid, which is excreted in the urine.
 B. Side Effects (Table 11–2)
   1. All salicylates and NSAIDs can interfere with normal
         renal function (an often unrecognized side effect)
         by inhibiting the synthesis of prostaglandins.
       a. In the presence of decreased renal blood flow, lo-
             cal synthesis of vasodilating prostaglandins has an
             important role in maintaining renal homeostasis.
       b. In well-hydrated patients with normal renal func-
             tion, prostaglandins play no apparent role in auto-
             regulation of renal blood flow, glomerular filtration
             rate, or renal tubular transport of ions and water.
   2. Increased blood pressure (or loss of blood pressure
         control in patients treated with antihypertensive
         drugs) has occurred in patients treated with NSAIDs
         (indomethacin, naproxen).
       a. This may reflect inhibition of prostaglandin syn-
             thesis (prostaglandins modulate arteriolar smooth
             muscle responses to vasoconstrictive effects of
             catecholamines and control extracellular fluid vol-
             ume by virtue of their natriuretic effects).
       b. The presence of low basal levels of prostaglandins
             in hypertensive patients suggests that a deficiency

Table 11–2
Side Effects Associated with Administration of Salicylates

Gastric irritation and ulceration (manifested by hematest-positive stools and iron deficiency anemia)

Prolongation of bleeding time (reflecting prevention of the formation of thromboxane)

Onset of hypertension

Central nervous system stimulation (plasma concentrations higher than 50 mg·dl^{-1})
  Hyperventilation
  Seizures
  Hyperthermia
  Dehydration
  Tinnitus (earliest sign of salicylate overdose)

Hepatic dysfunction

Renal dysfunction (inhibition of renal prostaglandin synthesis may interfere with maintenance of renal blood flow)

Metabolic alterations
  Hyperglycemia
  Metabolic acidosis (causes a shift of salicylic acid from plasma into the central nervous system; treated with sodium bicarbonate to facilitate renal excretion of salicylic acid)

Prolongation of labor

Allergic reactions (nasal polyps)

---

of vasodilating prostaglandins may be associated with essential hypertension.
3. Patients with asthma (especially if associated with nasal polyps) have an increased incidence of sensitivity to aspirin (also true for NSAIDs).

IV. DIFLUNISAL

A. Diflunisal is a fluorinated salicylic acid derivative that is effective orally and has prominent antiarthritic effects.
B. The effect of diflunisal on platelet function and bleeding time is dose-related but reversible.

V. PHENYLBUTAZONE

A. Phenylbutazone is an orally effective antiinflammatory drug that is useful in the treatment of acute gout (as an alternative to colchicine) and rheumatoid arthritis.

Table 11–3
Side Effects of Phenylbutazone

Anemia

Agranulocytosis

Nausea and vomiting

Rash

Sodium retention (pulmonary edema, dilutional anemia)

---

1. Oxyphenbutazone is a metabolite of phenylbutazone with antiinflammatory activity similar to the parent drug.
2. Extensive protein binding results in a slow elimination half-time, and significant concentrations of drug may remain in the synovial spaces of joints for up to 3 weeks after treatment is discontinued.

B. Side Effects (Table 11–3)

VI. PARA-AMINOPHENOL DERIVATIVES

A. Phenacetin and its active metabolite **acetaminophen** are orally effective alternatives to aspirin as analgesics and antipyretics.
   1. Gastric irritation and inhibition of platelet aggregation do not occur.
   2. Antiinflammatory effects are weak.

B. Metabolism. Approximately 75% of phenacetin is dealkylated to acetaminophen in the liver.

C. Side Effects
   1. **Methemoglobinemia and hemolytic anemia** may follow administration of phenacetin to patients with a genetic deficiency of glucose-6-phosphate enzyme in erythrocytes.
   2. **Hepatic necrosis** may accompany an overdose (more than 15 g) of acetaminophen.
      a. Renal failure and hypoglycemia may accompany an acetaminophen overdose.
      b. **Acetylcysteine,** when administered within the first 8 hours after an acetaminophen overdose, may be effective in restoring hepatic stores of glutathione and in preventing drug-induced hepatic necrosis.

VII. INDOMETHACIN

   A. Indomethacin is an orally effective, methylated indole derivative with analgesic, antipyretic, and antiinflammatory effects comparable to those of salicylates.

      1. This is the drug likely to be selected for treatment of ankylosing spondylitis.

      2. Antiinflammatory effects are comparable to those of colchicine for the treatment of acute attacks of gouty arthritis.

      3. Cardiac failure in neonates caused by patent ductus arteriosus may be controlled with a single dose of indomethacin, emphasizing the ability of this drug to selectively inhibit synthesis of prostaglandins.

   B. **Side effects** (gastrointestinal disturbances, hepatorenal toxicity, inhibition of platelet aggregation) limit the usefulness of this drug.

   C. All NSAIDs, but especially indomethacin, can interfere with the antihypertensive effects of diuretics and angiotensin converting enzyme inhibitors.

VIII. SULINDAC is a substituted analogue of indomethacin that has similar therapeutic actions and side effects.

   A. Ibuprofen, naproxen, fenoprofen, and ketoprofen are nonsteroidal propionic acid derivatives with prominent analgesic, antipyretic, and antiinflammatory effects, reflecting inhibition of cylcooxygenase and subsequent synthesis of prostaglandins (Fig. 11–2).

      1. These drugs are as useful as salicylates in treating various forms of arthritis (comparative trials of NSAIDs have rarely revealed clinically important differences between these drugs.)

         a. Sequestration of NSAIDs in synovial tissues of inflamed joints is facilitated by the weakly acidic (pK of 3–5) characteristics of these drugs.

         b. Most NSAIDs are extensively bound (greater than 95%) to albumin.

   B. **Side effects** of NSAIDs most commonly manifest as gastrointestinal disturbances (dyspepsia more common than gastric ulceration), decreased renal function, skin rashes, and central nervous system disturbances.

      1. Platelet function is altered, similar to that produced by salicylates.

      2. Any patient who is sensitive to salicylates may also be allergic to NSAIDs.

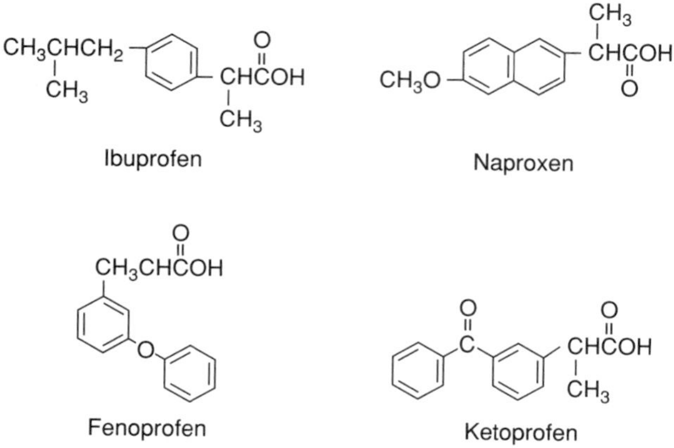

FIGURE 11–2.   Propionic acid derivatives.

    C. Naproxen is unique in that its long elimination half-time makes twice-daily administration effective.

IX. KETOROLAC

    A. Ketorolac is an NSAID that exhibits potent analgesic (30 mg IM is equivalent to 12 mg of morphine) but only moderate antiinflammatory activity.

        1. This drug may be used alone or in combination with opioids to treat postoperative pain (morphine-sparing effect).

        2. The major benefit of ketorolac is that it does not depress ventilation or the cardiovascular system.

        3. Ketorolac does not alter biliary tract dynamics and may be a logical choice for analgesia in those situations in which spasm of the biliary tract would be undesirable.

    B. Ketorolac inhibits platelet aggregation (increases bleeding time) by reversible inhibition of prostaglandin synthetase.

    C. Ketorolac may produce bronchospasm in patients who are sensitive to aspirin.

X. GOLD

    A. Gold may be preferred to glucocorticoids in the treatment of rheumatoid arthritis, producing symptomatic relief most likely by its uptake into macrophages and subsequent inhibition of phagocytosis and activities of lysosomal enzymes.

B. Side effects of gold therapy include glossitis, chrysiasis, thrombocytopenia, and proteinuria.

XI. COLCHICINE

A. Colchicine is unique in that its beneficial antiinflammatory effects are limited to the treatment of acute attacks of gout, as well as prophylaxis against such attacks.

B. Oral administration of colchicine must be discontinued as soon as gastrointestinal symptoms appear because hemorrhagic gastroenteritis can result in severe fluid and electrolyte losses.

XII. ALLOPURINOL

A. Allopurinol is the preferred drug for the treatment of primary hyperuricemia of gout and hyperuricemia that occurs during therapy with chemotherapeutic drugs.

  1. Allopurinol interferes with the terminal steps of uric acid synthesis by inhibiting xanthine oxidase, the enzyme that converts xanthine to uric acid.

  2. Drug-metabolizing enzymes are inhibited, which may result in unexpectedly prolonged effects produced by drugs that are extensively metabolized, including oral anticoagulants.

B. Side effects of allopurinol include hypersensitivity-like syndromes (fever, myalgia, rash, pruritus, nephritis) and hepatic dysfunction.

XIII. URICOSURIC DRUGS

A. Uricosuric drugs, such as probenecid and sulfinpyrazone, act directly on renal tubules to increase the rate of excretion of uric acid (antagonized by salicylates), as in patients treated with chemotherapeutic drugs.

B. Probenecid inhibits the renal tubular excretion of penicillin (plasma concentrations are at least twice the level achieved with the antibiotic alone).

C. Sulfinpyrazone inhibits platelet function and may induce hypoglycemia by decreasing the excretion of oral hypoglycemics.

Chapter

12

Sympathomimetics

Sympathomimetics include naturally occurring (endogenous) catecholamines, synthetic catecholamines, and synthetic noncatecholamines (indirect-acting and direct-acting) (Table 12-1). (Updated and revised from Stoelting RK. Sympathomimetics. In: Pharmacology and Physiology in Anesthetic Practice. 2nd ed. Philadelphia, JB Lippincott, 1991;264–84.)

I. CLINICAL USES (Table 12-2)

II. STRUCTURE ACTIVITY RELATIONSHIPS

A. All sympathomimetics are derived from beta-phenylethylamine (Fig. 12-1).
   1. The presence of hydroxyl groups on the 3 and 4 positions of the benzene ring (dihydroxybenzene) of beta-phenylethylamine is designated a catechol (drugs with this composition are designated **catecholamines**) (Fig. 12-1).
   2. Synthetic noncatecholamines include the beta-phenylethylamine structure, but lack hydroxyl groups on the 3 and/or 4 positions of the benzene ring (Fig. 12-2).

B. **Receptor Selectivity**
   1. Maximal alpha- and beta-adrenergic receptor activity depends on the presence of hydroxyl groups on the 3 and 4 positions of the benzene ring of beta-phenylethylamine (epinephrine has the optimal structure for producing alpha- and beta-adrenergic effects).
   2. Removal of the 4-hydroxyl group (phenylephrine) increases the alpha-1 selectivity of this drug.
   3. Hydroxyl groups in the 3 and 5 positions of the benzene ring confer beta-2 agonist activity on compounds with long chain substituents.

(text continues on page 217)

Table 12-1
Classification and Comparative Pharmacology of Sympathomimetics

| | Receptors Stimulated | | | Mechanism of Action | Cardiac Effects | | | Peripheral Vascular Resistance | Renal Blood Flow | Mean Arterial Pressure | Airway Resistance | Central Nervous System Stimulation | Single Intravenous Dose (70-kg adult) | Continuous Infusion Dose (70-kg adult) |
	Alpha	Beta-1	Beta-2		Cardiac Output	Heart Rate	Dysrhythmias							
Natural Catecholamines														
Epinephrine	+	++	++	Direct	++	++	+++	±	- -	+	- -	Yes	2-8 µg	1-20 µg·min⁻¹
Norepinephrine	+++	++	0	Direct	-	-	+	+++	- - -	+++	NC	No	Not used	4-16 µg·min⁻¹
Dopamine	++	++	+	Direct	+++	+	+	+	+++	+	NC	No	Not used	2-20 µg·kg⁻¹·min⁻¹
Synthetic Catecholamines														
Isoproterenol	0	+++	+++	Direct	+++	+++	+++	- -	- -	±	- - -	Yes	1-4 µg	1-5 µg·min⁻¹
Dobutamine	0	+++	0	Direct	+++	+	±	NC	++	±	NC	No	Not used	2-10 µg·kg⁻¹·min⁻¹
Synthetic Noncatecholamines														
Indirect-Acting														
Ephedrine	++	+	+	Indirect, some direct	++	++	++	+	- -	++	- -	Yes	10-25 mg	Not used
Mephentermine	++	+	+	Indirect	++	++	++	++	- -	++	-	Yes	10-25 mg	Not used
Amphetamines	++	+	+	Indirect	+	++	+	++	- -	+	NC	Yes	Not used	Not used
Metaraminol	++	+	+	Indirect, direct	-	-	+	+++	- - -	+++	NC	No	1.5-5 mg	40-500 µg·min⁻¹
Direct-Acting														
Phenylephrine	+++	0	0	Direct	-	-	NC	+++	- - -	+++	NC	No	50-100 µg	20-50 µg·min⁻¹
Methoxamine	+++	0	0	Direct	-	-	NC	+++	- - -	+++	NC	No	5-10 mg	

0, None; +, minimal increase; ++, moderate increase; +++, marked increase; -, minimal decrease; - -, moderate decrease; - - -, marked decrease; NC, no change

215

Table 12–2
Clinical Uses of Sympathomimetics

Increased myocardial contractility (response verified by measurements from pulmonary artery catheter)

Vasopressor (regional anesthesia; maintain perfusion pressure until excess volatile anesthetic is eliminated or hypovolemia is corrected)

Treatment of bronchospasm (albuterol)

Management of life-threatening allergic reactions (epinephrine)

Additive to local anesthetic solutions

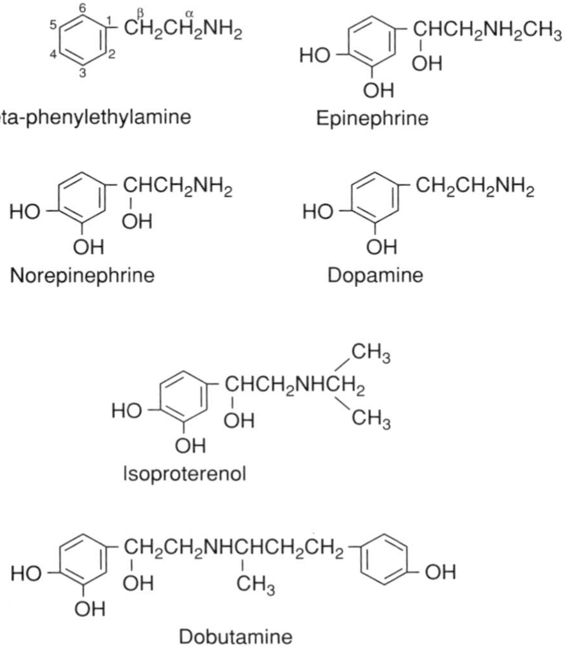

FIGURE 12–1. Sympathomimetics are derived from beta-phenylethylamine, with a catecholamine being any compound that has hydroxyl groups on the 3 and 4 positions of the benzene ring.

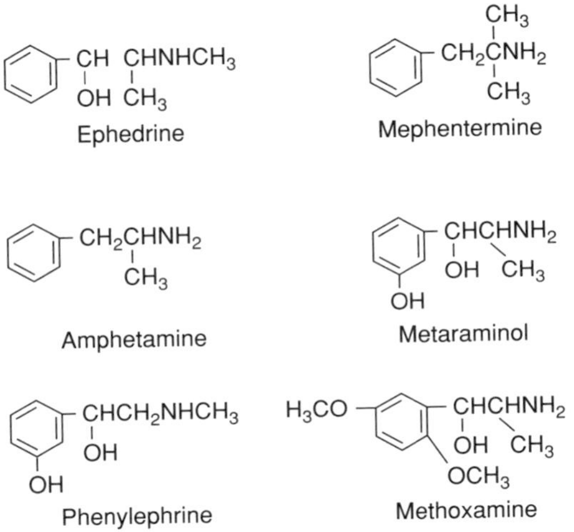

FIGURE 12–2. Indirect-acting and direct-acting synthetic noncatecholamines.

C. Central Nervous System Stimulation

1. Central nervous system stimulation is prominent with synthetic noncatecholamines that lack substituents on the benzene ring (methamphetamine).
2. Catecholamines have limited lipid solubility and thus are not likely to cross the blood–brain barrier in sufficient amounts to cause central nervous system stimulation.

III. MECHANISM OF ACTION

A. Sympathomimetics exert their pharmacologic effects by activating, either directly or indirectly, adrenoreceptors (alpha-adrenergic, beta-adrenergic) or dopaminergic receptors.
   1. Adrenoreceptors are members of the guanine (G)-protein–coupled receptor family.
   2. Genes encoding nine distinct adrenoreceptor subtypes (alpha-1a, alpha-1b, alpha-1c, alpha-2c2, alpha-2c4, alpha-2c10, beta-1, beta-2, beta-3) have been discovered.
   3. Elucidation of subtypes is the basis for development of selective agonists and antagonists.

B. In general, G-protein–coupled receptors are excitable proteins located in cell membranes, coupled via intermediary G proteins to effector systems (see Fig. 39–4).

　1. Production of cyclic adenosine monophosphate (cyclic AMP) (second messenger) is speculated to activate protein kinases and inward calcium ion (Ca^{2+}) flux, resulting in beta-1 effects (enhanced myocardial contraction).

　2. Beta-2 receptor activation reflects hyperpolarization of cell membranes and decreased inward Ca^{2+} flux (relaxation of vascular and bronchial smooth muscle).

　3. Alpha-1 receptor stimulation increases inward flux of Ca^{2+}.

　4. The density and anatomic distribution of alpha- and beta-adrenergic receptors is important in certain disease states, and influences the pharmacologic response evoked by sympathomimetics (Table 12–1; see also Chapter 39, Section V).

　5. Indirect-acting sympathomimetics are synthetic noncatecholamines that activate adrenoceptors by evoking the release of norepinephrine from postganglionic sympathetic nerve endings (Table 12–1).

　　a. Denervation or depletion of neurotransmitter (repeated doses of ephedrine) blunts the pharmacologic responses normally evoked by these drugs.

　　b. The blood pressure response to indirect-acting sympathomimetics is decreased by antihypertensive drugs that decrease central sympathetic nervous system activity.

　6. Direct-acting sympathomimetics activate adrenoceptors directly, and the response is not altered by denervation or depletion of neurotransmitter (Table 12–1).

IV. METABOLISM

A. Catecholamines are rapidly inactivated by the enzymes **monoamine oxidase (MAO)** and **catechol-O-methyltransferase (COMT).**

　1. The resulting inactive methylated metabolites are conjugated with glucuronic acid, appearing in the urine as 3-methoxy-4-hydroxymandelic acid, metanephrine (derived from epinephrine), and normetanephrine (derived from norepinephrine).

　2. Despite the importance of enzymatic degradation of

catecholamines, the biologic actions of these substances are terminated principally by uptake back into postganglionic sympathetic nerve endings.

   a. Inhibition of this uptake mechanism produces a greater potentiation of the effects of epinephrine than does inhibition of either enzyme.

   b. The completeness of this uptake mechanism and metabolism is emphasized by the appearance of only minimal amounts of unchanged catecholamines in the urine.

   3. Plasma concentrations of dopamine and epinephrine are not altered in passage across the lungs (arterial and venous concentrations are the same), whereas norepinephrine is removed to a large extent.

B. Synthetic Noncatecholamines

   1. Synthetic noncatecholamines lacking a 3-hydroxyl group are not affected by COMT and thus depend on MAO for their metabolism.

   2. Patients treated with MAO inhibitors may manifest exaggerated responses when treated with synthetic noncatecholamines.

V. ROUTE OF ADMINISTRATION

   A. Oral administration of catecholamines is not effective, presumably reflecting the metabolism of these compounds by enzymes in the gastrointestinal mucosa and liver before reaching the systemic circulation (epinephrine is given subcutaneously or IV; dopamine and norepinephrine are administered only IV).

   B. Absence of one or both of the 3,4-hydroxyl groups, as is characteristic of synthetic noncatecholamines, increases oral absorption of these drugs.

VI. NATURALLY OCCURRING CATECHOLAMINES
(Table 12-1; Fig. 12-1)

   A. Epinephrine is the most potent activator of alpha-adrenergic receptors (2 to 10 times more potent than norepinephrine), epinephrine also activates beta-1 and beta-2 receptors.

   1. Clinical Uses (Table 12-3)

   2. Cardiovascular Effects

   a. Epinephrine stimulates beta-1 receptors, causing

Table 12–3
Clinical Uses of Catecholamines

Epinephrine
    Additive to local anesthetic solutions
    Treatment of life-threatening allergic reactions
    Cardiopulmonary resuscitation
    Increased myocardial contractility

Dopamine
    Increased myocardial contractility, especially in the presence of
    low urine output

Isoproterenol
    Treatment of complete heart block (chemical pacemaker)
    Decreased pulmonary vascular resistance

Dobutamine
    Increased myocardial contractility, especially if heart rate and
    systemic vascular resistance are increased

an increase in systolic blood pressure, heart rate, and cardiac output.

b. There is a modest decrease in diastolic blood pressure, reflecting vasodilation in skeletal muscles due to activation of beta-2 receptors (preferential distribution of cardiac output to skeletal muscles).

c. Mean arterial pressure does not change greatly, so there is little likelihood that baroreceptor activation will occur to produce reflex bradycardia.

d. Epinephrine speeds heart rate by accelerating the rate of spontaneous phase 4 depolarization, which also increases the likelihood of cardiac dysrhythmias.

e. Epinephrine predominantly stimulates alpha-1 receptors in the skin, mucosa, and hepatorenal vasculature, producing intense vasoconstriction (renal blood flow is substantially decreased by epinephrine, even in the absence of changes in blood pressure).

f. Epinephrine, 10 $\mu g \cdot kg^{-1}$, when administered into the trachea of patients being mechanically ventilated, had no effect on heart rate or blood pressure (suggests that use of this route of administration during cardiopulmonary resuscitation may be ineffective).

3. **Airway smooth muscle** relaxation reflects epinephrine-induced activation of beta-2 receptors.
4. **Metabolic Effects**
   a. Beta-1 stimulation due to epinephrine increases liver glycogenolysis (activation of hepatic phosphorylase enzyme) and adipose tissue lipolysis (activation of triglyceride lipase).
   b. Alpha-1 stimulation produced by epinephrine inhibits insulin release (most likely explanation for the hyperglycemia that often occurs during the perioperative period).
   c. Beta-2 stimulation facilitates transfer of potassium into cells (hypokalemia), presumably reflecting activation of the sodium-potassium pump in skeletal muscles.
5. **Ocular effects** of epinephrine include mydriasis (contraction of the radial muscle of the iris).
6. **Coagulation** may be accelerated by epinephrine-induced activation of factor V (hypercoagulation may accompany surgical stimulation).

B. **Norepinephrine**
   1. Norepinephrine is the endogenous neurotransmitter released from postganglionic sympathetic nerve endings (potent beta-1 and alpha agonist effects, but little agonist effect at beta-2 receptors) (Table 12–1).
   2. **Cardiovascular Effects**
      a. Intravenous administration of norepinephrine results in intense vasoconstriction (skin, skeletal muscles, liver, kidneys) that may so decrease tissue blood flow that metabolic acidosis occurs.
      b. The resulting increase in systemic vascular resistance decreases venous return to the heart and increases systolic, diastolic, and mean arterial pressure.
      c. Decreased venous return to the heart, combined with baroreceptor-mediated reflex decreases in heart rate due to marked increases in blood pressure, tends to decrease cardiac output despite the beta-1 effects of norepinephrine.

C. **Dopamine**
   1. Depending on the dose, dopamine stimulates principally dopamine-1 receptors in the renal vasculature to produce renal vasodilation (0.5 to 3 $\mu g \cdot kg^{-1} \cdot min$ IV), beta-1 receptors in the heart (3 to 10 $\mu g \cdot kg^{-1} \cdot min^{-1}$ IV), and alpha receptors in the peripheral vasculature (at doses exceeding 10 $\mu g \cdot kg^{-1} \cdot min^{-1}$ IV).

      a. Nausea and vomiting produced by dopamine reflect stimulation of dopamine-2 receptors.

      b. Rapid metabolism of dopamine mandates its use as a continuous intravenous infusion so as to maintain therapeutic plasma concentrations.

      c. The lungs clear about 20% of the clinical doses of dopamine.

  2. Clinical Uses (Table 12–3)

      a. Dopamine is unique among the catecholamines in its ability to simultaneously increase myocardial contractility, renal blood flow, glomerular filtration rate, and urine output.

      b. Increased excretion of sodium may reflect inhibition of aldosterone secretion by dopamine.

      c. Hyperglycemia that is commonly present in patients receiving a continuous intravenous infusion of dopamine is likely to reflect drug-induced inhibition of insulin secretion.

  3. Cardiovascular Effects

      a. Dopamine increases cardiac output by activation of beta-1 receptors and stimulation of endogenous release of norepinephrine (may predispose patients to development of cardiac dysrhythmias but still less dysrhythmogenic than epinephrine).

      b. Increases in cardiac output produced by dopamine are usually accompanied by only modest increases in heart rate, blood pressure, and systemic vascular resistance.

  4. Ventilation Effects

      a. Intravenous infusion of dopamine interferes with the ventilatory response to hypoxemia, reflecting the role of dopamine as an inhibitory neurotransmitter at the carotid bodies.

      b. This may result in unexpected depression of ventilation (arterial blood gas levels) in patients who are being treated with dopamine to increase myocardial contractility.

VII. SYNTHETIC CATECHOLAMINES (Table 12–1; Fig. 12–1)

  A. Isoproterenol

    1. Isoproterenol is the most potent activator of all the sympathomimetics at beta-1 and beta-2 receptors (2 to 10 times more potent than epinephrine), but is devoid of alpha-agonist effects.

2. Metabolism of isoproterenol in the liver by COMT is rapid, necessitating a continuous intravenous infusion to maintain therapeutic plasma concentrations.

3. **Clinical Uses** (Table 12–3)

4. **Cardiovascular Effects**

   a. Cardiovascular effects of isoproterenol reflect activation of beta-1 receptors in the heart (increases in heart rate, myocardial contractility, and cardiac automaticity) and beta-2 receptors in the vasculature of skeletal muscles (decreased systemic vascular resistance).

   b. The net effect of these changes is an increase in cardiac output that is usually sufficient to increase systolic blood pressure.

   c. Mean arterial pressure may decline due to decreases in systemic vascular resistance and associated decreases in diastolic blood pressure.

   d. Decreased diastolic blood pressure that is induced by isoproterenol may decrease coronary blood flow at the same time that myocardial oxygen requirements are increased by tachycardia and increased myocardial contractility.

   e. Compensatory baroreceptor-mediated reflex slowing of the heart rate does not occur during infusion of isoproterenol because mean arterial pressure is not increased.

B. **Dobutamine**

   1. Dobutamine is a selective beta-1 agonist that must be administered by continuous intravenous infusion to offset its rapid metabolism.

   2. **Clinical Uses** (Table 12–3)

   3. **Cardiovascular Effects**

      a. Dobutamine produces dose-dependent increases in cardiac output and decreases in atrial filling pressure without marked increases in heart rate or blood pressure.

      b. Systemic vascular resistance may be decreased, but is usually not altered greatly.

      c. Unlike dopamine, dobutamine does not act indirectly by stimulating the release of norepinephrine from the heart, nor does this catecholamine activate dopaminergic receptors to increase renal blood flow.

Table 12–4
Clinical Uses of Synthetic Noncatecholamines

Ephedrine
   Treatment of hypotension
      Regional anesthesia (especially parturients)
      Overdose of inhaled or injected anesthetics
      Hypovolemia (maintenance of perfusion pressure until blood
        volume can be restored)

Phenylephrine
   Treatment of hypotension (same as ephedrine, except not likely
     to be recommended for parturients)
   Treatment of supraventricular cardiac tachydysrhythmias asso-
     ciated with hypotension
   Topical nasal decongestant or mydriatic

---

    d. Conduction velocity through the atrioventricular node is increased by dobutamine, raising the possibility that excessive increases in heart rate could occur in patients with atrial fibrillation.

VIII. SYNTHETIC NONCATECHOLAMINES (Table 12-1; Fig. 12-2)

A. Ephedrine

1. Ephedrine is an indirect-acting (endogenous release of norepinephrine) and direct-acting synthetic noncatecholamine that stimulates alpha- and beta-adrenergic receptors.

2. **Clinical Uses** (Table 12-4)

   a. Uterine blood flow is not greatly altered when ephedrine is administered to restore maternal blood pressure to normal following production of sympathetic nervous system blockade (in contrast to selective alpha-agonists, including phenylephrine, which restore blood pressure but, at the same time, decrease uterine blood flow because of vasoconstriction) (Fig. 12-3).

   b. Ephedrine can be used as a chronic oral medication to treat bronchial asthma, reflecting its bronchodilating effects by activation of beta-2 receptors.

3. **Cardiovascular Effects**

   a. Intravenous administration of ephedrine results in

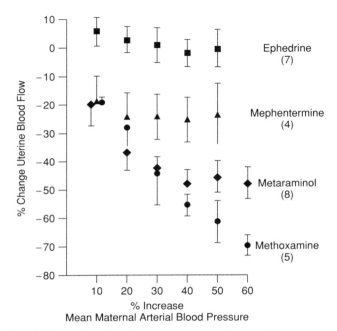

FIGURE 12–3. Ephedrine-induced increases in mean arterial pressure produce the smallest decreases in uterine blood flow. Mephentermine has an intermediate effect, and increases in blood pressure produced by metaraminol and methoxamine result in substantial decreases in uterine blood flow. (From Ralston DH, Shnider SM, deLorimer AA. Effects of equipotent ephedrine, metaraminol, mephentermine, and methoxamine on uterine blood flow in the pregnant ewe. Anesthesiology 1974;40:354–61; with permission.)

    increases in systolic and diastolic blood pressure, cardiac output, and skeletal muscle blood flow and decreases in renal blood flow (resembles epinephrine).

b. The principal mechanism for the cardiovascular effects of ephedrine is increased myocardial contractility owing to activation of beta-1 receptors (in the presence of beta blockade, the cardiovascular effects of ephedrine may resemble responses that are more typical of alpha receptor stimulation).

    c. A second dose of ephedrine produces a less intense blood pressure response than the first dose (tachyphylaxis), presumably reflecting persistent blockade of adrenoceptors or, alternatively, depletion of norepinephrine stores.

B. Mephentermine is an indirect-acting synthetic noncatecholamine that stimulates alpha- and beta-adrenergic receptors.

C. Amphetamine, along with related sympathomimetics dextroamphetamine and methamphetamine, produces cardiovascular effects that resemble those of ephedrine but that differ in also producing significant central nervous system stimulation.

D. Metaraminol is a synthetic noncatecholamine that stimulates alpha- and beta-adrenergic receptors by indirect and direct effects (produces more intense peripheral vasoconstriction and less of an increase in myocardial contractility than ephedrine).

E. Phenylephrine

    1. Phenylephrine is a direct-acting synthetic noncatecholamine that stimulates principally alpha-1 adrenergic receptors (mimicking norepinephrine).

        a. The dose of phenylephrine necessary to stimulate alpha-1 receptors (venoconstriction) is less than that which is necessary to stimulate alpha-2 receptors.

        b. Phenylephrine-induced venoconstriction may deserve consideration in patients who have recently undergone saphenous vein to coronary artery bypass grafts.

    2. Clinical Uses (Table 12–4)

    3. Cardiovascular Effects

        a. Rapid intravenous injection of phenylephrine produces dose-dependent peripheral vasoconstriction and increases in blood pressure that are accompanied by decreases in cardiac output.

        b. Decreased cardiac output most likely reflects reflex bradycardia in response to drug-induced increases in diastolic blood pressure (stimulation of the carotid sinus).

F. Methoxamine is a synthetic noncatecholamine that acts selectively on alpha-adrenergic receptors to produce intense arterial vasoconstriction and reflex bradycardia.

Table 12–5
Comparative Pharmacology of Selective Beta-2 Agonists

	Beta-2 Selectivity	Peak Effect (min)	Duration of Action (h)	Method of Administration
Metaproterenol	+++	30–60	3–4	MDI, nebulization, oral
Terbutaline	++++	60	4	MDI, nebulization, subcutaneous
Albuterol	++++	30–60	4	MDI, oral
Bitolterol	++++	30–60	5	MDI
Isoetharine	++	15–60	2–3	MDI, nebulization
Ritodrine	++++			Intravenous, oral

++, minimal stimulation; +++, moderate stimulation; ++++, marked stimulation; *MDI,* metered-dose inhaler

IX. SELECTIVE BETA-2 AGONISTS

A. Selective beta-2 agonists specifically relax bronchiole and uterine smooth muscle without exerting significant beta-1 effects on the heart (Table 12–5).

B. **Clinical Uses**
   1. **Reversible Bronchospasm**
      a. Inhalation of beta-2 agonists by metered dose inhaler is as effective in treating bronchospasm as the subcutaneous injection of epinephrine.
      b. **Albuterol** is a likely selection for the treatment of bronchospasm in anesthetized patients (metered dose inhaler can be placed in the inspiratory limb of the anesthetic delivery system).
   2. **Tocolysis**
      a. **Ritodrine** is the beta-2 agonist most often used to stop uterine contractions of premature labor.
      b. Ritodrine readily crosses the placenta and thus may cause cardiovascular and metabolic side effects in the mother and fetus (Table 12–6).

C. **Theophylline**
   1. Theophylline (aminophylline is theophylline in complex with ethylenediamine to increase solubility) is a bronchodilating drug with an efficacy that is similar to that of beta-2 agonists.

Table 12–6
Side Effects of Ritodrine

Tachycardia (beta-1 stimulation)

Increased cardiac output

Pulmonary edema (especially if hydration is aggressive)

Exaggerated hypotension in presence of volatile anesthetics

Hypokalemia

Hyperglycemia (ketoacidosis a risk in insulin-dependent diabetics)

2. Side effects of aminophylline (cardiac dysrhythmias, central nervous system stimulation, especially when plasma concentrations exceed 20 $\mu g \cdot ml^{-1}$) limit the use of this drug in preference to selective beta-2 agonists for the treatment of reversible bronchospasm.

D. **Pentoxifylline** is a methylxanthine derivative that decreases viscosity of blood and may improve tissue oxygenation in patients with chronic occlusive arterial disease of the limbs.

13
Digitalis and Related Drugs

Digitalis is the term used for cardiac glycosides that occur naturally in many plants, including the foxglove plant (Fig. 13-1). (Updated and revised from Stoelting RK. Digitalis and related drugs. In: Pharmacology and Physiology in Anesthetic Practice. 2nd ed. Philadelphia, JB Lippincott, 1991;285-94.)

I. CLINICAL USES (Table 13-1)

A. Digitalis preparations may not be of benefit in high output cardiac failure (hyperthyroidism, thiamine deficiency). There is even uncertainty that digoxin maintains beneficial effects in cardiac failure as judged by mortality studies.

B. Before administering a cardiac glycoside to treat a supraventricular cardiac dysrhythmia, it is important to confirm that the dysrhythmia is not due to digitalis toxicity.

C. Administration of propranolol or esmolol, combined with digoxin, may provide more rapid control of supraventricular tachydysrhythmias and minimize the likelihood of toxicity by permitting decreases in the dose of both drugs.

D. In approximately 30% of patients with Wolff-Parkinson-White syndrome, digitalis reduces refractoriness in the accessory conduction pathway to the point that rapid atrial impulses can cause ventricular fibrillation.

E. Digitalis may be harmful in patients with hypertrophic subaortic stenosis because increased myocardial contractility intensifies the resistance to ventricular ejection.

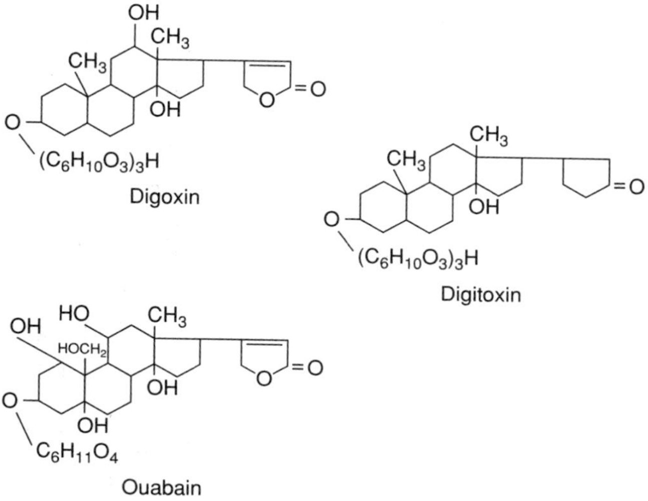

FIGURE 13–1.   Cardiac glycosides.

Table 13–1
Clinical Uses of Digitalis

Treatment of Cardiac Failure
 Essential hypertension
 Valvular heart disease
 Atherosclerotic heart disease

Slowing of Ventricular Response Rate
 Paroxysmal atrial tachycardia
 Atrial fibrillation
 Atrial flutter

II. STRUCTURE ACTIVITY RELATIONSHIPS

 A. The basic structure of cardiac glycosides is that of a steroid nucleus that consists of a glycone (sugar, such as glucose) and an aglycone portion (Fig. 13–1).

 B. Glycones are necessary to ensure fixation of cardiac glycosides to cardiac muscle and production of the pharmacologic effect that is characterized as "digitalis-like."

III. MECHANISM OF ACTION

A. Direct Effects on the Heart

1. The most likely explanation for the direct positive inotropic effect of cardiac glycosides is drug-induced inhibition of the sodium pump mechanism located in cardiac cell membranes, leading to decreased extrusion of calcium ions (Ca^{2+}) from cardiac cells.

2. It is presumed that this increased intracellular concentration of Ca^{2+} is responsible for the positive inotropic effects of cardiac glycosides (increased amounts of Ca^{2+} are available to react with cardiac contractile proteins).

B. Alterations in Autonomic Nervous System Activity

1. Cardiac glycosides increase parasympathetic nervous system activity (due to sensitization of the carotid sinus and activation of vagal nuclei).

2. The manifestation of these effects is a slowed heart rate (decreased activity of the sinoatrial node and prolonged effective refractory period), especially in the presence of atrial fibrillation.

IV. PHARMACOKINETICS (Table 13-2)

A. At equilibrium, the concentration of cardiac glycosides in the heart is 15 to 30 times greater than that in plasma.

B. Digoxin

1. The maintenance dose of digoxin is adjusted to the individual patient's response, electrocardiogram, and the plasma concentration of digoxin.

   a. The maintenance dose must be equal to the daily loss (clearance) of drug.

   b. In the presence of renal dysfunction, the elimination half-time of digoxin is decreased in proportion to creatinine clearance (digoxin dose should be decreased 50% when the serum creatinine concentration is 3 to 5 mg·dl^{-1}).

2. The principal inactive tissue reservoir site for digoxin is skeletal muscle (decreased in elderly patients).

C. Digitoxin. The long elimination half-time of digitoxin is an advantage for maintaining therapeutic concentrations should a patient miss several doses.

D. Ouabain

1. Ouabain is administered in doses of 1.5 to 3 µg·kg^{-1} IV (oral administration is ineffective) to provide rapid increases in myocardial contractility or to decrease

Table 13–2
Comparison of Digoxin and Digitoxin

	Digoxin	*Digitoxin*
Average Digitalizing Dose		
Oral	0.75–1.5 mg	0.8–1.2 mg
Intravenous	0.5–1 mg	0.8–1.2 mg
Average Daily Maintenance Dose		
Oral	0.125–0.5 mg	0.05–0.2 mg
Intravenous	0.25 mg	0.1 mg
Onset of Effect		
Oral	1.5–6 h	3–6 h
Intravenous	5–30 min	30–120 min
Absorption from Gastrointestinal Tract	75%	90%–100%
Plasma Protein Binding	25%	95%
Route of Elimination	Renal	Hepatic
Enterokepatic Circulation	Minimal	Marked
Elimination Half-Time	31–33 h	5–7 days
Therapeutic Plasma Concentration	0.5–2 ng·ml^{-1}	10–35 ng·ml^{-1}

(Data from Hoffman BF, Bigger JT. Digitalis and allied cardiac glycosides. In: Gilman AG, Goodman LS, Rall TW, Murad F, eds. The Pharmacological Basis of Therapeutics. 7th ed. New York. Macmillan Publishing Co. 1985, 716; with permission.)

the heart rate in uncontrolled atrial fibrillation (unlikely that ouabain offers any advantages over digoxin).

2. A longer-acting digitalis preparation is substituted for ouabain when maintenance therapy is indicated (50% of unchanged ouabain can be recovered in the urine in the first 8 hours).

V. CARDIOVASCULAR EFFECTS

A. The principal cardiovascular effect of digitalis glycosides is a dose-related **increase in myocardial contractility**

Table 13–3
Electrocardiographic Effects of Cardiac Glycosides at Therapeutic Plasma Concentrations*

Prolonged P-R interval (rarely >0.25 second)

Shortened Q-T interval

ST-T segment depression (may suggest myocardial ischemia)

Diminished amplitude or inversion of the T-wave

*Changes on the electrocardiogram disappear approximately 20 days after digitalis is discontinued.

(increased stroke volume, decreased heart size, decreased left ventricular end-diastolic pressure) that becomes significant with less than fully digitalizing doses.

1. Improved renal perfusion favors mobilization and excretion of edema fluid (diuresis often accompanies administration of cardiac glycosides to patients in cardiac failure).

2. Excessive sympathetic nervous system activity that occurs as a compensatory response to cardiac failure is decreased with the improved circulation that accompanies administration of cardiac glycosides.

B. In addition to their positive inotropic effects, cardiac glycosides enhance parasympathetic nervous system activity, leading to delayed conduction of cardiac impulses through the atrioventricular node and decreases in heart rate.

VI. ELECTROCARDIOGRAPHIC EFFECTS (Table 13–3)

VII. DIGITALIS TOXICITY

A. Causes

1. The most frequent cause of digitalis toxicity in the absence of renal dysfunction is the concurrent administration of diuretics that cause potassium ion (K^+) depletion (hypokalemia probably increases myocardial binding of cardiac glycosides, resulting in excess drug effect).

a. Hyperventilation of the lungs during anesthesia can abruptly decrease serum K^+ concentrations

Table 13–4
Diagnosis of Digitalis Toxicity

Plasma digoxin concentration (toxicity is likely when higher than 3 ng·ml^{-1})

Anorexia, nausea, and vomiting

Atrial or ventricular cardiac dysrhythmias

Prolonged P-R interval (QRS not prolonged)

        an average of 0.5 mEq·L^{-1} for every 10 mmHg decrease in PaCO$_2$.

    b. Other electrolyte abnormalities that contribute to digitalis toxicity include **hypercalcemia** and **hypomagnesemia.**

  2. An increase in sympathetic nervous system activity, as produced by arterial hypoxemia, increases the likelihood of digitalis toxicity.

  3. Elderly patients with decreased skeletal muscle mass and decreased renal function are vulnerable to digitalis toxicity if the usual doses of a digitalis drug are administered.

 B. Diagnosis (Table 13-4)

 C. Treatment (Table 13-5)

Table 13–5
Treatment of Digitalis Toxicity

Correction of Predisposing Causes
  Hypokalemia (measure serum potassium concentration and, if normal, administer potassium, 0.025 to 0.05 mEq·kg^{-1} IV, to treat life-threatening cardiac dysrhythmias)
  Arterial hypoxemia

Suppression of Cardiac Dysrhythmias
  Phenytoin (0.5 to 1.5 mg·kg^{-1} IV over 5 minutes)
  Lidocaine (1 to 2 mg·kg^{-1} IV)
  Propranolol

Control of Excessive Parasympathetic Nervous System Activity
  Atropine (35 to 70 µg·kg^{-1} IV)

Administration of Antibodies (Fab Fragments)

Table 13–6
Digitalis Therapy and Drug Interactions

Quinidine (displaces digoxin from binding sites in tissues)

Succinylcholine (could enhance parasympathetic activity of digitalis, but there is no clinical evidence that this occurs)

Pancuronium (may increase the likelihood of cardiac dysrhythmias)

Calcium (enhances digitalis effects)

Diuretics (if contributing to hypokalemia)

Volatile anesthetics (decrease the likelihood of digitalis-induced cardiac dysrhythmias)

VIII. PREOPERATIVE PROPHYLACTIC DIGITALIS

A. The disadvantage of prophylactic administration of digitalis is the administration of a drug with a narrow therapeutic-to-toxic dose difference (intraoperative events may lead to hypokalemia or increased sympathetic nervous system activity) to patients with no obvious need for the drug.

B. Despite theoretical disadvantages, there is evidence that **selected patients** (elderly patients undergoing thoracic or abdominal surgery) may benefit (decreased occurrence of postoperative supraventricular cardiac dysrhythmias) from prophylactic digitalis.

C. There is no evidence to support discontinuing digitalis in any patient preoperatively, especially if the drug is being administered for heart rate control.

IX. DRUG INTERACTIONS (Table 13-6)

X. NONCATECHOLAMINE NONGLYCOSIDE CARDIAC INOTROPES

A. Calcium

1. Calcium chloride, 5 to 10 mg·kg^{-1} IV, produces an intense positive inotropic effect (increased stroke volume, decreased left ventricular end-diastolic pressure) lasting 10 to 20 minutes.

2. The inotropic effects of calcium are enhanced in the presence of hypocalcemia, as may be present at the conclusion of cardiopulmonary bypass.

Table 13–7
Side Effects of Glucagon

Tachycardia

Nausea and vomiting

Paradoxical hypoglycemia (insufficient glycogen stores to offset increased insulin release)

Hypokalemia (insulin facilitates transfer of potassium into cells)

Hypertension (catecholamine release)

B. Glucagon
1. Glucagon, like catecholamines, enhances formation of cyclic adenosine monophosphate (AMP) but, unlike catecholamines, does not act via beta-adrenergic receptors.
2. **Cardiovascular Effects**
   a. Glucagon (1 to 5 mg IV to adults) reliably increases stroke volume and heart rate, independent of adrenergic receptor activation (most likely indication for glucagon is treatment of excessive beta-adrenergic blockade).
   b. The renal effect is similar to that of dopamine, but glucagon is less potent.
3. **Side Effects** (Table 13–7)
C. Selective Phosphodiesterase Inhibitors (Figure 13–2). These heterogenous compounds appear to have a competitive inhibitory action on the isoenzymes of phosphodiesterase, decreasing the hydrolysis and thereby increasing the intracellular concentrations of cyclic AMP in the myocardium and vascular smooth muscle.
1. **Amrinone**
   a. Amrinone is a noncatecholamine nonglycoside derivative that produces dose-dependent positive

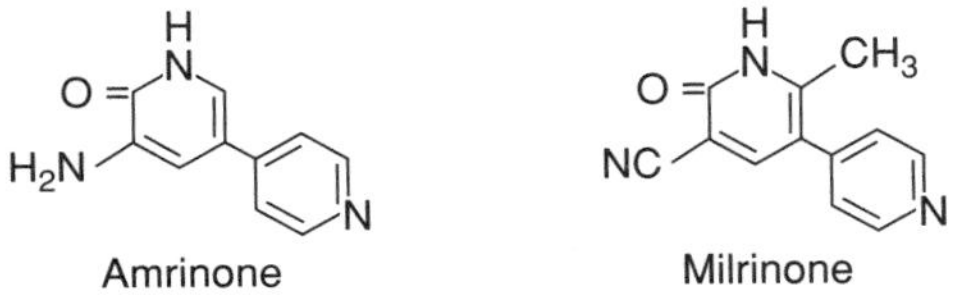

FIGURE 13–2.   Selective phosphodiesterase inhibitors.

inotropic and vasodilator effects (0.5 to 1.5 mg·kg^{-1} IV, followed by a continuous infusion of 2 to 10 µg·kg^{-1}·min^{-1}) manifesting as increased cardiac output and decreased left ventricular end-diastolic pressure.

   b. Amrinone can be used in conjunction with digitalis without provoking digitalis toxicity, suggesting that the mechanism of action of these two drugs is different.

   c. Patients experiencing left ventricular dysfunction and those who have failed to respond to catecholamines may respond to amrinone.

2. **Milrinone** is a bypyridine derivative that, like amrinone, produces positive inotropic and vasodilating effects. Despite its beneficial hemodynamic actions, long-term therapy with oral milrinone increases the morbidity and mortality (mechanism unknown) of patients with severe chronic heart failure.

14

Alpha- and Beta-Adrenergic Receptor Antagonists

Alpha- and beta-adrenergic receptor antagonists prevent the inter-action of the endogenous neurotransmitter norepinephrine, or sympathomimetics, with the corresponding adrenergic receptor, producing predictable decreases in sympathetic nervous system activity. (Updated and revised from Stoelting RK. Alpha- and beta-adrenergic receptor antagonists. In: Pharmacology and Physiology in Anesthetic Practice. 2nd ed. Philadelphia, JB Lippincott, 1991;295-310.)

I. ALPHA-ADRENERGIC RECEPTOR ANTAGONISTS
(Table 14-1)

A. Drug-induced alpha-adrenergic blockade prevents the effects of catecholamines and sympathomimetics on the heart and offsets the inhibitory effects of epinephrine on insulin secretion.

B. Orthostatic hypotension, reflex tachycardia, and impotence are predictable side effects of alpha-adrenergic blockade.

C. Mechanism of Action

1. Binding with alpha-adrenergic receptors may be **reversible** (phentolamine, prazosin, yohimbine) or **irreversible** (phenoxybenzamine).

2. Binding with alpha-adrenergic receptors may be **nonselective** at postsynaptic alpha-1 receptors and presynaptic alpha-2 receptors (phentolamine, phenoxybenzamine) or **selective** at alpha-1 receptors (prazosin) and alpha-2 receptors (yohimbine).

Table 14–1
Alpha-Adrenergic Receptor Antagonists

Phentolamine
Treatment of acute hypertensive emergencies (30 to 70 µg·kg⁻¹ IV)
Local infiltration when a sympathomimetic is accidentally administered extravascularly.

Phenoxybenzamine
Chronic control of blood pressure in patients with pheochromocytoma

Yohimbine
Treatment of impotence

Prazosin
Chronic control of blood pressure in patients with pheochromocytoma (reflex tachycardia unlikely because of selective alpha-1 antagonist effect)

II. BETA-ADRENERGIC RECEPTOR ANTAGONISTS
(Fig. 14–1)

A. Drug-induced beta-adrenergic blockade prevents effects of catecholamines and sympathomimetics on the heart and smooth muscle of the airways and blood vessels.

B. Beta-antagonist drug therapy should be continued throughout the perioperative period to maintain desirable effects and to avoid the risk of sympathetic nervous system hyperactivity associated with abrupt discontinuation of these drugs.

C. **Mechanism of Action**
1. **Binding** of beta-adrenergic receptor antagonists to beta-adrenergic receptors is reversible, such that the antagonist drug can be displaced from receptors if sufficiently large amounts of agonists become available **(competitive antagonism).**
2. Chronic administration of beta-adrenergic antagonists is associated with an increase in the number of beta-adrenergic receptors **(up-regulation).**

D. **Classification**
1. Beta-adrenergic receptor antagonists are classified as **nonselective** antagonists and **selective** antagonists on beta-1 (metoprolol, atenolol) and beta-2 receptors (Table 14–2).

cially in the presence of increased sympathetic nervous system activity.

b. Heart rate slowing induced by propranolol lasts longer than the negative inotropic effects, suggesting a possible subdivision of beta-1 receptors.

c. Beta-2 antagonist effects of propranolol manifest as increased peripheral vascular resistance, including coronary vascular resistance.

d. Propranolol relieves myocardial ischemia because changes that decrease myocardial oxygen requirements (decreased heart rate and myocardial contractility) more than offset those changes that increase myocardial oxygen requirements (prolongation of systolic ejection and dilatation of the cardiac ventricles) or decrease coronary blood flow (increased coronary vascular resistance).

2. Pharmacokinetics

a. Hepatic first-pass metabolism is the reason the oral dose of propranolol must be substantially greater than the intravenous dose.

b. Protein binding of propranolol is extensive (may be decreased by heparin or the hemodilution that occurs when cardiopulmonary bypass is initiated).

c. Metabolism of propranolol is in the liver (decreases in hepatic blood flow decrease clearance) to the active metabolite, 4-hydroxypropranolol (especially after oral administration of propranolol).

d. Clearance of local anesthetics may be decreased owing to propranolol-induced decreases in hepatic blood flow (although bupivacaine clearance is relatively insensitive to changes in hepatic blood flow).

e. Clearance of opioids via the pulmonary first-pass effect (fentanyl, especially) is decreased by chronic propranolol treatment (presumably reflecting the ability of one basophilic amine [propranolol] to inhibit the pulmonary uptake of a second basic lipophilic amine [fentanyl]).

F. Nadolol is a nonselective beta-adrenergic receptor antagonist that is unique in that its long duration of action (metabolism does not occur and unchanged drug is excreted in the bile and urine) permits once-daily oral administration.

G. Pindolol is a nonselective beta-adrenergic receptor antagonist with intrinsic sympathomimetic activity (causes minimal resting bradycardia).

H. Timolol is a nonselective beta-adrenergic receptor antagonist that is effective in the treatment of glaucoma (applied topically to the cornea, it results in decreased production of aqueous humor).

1. Systemic absorption after topical application may manifest as hypotension and bradycardia that may be resistant to treatment with atropine.
2. Unexpected postoperative apnea has been observed in neonates treated with timolol.

I. Metoprolol is a selective beta-1 antagonist that prevents inotropic and chronotropic responses to beta-adrenergic stimulation but leaves intact bronchodilator, vasodilator, and metabolic effects of beta-2 receptors (large doses may convert metoprolol to a nonselective beta-adrenergic antagonist).

J. Atenolol is a long-acting (once-daily oral administration for treatment of essential hypertension) selective beta-1 receptor antagonist that depends on renal excretion of unchanged drug.

K. Esmolol is a rapid-onset and short-acting selective beta-1 receptor antagonist (heart rate returns to predrug levels within 15 minutes).

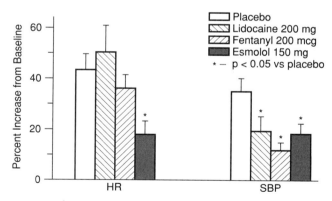

FIGURE 14–2. Maximum percent increase in heart rate (HR) and systolic blood pressure (SBP) in response to direct laryngoscopy and tracheal intubation, with or without prior administration of lidocaine, fentanyl, or esmolol. All three drugs blunted the increase in SBP, but only esmolol also protected against an increase in HR. (Helfman SM, Gold MI, DeLesser EA, Herrington CA. Which drug prevents tachycardia and hypertension associated with tracheal intubation: lidocaine, fentanyl, or esmolol? Anesth Analg 1991;72:482–6; with permission.)

Table 14–5
Clinical Uses of Beta-Antagonists

Treatment of Essential Hypertension
   Decreased cardiac output owing to decreased heart rate
   Decreased renin secretion (also results in decreased aldosterone
      secretion such that beta-antagonists prevent the compensatory
      sodium and water retention that accompanies treatment with a
      vasodilator)

Management of Angina Pectoris
   Decreased myocardial oxygen requirements secondary to
      decreased heart rate and cardiac output

Treatment of Postmyocardial Infarction

**Preoperative Preparation (Elective or Emergency) of
   Hyperthyroid Patients**

Suppression of Cardiac Dysrhythmias
   Decreased sympathetic nervous system activity to the heart with a
      resultant decrease in the rate of spontaneous phase 4
      depolarization of ectopic cardiac pacemakers (especially if due
      to digitalis toxicity)

Prevention of Excess Sympathetic Nervous System Activity
   During direct laryngoscopy and tracheal intubation
   Hypertrophic obstructive cardiomyopathies
   Pheochromocytoma
   Hyperthyroidism
   Cyanotic episodes in patients with tetralogy of Fallot
   Reflex baroreceptor-mediated increases in heart rate in patients
      treated with vasodilators
   Anxiety (public speaking)

III. SIDE EFFECTS OF BETA-ANTAGONISTS (Table 14–3)

   A. The principal contraindication to administration of beta-
      antagonists is preexisting atrioventricular heart block or
      cardiac failure not caused by tachycardia.
   B. Nonselective beta-antagonists or high doses of selective
      beta-antagonists should not be administered to patients
      with chronic obstructive airway disease.
   C. **Treatment of Excess Myocardial Depression** (Table
      14–4)

IV. CLINICAL USES OF BETA-ANTAGONISTS (Table 14–5)

Table 14–6
Clinical Uses of Labetalol

Attenuation of any increases in blood pressure and heart rate that occur during and following surgery

Rebound hypertension following withdrawal of clonidine

Pheochromocytoma

Controlled hypotension (unlike nitroprusside, it is not associated with increases in heart rate, intrapulmonary shunt, or cardiac output)

V. COMBINED ALPHA- AND BETA-ADRENERGIC RECEPTOR ANTAGONISTS

A. Labetalol

1. Labetalol exhibits **selective alpha-1 antagonist** and **nonselective beta-1 and beta-2 antagonist** effects following oral or intravenous administration.

   a. Presynaptic alpha-2 receptors are spared by labetalol.

   b. Labetalol is one fifth to one tenth as potent as phentolamine in its ability to block alpha receptors and is approximately one fourth to one third as potent as propranolol in blocking beta receptors.

2. **Cardiovascular Effects.** Labetalol, 0.1 to 0.5 mg·kg^{-1} IV, acutely lowers blood pressure by decreasing systemic vascular resistance (alpha-1 blockade), whereas reflex tachycardia triggered by vasodilation is attenuated by simultaneous beta blockade.

3. **Clinical Uses** (Table 14-6)

4. **Side Effects**

   a. Orthostatic hypotension is the most prominent side effect.

   b. Fluid retention is the reason for combining chronic labetalol therapy with a diuretic.

   c. Bronchospasm, cardiac failure, and heart block are possible, but less likely than in patients treated with beta-receptor antagonists.

Chapter

15

Antihypertensive Drugs

All available antihypertensive drugs act, to some extent, by interfering with normal homeostatic mechanisms. (Updated and revised from Stoelting RK. Antihypertensive drugs. In: Pharmacology and Physiology in Anesthetic Practice. 2nd ed. Philadelphia, JB Lippincott, 1991;311–23.)

I. INTRODUCTION

A. Potential adverse interactions between antihypertensive drugs and anesthetics have been exaggerated.

1. When interactions are likely, they are usually predictable and can thus be avoided or their significance minimized.

2. Specific concerns during administration of anesthesia to patients being treated with antihypertensive drugs include **attenuation of sympathetic nervous system activity, modification of the response to sympathomimetic drugs,** and **sedation.**

    a. Attenuation of sympathetic nervous system activity is reflected by orthostatic hypotension and exaggerated blood pressure decreases during anesthesia in response to blood loss, body position change, or decreased venous return owing to positive pressure ventilation of the lungs.

    b. Antihypertensive drugs that deplete norepinephrine or that act on peripheral vascular smooth muscle decrease the sensitivity to indirect-acting sympathomimetic drugs.

    c. Sympathetic nervous system blockade that deprives the alpha-adrenergic receptors of tonic impulses results in exaggerated responses to catecholamines and direct-acting sympathomimetic drugs.

Table 15–1
Side Effects of Treatment with Methyldopa

Bradycardia (predominance of parasympathetic nervous system activity)

Sedation

Hepatic dysfunction

Positive Coombs' test

Rebound hypertension (incidence less than that observed after discontinuation of other centrally acting antihypertensive drugs)

B. Patients remaining on antihypertensive drug therapy show less extreme swings in blood pressure and heart rate during anesthesia and are less likely to exhibit cardiac dysrhythmias.

    1. It is an inescapable conclusion that antihypertensive drugs should be continued throughout the perioperative period.

    2. The usual dose and unique pharmacology of each antihypertensive drug, as well as the physiologic reflexes that occur in response to drug-induced blood pressure changes, must be considered when planning the management of anesthesia (Table 15–1).

C. Nonsteroidal antiinflammatory drugs may interfere with the blood-pressure–lowering effects of antihypertensive drugs (see Chapter 11).

II. METHYLDOPA is a centrally acting antihypertensive drug that is altered in the central nervous system to alpha-methyl-norepinephrine, which stimulates inhibitory alpha-2 adrenergic receptors in the hypothalamus (inhibits sympathetic nervous system outflow from the vasomotor center to the periphery).

    A. Cardiovascular effects of methyldopa include decreases in systemic vascular resistance and blood pressure, whereas cardiac output (renal, cerebral, and myocardial blood flow) are maintained.

    B. Side Effects (Table 15–1)

III. CLONIDINE is a centrally acting antihypertensive drug that selectively stimulates alpha-2 inhibitory neurons (ratio of 200 : 1 [alpha-2 : alpha-1]) in the medullary vasomotor center,

Table 15–2
Clinical Uses of Clonidine

Treatment of essential hypertension

Diagnosis of pheochromocytoma (causes a decrease in the plasma
  concentration of catecholamines only in normal patients)

Suppression of symptoms of opioid withdrawal (presumed to
  replace opioid-mediated inhibition with alpha-2–mediated
  inhibition of central nervous system sympathetic activity)

Neuraxial analgesia (without depression of ventilation)

Preoperative medication
  Decreases heart rate response to tracheal intubation
  Decreases intraoperative liability of blood pressure and heart rate
  Facilitates production of controlled hypotension intraoperatively
  Decreases plasma catecholamine concentrations
  Decreases anesthetic requirements for inhaled and injected
    anesthetics

resulting in a decrease in sympathetic nervous system outflow from the central nervous system to peripheral tissues.

- **A. Clinical Uses** (Table 15-2)
    1. Clonidine stabilizes perioperative hemodynamic re-
       sponses to stimuli (direct laryngoscopy, tracheal intu-
       bation, surgical skin incision) by inhibiting catechola-
       mine release centrally and peripherally (plasma
       catecholamine concentrations are decreased up to
       50%).
    2. Clonidine decreases anesthetic requirements for in-
       haled anesthetics (MAC decreased up to 50%) seda-
       tive-hypnotics, and opioids.
- **B. Cardiovascular Effects**
    1. Homeostatic cardiovascular reflexes are maintained,
       thus avoiding the problems of orthostatic hypoten-
       sion.
    2. Renal blood flow is maintained.
- **C. Side Effects**
    1. The most frequent side effects of clonidine therapy
       are sedation, anxiolysis, and xerostomia.
    2. **Bradycardia** may accompany the use of clonidine
       as a preoperative medication.
    3. **Rebound hypertension** is most likely to accom-
       pany discontinuation of clonidine therapy in patients
       receiving more than 1.2 mg of clonidine daily.

    a. The increase in blood pressure is associated with intense peripheral vasoconstriction and increased plasma concentrations of catecholamines (beta-adrenergic blockade may exaggerate the rebound hypertension).

    b. Rebound hypertension can usually be controlled by reinstituting clonidine therapy or by administering a vasodilating drug, such as hydralazine or nitroprusside.

    c. Rebound hypertension following abrupt discontinuation of antihypertensive drugs is not unique to clonidine (beta-adrenergic antagonists, methyldopa), but has not been observed in association with abrupt discontinuation of drugs that act independently of central and peripheral sympathetic nervous system mechanisms (direct vasodilators, angiotensin-converting enzyme inhibitors).

  4. The use of clonidine is limited at higher doses by the ceiling effect, and by alpha-1 actions, such as vasoconstriction.

IV. HYDRALAZINE decreases blood pressure by exerting a direct relaxant effect on vascular smooth muscle (arterioles greater than veins).

  A. Treatment of abrupt increases in blood pressure with hydralazine, 2.5 to 10 mg IV, may evoke baroreceptor-mediated reflex increases in heart rate (concomitant administration of a beta-adrenergic antagonist may be required).

  B. Acetylation is the major route of metabolism of hydralazine (rapid acetylators have lower plasma concentrations than do slow acetylators).

  C. Cardiovascular Effects

    1. The preferential dilatation of arterioles compared with veins minimizes orthostatic hypotension and promotes an increase in cardiac output.

    2. Heart rate, stroke volume, and cardiac output increase, reflecting reflex baroreceptor-mediated increases in sympathetic nervous system activity owing to decreases in blood pressure.

  D. Side Effects (Table 15–3)

V. PRAZOSIN produces peripheral vasodilation via selective and competitive postsynaptic alpha-1 receptor blockade (ab-

Table 15–3
Side Effects of Hydralazine Therapy

Reflex tachycardia

Sodium and water retention (if a diuretic is not administered concomitantly)

Vertigo

Myocardial stimulation (angina pectoris)

Peripheral neuropathies

Enhanced defluorination of volatile anesthetics

Lupus erythematosus–like syndrome (associated with chronic therapy in slow acetylators)

sence of presynaptic alpha-2 effects leaves the normal inhibition of norepinephrine release intact).

A. Clinical Uses (Table 15–4)
B. Cardiovascular Effects
   1. Prazosin decreases systemic vascular resistance without causing reflex-induced tachycardia or increases in renin activity, as occur with hydralazine or minoxidil.
      a. Failure to alter plasma renin activity reflects the continued activity of alpha-2 receptors that normally inhibit release of renin.
      b. Vascular tone in both resistance and capacitance vessels is decreased, resulting in decreased venous return and cardiac output.
   2. Because of its greater affinity for alpha receptors in veins than in arteries, prazosin produces hemodynamic changes (orthostatic hypotension) that resemble those of nitroglycerin more than hydralazine.
C. Side effects of prazosin may cause vertigo, fluid reten-

Table 15–4
Clinical Uses of Prazosin

Treatment of essential hypertension

Reduction of afterload in the treatment of cardiac failure

Cardiac antidysrhythmic

Preoperative preparation of patients with pheochromocytoma

tion (necessitating concomitant administration of a diuretic), and orthostatic hypotension (may manifest as syncope).

D. Vasodilation and decreases in systemic vascular resistance may be exaggerated, resulting in hypotension during regional anesthesia in the prazosin-treated patient.

    1. Phenylephrine (selective alpha-1 agonist) may not be effective in reversing hypotension due to regional anesthesia in the presence of prazosin.

    2. A more potent alpha-agonist (epinephrine) or a beta-1 agonist (epinephrine or ephedrine) may be needed to correct hypotension.

VI. MINOXIDIL is an orally active antihypertensive drug that decreases blood pressure by direct relaxation of arteriolar smooth muscle.

  A. Cardiovascular Effects

    1. Minoxidil is used in combination with a beta-adrenergic antagonist and a diuretic to decrease the magnitude of cardiovascular stimulation (increased heart rate and cardiac output) and fluid retention that may accompany therapy with this drug.

    2. Orthostatic hypotension is not prominent in patients treated with minoxidil.

  B. Side effects of minoxidil include fluid retention (pulmonary hypertension may occur), pericardial effusion and cardiac tamponade, changes on the electrocardiogram (flattening or inversion of the T wave and increased voltage of the QRS complex), and hypertrichosis (affecting the face and arms of patients treated longer than 1 month).

VII. GUANETHIDINE acts exclusively on the peripheral sympathetic nervous system and produces its antihypertensive effect by inhibiting the presynaptic release of the neurotransmitter, norepinephrine, in response to sympathetic nervous system stimulation.

  A. A rare use of guanethidine (and reserpine) is its intravenous injection into an extremity isolated from the circulation for treatment of reflex sympathetic dystrophy.

  B. Cardiovascular Effects

    1. Orthostatic hypotension is the most prominent side effect of treatment with guanethidine.

Table 15–5
Pharmacologic Effects of Single Doses of Angiotensin-Converting Enzyme Inhibitors

	Oral Dose (mg)	Prodrug	Onset (min)	Peak Effect	Duration (h)
Captopril	100	No	15–30	1–2	6–10
Enalapril	20	Yes	60–120	4–8	18–30
Lisinopril	10	No	60	2–4	18–30

Adapted from Mirenda JV, Grissom TE. Anesthetic implications of the renin-angiotensin system and angiotensin-converting enzyme inhibitors. Anesth Analg 1991;72:667–83.

    2. The antihypertensive effect of guanethidine is prevented by drugs (tricyclic antidepressants, amphetamines, cocaine) that prevent passage of norepinephrine, as well as this drug, into postganglionic sympathetic nerve endings.

  C. Sedation and decreases in anesthetic requirements are not produced by guanethidine, reflecting the limited ability of this poorly lipid-soluble drug to cross the blood–brain barrier.

VIII. CAPTOPRIL is an orally effective antihypertensive drug that acts by competitive inhibition of angiotensin I-converting enzyme (ACE inhibitor) (Table 15–5).

  A. Measures of general well-being (cognitive function, work performance, physical symptoms, sexual function) are better maintained in patients treated with captopril (and other ACE inhibitors) than in those treated with drugs acting on the central nervous system; this, in turn, leads to improved patient compliance with drug therapy.

  B. Cardiovascular Effects

    1. The antihypertensive effect of captopril is due to a decrease in systemic vascular resistance as a result of decreased sodium ion (Na^+) and water retention.

      a. Inhibition of angiotensin I-converting enzyme prevents conversion of angiotensin I to angiotensin II, which prevents angiotensin-II–mediated vasoconstriction, activation of the sympathetic ner-

Table 15–6
Side Effects of Captopril

Skin rash (may be accompanied by fever and joint discomfort)

Loss of taste sensation

Angioedema (rare)

Hyperkalemia (especially in patients with impaired renal function or when a potassium-sparing diuretic is given simultaneously)

Cough (may reflect potentiation of the effects of kinins)

Proteinuria

Neutropenia (rare)

---

       vous system, and stimulation of aldosterone secretion from the adrenal cortex.

   b. The decrease in aldosterone secretion results in a slight increase in serum potassium levels.

   c. The increase in plasma concentrations of renin reflects the loss of negative feedback control normally provided by angiotensin II on renin secretion.

  2. Orthostatic hypotension is unlikely because this drug does not interfere with sympathetic nervous system activity.

  3. The absence of a compensatory reflex-mediated increase in heart rate when blood pressure is decreased suggests that captopril may cause changes in baroreceptor sensitivity.

  4. Unlike beta-adrenergic antagonists, this antihypertensive drug lacks metabolic effects and is acceptable for patients with diabetes mellitus.

  5. Captopril may improve the efficacy of vasodilators in treating cardiac failure, presumably by blocking vasodilation-induced increases in renin output.

  6. Rebound hypertension seen with clonidine has not been observed with ACE inhibitors.

  7. The probability of hypertension during the induction of anesthesia may be increased in hypertensive patients treated chronically with an ACE inhibitor.

C. Side Effects (Table 15-6)

IX. ENALAPRIL is an ACE inhibitor (a prodrug that is converted in the liver to its active form) that resembles captopril and is effective as a single daily oral dose (Table 15-5). The *in* *vivo* active metabolite (diacid) of enalapril is effective as an intravenous preparation.

X. SARALASIN and related drugs preferentially competes with angiotensin II for receptors on vascular smooth muscle, resulting in a decrease in systemic vascular resistance and blood pressure.

XI. METYROSINE blocks catecholamine synthesis by inhibiting tyrosine hydroxylase, the enzyme that catalyzes the conversion of tyrosine to dopa (may be useful for preoperative treatment of patients with pheochromocytoma).

Chapter

16

Peripheral Vasodilators

Peripheral vasodilators are used clinically to treat hypertensive crises, produce controlled hypotension, and facilitate forward left ventricular stroke volume, as in patients with regurgitant valvular heart lesions or acute cardiac failure (Fig. 16-1). (Updated and revised from Stoelting RK. Peripheral vasodilators. In: Pharmacology and Physiology in Anesthetic Practice. 2nd ed. Philadelphia, JB Lippincott, 1991;324–39.)

I. NITROPRUSSIDE

A. Nitroprusside is a direct-acting, nonselective peripheral vasodilator that causes relaxation of arterial and venous vascular smooth muscle.

1. Onset of action is almost immediate and the duration of action is transient, requiring continuous intravenous infusion to maintain a therapeutic effect.

2. The extreme potency of nitroprusside necessitates careful titration of dosage as provided by continuous infusion devices and frequent monitoring of blood pressure.

B. **Clinical Uses** (Table 16-1)

1. Nitrovasodilators (nitroprusside, nitroglycerin) produce nitric oxide (NO) which activates the enzyme guanylate cyclase.

2. Guanylate cyclase results in increased concentrations of cyclic guanosine monophosphate (cyclic GMP) in vascular smooth muscle, leading to vasodilation in veins and arteries (see Section VIII).

3. Prophylactic nitroglycerin (0.9 $\mu g \cdot kg^{-1} \cdot min^{-1}$ IV) does not decrease the incidence of perioperative myocardial ischemia in patients with known or suspected coronary artery disease who are undergoing noncardiac surgery.

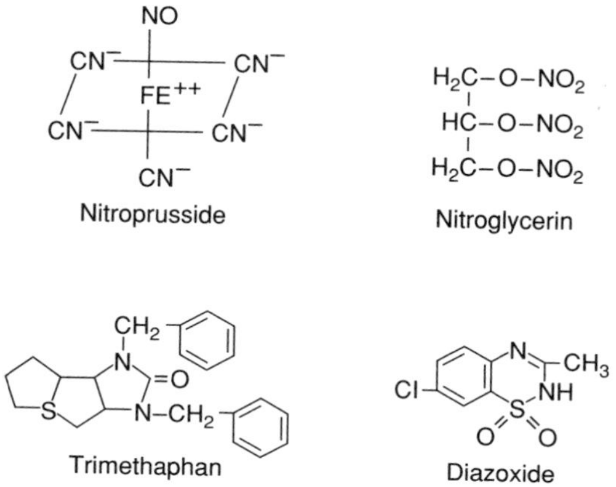

FIGURE 16–1. Peripheral vasodilators.

C. Metabolism

1. Metabolism of nitroprusside begins with transfer (independent of enzyme activity) of an electron from the iron of oxyhemoglobin to nitroprusside, yielding methemoglobin and an unstable nitroprusside radical (Fig. 16–2).

2. The unstable nitroprusside radical releases five cyanide ions, one of which reacts with methemoglobin to form cyanmethemoglobin.

   a. The remaining free cyanide ions are available to

Table 16–1
Clinical Uses of Nitroprusside

Treatment of hypertensive crises

Controlled hypotension

Improvement of cardiac output in patients with acute cardiac failure due to myocardial ischemia or regurgitant valvular heart disease

Blunting of circulatory responses to tracheal intubation

Facilitation of rewarming following conclusion of cardiopulmonary bypass

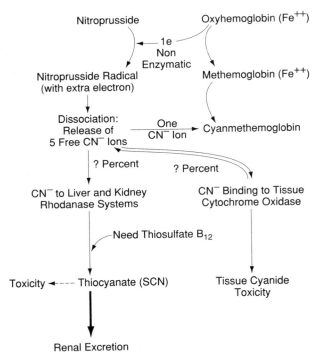

FIGURE 16–2. Metabolism of nitroprusside begins with the transfer of an electron from the iron of oxyhemoglobin to nitroprusside, yielding methemoglobin and an unstable nitroprusside radical. (From Tinker JH, Michenfelder, JD. Sodium nitroprusside: Pharmacology, toxicity and therapeutics. Anesthesiology 1976;45:340–54; with permission.)

rhodanase enzyme in the liver and kidneys for conversion to thiocyanate (rate of conversion dependent on availability of a sulfur donor for the enzyme).
  b. Any free cyanide that is not rapidly converted to thiocyanate can bind to cytochrome oxidase, impairing aerobic respiration (cyanide toxicity).
  c. The amount of cyanide release from nitroprusside depends entirely on the total dose of drug that is administered.

Table 16–2
Treatment of Cyanide Toxicity

Immediate discontinuation of nitroprusside administration with the appearance of tachyphylaxis in association with metabolic acidosis and increased mixed venous PO_2

Sodium thiosulfate, 150 mg·kg^{-1} IV (acts as a sulfur donor to convert cyanide to thiocyanate)

3. Thiocyanate is cleared slowly by the kidneys and may accumulate with prolonged therapy or in the presence of renal failure.
   a. Skeletal muscle weakness and mental confusion may occur if the plasma thiocyanate concentration is higher than 10 mg·dl^{-1}.
   b. Prolonged increases of plasma thiocyanate concentrations can result in hypothyroidism because thiocyanate inhibits uptake of iodide ions by the thyroid gland.
4. Solutions of nitroprusside exposed to light may release cyanide *in vitro.*

D. **Cyanide Toxicity**
   1. Cyanide toxicity from spontaneous breakdown of nitroprusside should be suspected in any patient who is resistant to the hypotensive effects of the drug despite adequate infusion rates or in a previously responsive patient who becomes unresponsive to the blood pressure–lowering effects of the drug (tachyphylaxis).
      a. Mixed venous PO_2 is increased in the presence of cyanide toxicity, indicating paralysis of cytochrome oxidase and inability of the tissues to use oxygen.
      b. Metabolic acidosis develops as a reflection of anaerobic metabolism in the tissues.
      c. There is no evidence that preexisting hepatic or renal disease increases the likelihood of cyanide toxicity.
   2. **Treatment of Cyanide Toxicity** (Table 16-2)

E. **Dose**
   1. Nitroprusside should be administered on the basis of total dose (maximum acceptable suggested dose is 8 µg·kg^{-1}· min^{-1} IV for 1 to 3 hours) and not the blood pressure effect that is achieved.

    a. Most anesthetized patients do not require a dose near this maximum amount, with the usual continuous intraoperative infusion rate being 0.5 to 2 $\mu g \cdot kg^{-1} \cdot min^{-1}$ IV.

    b. Propranolol can also be used to blunt baroreceptor reflex responses, thus minimizing the dose of nitroprusside required to produce desirable degrees of blood pressure reduction.

  2. Whenever the dose of nitroprusside approaches the maximum infusion rate, it is important to monitor arterial pH for evidence of metabolic acidosis as a manifestation of cyanide toxicity.

F. Effects on Organ Systems

  1. Cardiovascular System

    a. Nitroprusside produces prompt decreases in blood pressure as a result of arterial and venous vasodilation.

    b. Baroreceptor-mediated reflex responses to nitroprusside-induced decreases in blood pressure manifest as tachycardia and increased myocardial contractility, which may offset the blood pressure–lowering effects of nitroprusside.

    c. **Coronary steal** occurs because nitroprusside dilates resistance vessels in nonischemic myocardium, resulting in diversion of blood flow from ischemic areas where vessels are already maximally dilated.

  2. Cerebral Blood Flow

    a. Nitroprusside is a direct cerebral vasodilator that increases cerebral blood flow and cerebral blood volume (in patients with decreased intracranial compliance, these changes may cause undesirable increases in intracranial pressure).

    b. Decreasing blood pressure over 5 minutes with nitroprusside in the presence of hypocarbia and hyperoxia may negate the increase in intracranial pressure that accompanies the rapid infusion of nitroprusside.

  3. Hypoxic Pulmonary Vasoconstriction

    a. Decreases in PaO_2 levels that may accompany the infusion of nitroprusside and other peripheral vasodilators are presumed to reflect drug-induced attenuation of hypoxic pulmonary vasoconstriction.

    b. Peripheral vasodilator-induced decreases in blood pressure may be more likely to increase shunt

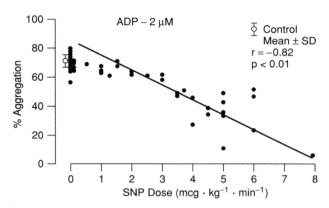

FIGURE 16–3. Platelet aggregation (%) at varying intravenous infusion rates of sodium nitroprusside (SNP). (From Hines R, Barash PG. Infusion of sodium nitroprusside induces platelet dysfunction in vitro. Anesthesiology 1989;70:611-5; with permission.)

fraction in patients with normal lungs than in those with chronic obstructive airway disease.

4. **Platelet aggregation** may be impaired by nitroprusside, especially at infusion rates higher than 3 $\mu g \cdot kg^{-1} \cdot min^{-1}$ IV (Fig. 16-3).

II. NITROGLYCERIN

A. Nitroglycerin is an organic nitrate that acts principally on venous capacitance vessels to produce peripheral pooling of blood, reduction in heart size, and decreased cardiac ventricular wall tension.

1. The most common use of nitroglycerin is treatment of angina pectoris owing to either atherosclerosis of the coronary arteries or intermittent vasospasm of these vessels.

2. Production of controlled hypotension has also been achieved with continuous intravenous infusion of nitroglycerin.

B. **Route of Administration**

1. Sublingual administration limits the initial first-pass hepatic metabolism of nitroglycerin.

2. Transdermal absorption of nitroglycerin may provide sustained protection against myocardial ischemia.

Table 16–3
Clinical Uses of Nitroglycerin

Treatment of angina pectoris (ineffectiveness of three sublingual tablets administered in a 15-minute period may reflect myocardial infarction)

Treatment of cardiac failure

Controlled hypotension (its predominant action on venous capacitance vessels means that blood volume is important in achieving a blood pressure decrease)

Treatment of acute hypertension (as may accompany noxious stimulation in the parturient with coronary artery disease)

    3. Continuous intravenous infusion of nitroglycerin via special delivery tubing (to decrease absorption of the drug into the plastic) is a useful approach to maintain a constant plasma concentration of nitroglycerin.

C. Mechanism of Action (see Section IB)
    1. The ability of nitroglycerin to decrease myocardial oxygen requirements is the most likely mechanism by which this drug relieves angina pectoris in patients with atherosclerotic disease of the coronary arteries (coronary blood flow is not increased).
    2. The ability of nitroglycerin to dilate selectively large conductive coronary arteries (redistribution of coronary blood flow to ischemic areas of subendocardium) may be an important mechanism in the relief of angina pectoris owing to vasospasm.

D. Metabolism
    1. Nitroglycerin is metabolized in the liver by nitrate reductase to glycerol dinitrate and nitrite, which are about 10 times less potent as vasodilators.
    2. The nitrite metabolite of nitroglycerin is capable of oxidizing the ferrous ion in hemoglobin to the ferric state with the production of methemoglobin.

E. Clinical Uses (Table 16–3)

F. Effects on Organ Systems
    1. Smooth muscle of the biliary tract is relaxed such that pain that mimics angina pectoris but is due to opioid-induced biliary tract spasm will often be relieved by nitroglycerin.
    2. Nitroglycerin is a cerebral vasodilator (headache may be severe after sublingual administration) and may

increase intracranial pressure in patients with decreased intracranial compliance.

3. **Cardiovascular Effects**

   a. Nitroglycerin doses of up to 2 $\mu g \cdot kg^{-1} \cdot min^{-1}$ IV produce dilatation of veins that predominates over that produced in arterioles (decreased venous return results in decreased cardiac output).

   b. Heart rate is often not changed or is only slightly increased during administration of nitroglycerin.

   c. Nitroglycerin-induced decreases in blood pressure are more dependent on blood volume than are blood pressure changes produced by nitroprusside.

   d. Pulmonary vascular resistance is decreased, presumably reflecting a direct relaxant effect of nitroglycerin on pulmonary vasculature.

   e. Nitroglycerin dilates larger conductance vessels in the coronary circulation, often leading to an increase in coronary blood flow for ischemic subendocardial areas (reason nitroglycerin recommended in favor of nitroprusside for treatment of acute hypertension in patients with coronary artery disease).

   f. Platelet aggregation is not altered, suggesting that prolonged bleeding time is due to vasodilation and increased venous capacitance.

III. TRIMETHAPHAN

A. Trimethaphan directly relaxes capacitance vessels and produces autonomic nervous system ganglionic blockade, resulting in decreased blood pressure because of decreases in cardiac output and systemic vascular resistance (histamine release does not contribute to hypotension).

   1. Increases in heart rate secondary to administration of trimethaphan most likely reflect parasympathetic nervous system ganglionic blockade.

   2. The route of metabolism of trimethaphan is unclear, but may include hydrolysis by plasma cholinesterase.

   3. As a quaternary ammonium drug, trimethaphan has a limited passage across the blood–brain barrier, and central nervous system effects are unlikely.

Table 16–4
Side Effects of Trimethaphan

Ganglionic blockade
  Mydriasis (may interfere with neurologic evaluation)
  Ileus
  Urinary retention
  Tachycardia
Inhibition of plasma cholinesterase
Histamine release (limits use in presence of pheochromocytoma)

B. Clinical Uses
    1. Trimethaphan is most often used as a continuous intravenous infusion to produce controlled hypotension.
    2. Associated tachycardia may offset the blood pressure-lowering effects of trimethaphan, requiring the administration of propranolol.
C. Side Effects (Table 16-4)
    1. Trimethaphan may evoke smaller increases in intracranial pressure than those associated with comparable degrees of hypotension produced by nitroprusside or nitroglycerin.
    2. In animals, trimethaphan, but not nitroprusside, has been found to decrease cerebral blood flow despite an unchanged cerebral metabolic rate for oxygen.

IV. DIAZOXIDE

    A. Diazoxide is related chemically to the thiazide diuretics, and is used to treat acute blood pressure increases as occur in patients with accelerated and severe hypertension associated with glomerulonephritis (1 to 3 mg·kg^{-1} IV decreases blood pressure within 1 to 2 minutes and lasts 6 to 7 hours).
    1. Diozoxide is eliminated principally unchanged by the kidneys.
    2. Although excessive blood pressure decreases are unlikely, a disadvantage of diazoxide compared with other peripheral vasodilator drugs is the inability to titrate the dose of this drug in accordance with the patient's blood pressure response.
B. Cardiovascular Effects
    1. Diazoxide-induced decreases in blood pressure are associated with significant increases in cardiac out-

put and heart rate (unsuitable for treatment of hypertension associated with a dissecting aortic aneurysm or pheochromocytoma).
   2. Hypotensive effects of diazoxide may be accentuated in patients receiving beta-adrenergic antagonists because baroreceptor-mediated reflex increases in sympathetic nervous system activity (increased heart rate and cardiac output) are prevented.
   C. **Side effects** of diazoxide include sodium and water retention, uterine relaxation, and hyperglycemia.

V. **ISOSORBIDE DINITRATE** is the most commonly administered oral nitrate for the prophylaxis of angina pectoris (low doses are not more effective than placebo). Orthostatic hypotension may accompany acute administration of isosorbide dinitrate, but tolerance to this effect seems to develop with chronic therapy.

VI. **DIPYRIDAMOLE**

   A. Dipyridamole is administered orally as prophylaxis against angina pectoris and, in combination with warfarin, may be administered to patients with prosthetic heart valves as prophylaxis against thromboemboli (like aspirin, this drug inhibits platelet aggregation).
   B. Dipyridamole inhibits cellular uptake of adenosine, which serves as a vasodilator and an important signal for the autoregulation of coronary blood flow.

VII. **PURINES**

   A. **Adenosine**
      1. Adenosine is an endogenous nucleotide occurring in all cells of the body.
         a. The half-time of adenosine in plasma is brief (0.6 to 1.5 seconds) because of its deamination to inosine and its uptake by erythrocytes.
         b. Vasodilator actions of adenosine tend to maintain the balance between oxygen delivery and oxygen demand in the heart and other organs (during periods of hypoxia or ischemia, the production of adenosine by cardiac myocytes increases).
      2. **Antidysrhythmic Action**
         a. Administration of adenosine, 6 to 12 mg IV, by rapid injection (as an alternative to verapamil) usually converts paroxysmal supraventricular

Table 16–5
Side Effects of Adenosine

Sinus bradycardia

Transient atrioventricular heart block

Asystole

Coronary artery steal (angina pectoris)

Dyspnea

Flushing

Nausea

Headache

Bronchospasm (most common with aerosolized delivery)

tachycardia (not effective for treatment of atrial flutter, atrial fibrillation, or ventricular tachycardia) to normal sinus rhythm within 1 minute.

b. In the absence of a functioning artificial cardiac pacemaker, adenosine should not be administered in the presence of second- or third-degree atrioventricular heart block or in the presence of sick sinus syndrome.

c. The ability of adenosine to cause selective atrioventricular nodal conduction blockade reflects hyperpolarization of atrial myocytes (adenosine-sensitive potassium channels which are not present in ventricular myocytes).

3. **Controlled Hypotension**

a. Adenosine-induced controlled hypotension is characterized by rapid onset and prompt reversal when the drug is discontinued.

b. Doses of adenosine required to produce controlled hypotension are unlikely to alter cardiac automaticity or conduction of cardiac impulses.

c. Tachycardia, acid-base disturbances, and tachyphylaxis do not occur when adenosine is administered to produce controlled hypotension.

d. Uric acid levels may increase when adenosine is used for controlled hypotension, suggesting the need for caution in selecting this drug for patients with gout.

4. **Side Effects** (Table 16-5)

Table 16–6
Physiologic Functions of Nitric Oxide

Endogenous vasodilator (synthesis of nitric oxide [endothelium-derived relaxing factor] is essential for regulation of blood pressure)

Inhibitor of platelet aggregation

Neurotransmitter (memory)

Sensory transmission in the peripheral nervous system

Antitumor functions

Penile erection

Secretion of insulin

VIII. NITRIC OXIDE (NO) (see Section IB)

    A. NO is synthesized from the amino acid L-arginine by a family of enzymes, the nitric oxide syntheses.

        1. NO diffuses out of the producing cells into target cells, where it activates cyclic GMP (half-time is less than 5 seconds, which ensures a relatively localized action).

        2. NO acts as a mediator of diverse physiologic functions (Table 16–6).

    B. Inhaled NO (5 to 80 ppm) produces selective pulmonary vasodilation in patients with preexisting pulmonary hypertension (adult respiratory distress syndrome, persistent pulmonary hypertension of the newborn).

        1. Selective and transient effects of inhaled NO on pulmonary vasculature reflect its conversion by hemoglobin to nitrate.

        2. Systemic vasodilation does not accompany the inhalation of NO.

    C. Toxicity from inhaled NO may be due either to NO (unlikely when below 40 ppm) or its reactive metabolite, nitrogen dioxide (NO_2).

        1. The potential for NO or NO_2 to induce pulmonary toxicity (particularly in conjunction with high inhaled concentrations of oxygen) in injured lungs is not known.

        2. Soda lime does not reliably decrease the concentration of NO_2.

Chapter

17

Cardiac Antidysrhythmic Drugs

Treatment of cardiac dysrhythmias and disturbances in conduction of cardiac impulses with antidysrhythmic drugs is based on an understanding of the electrophysiologic basis of the abnormality and the mechanism of action of the therapeutic drug to be employed. (Updated and revised from Stoelting RK. Cardiac antidysrhythmic drugs. In: Pharmacology and Physiology in Anesthetic Practice. 2nd ed. Philadelphia, JB Lippincott, 1991;340–52.)

I. INTRODUCTION

   A. Antidysrhythmic drugs pose little threat to the uneventful course of anesthesia and should be continued up to the time of induction of anesthesia.
   B. Cardiac dysrhythmias during anesthesia may reflect **emergence of latent pacemakers** in the presence of **suppression of the sinoatrial node** or development of **reentry circuits**.

II. CLASSIFICATION

   A. Antidysrhythmic drugs are classified into four groups based on their mechanism of action (Table 17-1).
   B. Antidysrhythmic drugs differ in their pharmacokinetics and efficacy in treating specific types of cardiac dysrhythmias (Tables 17-2 and 17-3).

III. MEMBRANE STABILIZERS

   A. Quinidine
      1. Indications for administration of quinidine include prevention of recurrence of supraventricular tachydys-

269

Table 17–1
Classification of Antidysrhythmic Drugs

Class		Mechanism	Examples
I		Membrane stabilizers (sodium channel blockade)	
	IA	Slow conduction—moderate	Quinidine
			Procainamide
			Disopyramide
	IB	Slow conduction—mild	Lidocaine
			Tocainide
			Mexiletine
			Phenytoin
	IC	Slow conduction—marked	Flecainide
			Encainide
			Lorcainide
II		Beta-adrenergic antagonists	Propranolol
III		Prolonged repolarization	Bretylium
			Amiodarone
IV		Calcium entry blockers	Verapamil
			Diltiazem

rhythmias (Wolff-Parkinson-White syndrome), suppression of ventricular premature contractions, and slowing of the atrial rate in the presence of atrial fibrillation (about 25% of patients convert to normal sinus rhythm).

2. It is common to administer digitalis before treating atrial fibrillation with quinidine because an occasional patient will manifest a paradoxical increase in the ventricular response rate.

3. Intravenous administration of quinidine may cause peripheral vasodilation (alpha-adrenergic blockade) and myocardial depression.

4. **Side Effects** (Table 17–4)

B. Procainamide

1. Procainamide has therapeutic uses similar to those of quinidine (procainamide, 1.5 mg·kg^{-1} IV, is administered over 1 minute and repeated every 5 minutes until the cardiac dysrhythmia is controlled, followed by a constant rate of intravenous infusion).

(text continues on page 273)

Table 17–2
Pharmacokinetics of Cardiac Antidysrhythmic Drugs

	Principal Clearance Mechanism	Protein Binding (percent)	Elimination Half-Time (h)	Therapeutic Plasma Concentration
Quinidine	Hepatic	80–90	5–12	2–8 μg·ml^{-1}
Procainamide	Renal/hepatic	15	2.5–5	4–10 μg·ml^{-1}
Disopyramide	Renal/hepatic	15	8–12	2–4 μg·ml^{-1}
Lidocaine	Hepatic	55	1.4–1.8	1–5 μg·ml^{-1}
Tocainide	Hepatic/renal	10–30	12–15	4–10 μg·ml^{-1}
Mexiletine	Hepatic/renal	60–75	6–12	0.75–2 μg·ml^{-1}
Phenytoin	Hepatic	93	8–60	10–20 μg·ml^{-1}
Flecainide	Hepatic	35–45	13–30	0.3–1.5 μg·ml^{-1}
Encainide	Hepatic/renal	70	1–3	0.3–0.6 μg·ml^{-1}
Propranolol	Hepatic	90–95	2–4	10–30 ng·ml^{-1}
Bretylium	Renal	<10	8–12	75–100 ng·ml^{-1}
Amiodarone	Hepatic	96	8–107 days	1.5–2 μg·ml^{-1}
Verapamil	Hepatic	90	4.5–12	100–300 ng·ml^{-1}

Table 17-3
Efficacy of Antidysrhythmic Drugs for Treatment of Specific Cardiac Dysrhythmias

	Conversion of Atrial Fibrillation	Paroxysmal Supraventricular Tachycardia	Premature Ventricular Contractions	Ventricular Tachycardia
Quinidine	+	++	++	+
Procainamide	+	++	++	++
Disopyramide	+	++	++	++
Lidocaine	0	0	++	++
Tocainide	0	0	++	++
Mexiletine	0	0	++	++
Phenytoin	0	0	++	++
Flecainide	0	+	++	++
Encainide	0	+	++	++
Propranolol	+	++	+	+
Bretylium	0	0	+	++
Amiodarone	+	++	++	++
Verapamil	+	++	0	0

0, no effect; +, effective; ++, highly effective

Table 17–4
Side Effects of Quinidine

Heart block (EEG monitoring is important to detect associated prolongation of P-R interval, QRS complex, and Q-T interval.)

Sudden death

Hypotension (alpha-adrenergic receptor blockade)

Direct myocardial depression (exaggerated by hyperkalemia)

Tachycardia

Fever

Cinchonism (tinnitis, blurring of vision, decreased hearing acuity)

Displacement of digoxin from tissue binding sites

Potentiator of neuromuscular blocking drugs

2. Although procainamide and quinidine have a broader spectrum of antidysrhythmic effects than lidocaine, they are rarely used during anesthesia because of their propensity to produce hypotension.

3. **Side Effects** (Table 17–5)

C. **Disopyramide**

1. Disopyramide has similar therapeutic uses as quinidine.

2. The anticholinergic action of disopyramide produces a dry mouth, blurred vision, and occasionally, urinary retention.

3. The potential for direct myocardial depression, especially in patients with preexisting left ventricular dysfunction, seems to be greater with this drug than with quinidine or procainamide.

D. **Lidocaine**

1. Lidocaine is used principally for suppression of ventric-

Table 17–5
Side Effects of Procainamide

Hypotension (rapid intravenous injection)

Heart block

Direct myocardial depression (exaggerated by hyperkalemia)

Lupus erythematosus–like syndrome (accompanying chronic therapy in slow acetylators)

Fever

ular dysrhythmias (suppression of reentry mechanisms), having minimal effects on supraventricular dysrhythmias.

   a. Rapid administration of lidocaine, 1 to 1.5 mg·kg^{-1} IV, provides antidysrhythmic effects lasting 15 to 60 minutes (short duration of action is related to rapid tissue redistribution and metabolism).

   b. Maintenance of a therapeutic plasma lidocaine concentration of 1 to 5 µg·ml^{-1} following a single initial intravenous injection is most often achieved by the continuous intravenous infusion of 15 to 60 µg·kg^{-1}·min^{-1} (1 to 4 mg·min^{-1} IV in an adult).

   c. Decreased hepatic blood flow, as produced by anesthetics or cardiac failure, may decrease by 50% the rate of intravenous lidocaine infusion necessary to maintain therapeutic plasma levels.

2. Advantages of lidocaine compared with quinidine and procainamide include a more rapid onset and prompt disappearance of effects when the intravenous infusion is terminated (permitting a moment-to-moment titration of the infusion rate as necessary to suppress the cardiac dysrhythmia).

3. Lidocaine for intravenous injection differs from that used for local anesthesia in that it contains no preservative.

4. Mechanism of Action

   a. Effectiveness of lidocaine in suppressing premature ventricular contractions reflects its ability to decrease the rate of spontaneous phase 4 depolarization in ventricular cardiac tissue.

   b. Lidocaine reduces the disparity in the duration of action potentials in normal and ischemic myocardial cells and thus improves the chances of uniform spread of depolarization through the myocardium.

5. Side Effects

   a. Lidocaine is essentially devoid of effects on the electrocardiogram (ECG) or cardiovascular system when the plasma concentration remains lower than 5 µg·ml^{-1}.

   b. The principal possible side effects of lidocaine are on the central nervous system (seizures when plasma concentrations are 5 to 10 µg·ml^{-1} and central nervous system depression, apnea, and cardiac arrest when plasma concentrations are higher than 10 µg·ml^{-1}).

   c. The convulsive threshold for lidocaine is decreased

during arterial hypoxemia, hyperkalemia, or acidosis, emphasizing the importance of monitoring these parameters during the continuous intravenous infusion of lidocaine to patients for suppression of ventricular cardiac dysrhythmias.

E. Tocainide and mexiletine are orally effective analogues of lidocaine used for suppression of symptomatic cardiac ventricular dysrhythmias.

F. Phenytoin

1. Phenytoin is particularly effective in suppressing cardiac ventricular dysrhythmias associated with digitalis toxicity (1.5 mg·kg^{-1} IV every 5 minutes until the cardiac dysrhythmia is controlled).

2. **Side effects** of phenytoin, as administered during acute treatment of cardiac dysrhythmias, principally involve the central nervous system (nystagmus, sedation, ataxia).

G. Flecainide is a fluorinated local anesthetic analogue of procainamide that is effective in suppressing nonsustained ventricular cardiac dysrhythmias. An increased incidence of sudden death has been observed in patients who experience sustained ventricular cardiac dysrhythmias or ventricular dysrhythmias following myocardial infarction and in whom flecainide was also being administered for dysrhythmia suppression.

H. Encainide is a unique antidysrhythmic drug that combines the electrophysiologic effects of quinidine and lidocaine to suppress ventricular cardiac dysrhythmias (sudden death may occur, as described for flecainide).

IV. BETA-ADRENERGIC ANTAGONISTS

A. Beta-adrenergic antagonists depress both automaticity and conduction of cardiac impulses (highly dependent on the degree of underlying sympathetic nervous system activity) and, at high doses, certain of these drugs exhibit membrane-depressant actions (propranolol).

B. Propranolol is used principally to slow the ventricular response to atrial fibrillation or paroxysmal supraventricular tachycardia.

1. Cardiac antidysrhythmic effects of propranolol most likely reflect blockade of responses of beta-receptors in the heart to sympathetic nervous system stimulation and circulating catecholamines (decreasing the rate of spontaneous phase 4 depolarization and rate of discharge of the sinoatrial node).

2. **Metabolism and excretion** is extensive in the liver, resulting in an active metabolite, 4-hydroxypropranolol, which contributes to the cardiac antidysrhythmic activity following oral administration of propranolol.
3. **Side Effects** of propranolol include prolongation of the P-R interval on the ECG with a minimal effect on the QRS complex and Q-T interval.
   a. In patients with chronic cardiac failure, administration of propranolol may blunt compensatory sympathetic nervous system activity necessary for continued cardiac compensation.
   b. Propranolol is not recommended for treatment of patients with preexisting atrioventricular heart block.

V. DRUGS THAT PROLONG REPOLARIZATION

A. Antiadrenergic drugs that prolong repolarization by increasing the duration of action potentials in atrial, ventricular, and Purkinje fibers are effective in treating atrial and ventricular cardiac dysrhythmias.
B. **Bretylium** is uniquely effective in the treatment of ventricular tachycardia and ventricular fibrillation (5 to 10 $mg \cdot kg^{-1}$ IV).
C. **Amiodarone** is administered to prevent recurrent paroxysmal supraventricular tachydysrhythmias (atrial fibrillation that accompanies Wolff-Parkinson-White syndrome) and recurrent ventricular tachycardia or fibrillation.
   1. Therapeutic effects of amiodarone may persist for prolonged periods after discontinuation of the drug (up to 45 days).
   2. **Mechanism of Action**
      a. Amiodarone prolongs the duration of action potentials in atrial and ventricular muscle and increases the refractory period of the accessory pathway in most patients with Wolff-Parkinson-White syndrome.
      b. Amiodarone acts as an effective antianginal drug by dilating coronary arteries and increasing coronary blood flow.
   3. **Metabolism and Excretion**
      a. Amiodarone is minimally dependent on renal excretion, as reflected by an unchanged elimination half-time in the absence of renal function.
      b. There is an inconsistent relationship between the

Table 17–6
Side Effects of Amiodarone

Bradycardia (resistance to atropine)

Heart block (may be more likely in patients undergoing anesthesia, in whom the need for a temporary artificial cardiac pacemaker or intravenous infusion of isoproterenol should be considered)

Neurologic abnormalities (skeletal muscle weakness, ataxia, peripheral neuropathies)

Pulmonary fibrosis (may be at risk for adult respiratory distress syndrome following cardiopulmonary bypass)

Hypothyroidism or hyperthyroidism

Corneal microdeposits

Photosensitivity

Cyanotic discoloration of the face (rare)

Increased plasma transaminase enzymes

Displacement of digoxin from protein binding sites

plasma concentration of amiodarone and its pharmacologic effects (concentration of drug in the myocardium is 10 to 50 times that in the plasma).
4. **Side Effects** (Table 17–6)

VI. CALCIUM ENTRY BLOCKERS

A. **Verapamil** is uniquely effective in the suppression of reentrant supraventricular tachydysrhythmias (75 to 150 $\mu g \cdot kg^{-1}$ IV, followed by a continuous infusion of about 5 $\mu g \cdot kg^{-1} \cdot min^{-1}$).
   1. **Mechanism of Action.** Verapamil slows the rate of spontaneous phase 4 depolarization (related to inhibition of inward flux of calcium ions) in sinoatrial and atrioventricular nodal tissue.
   2. **Side Effects** (see Chapter 18)

18

Calcium Entry Blockers

Calcium entry blockers (also known as calcium antagonists and calcium channel blockers) are a diverse group of structurally unrelated compounds that selectively interfere with inward calcium ion (Ca^{2+}) movement across cell membranes (Fig. 18-1). (Updated and revised from Stoelting RK. Calcium entry blockers. In: Pharmacology and Physiology in Anesthetic Practice. 2nd ed. Philadelphia, JB Lippincott, 1991;353-64.)

I. MECHANISM OF ACTION

A. Channels with a system of gates exist in membranes of excitable cells for the inward transfer of Ca^{2+}, sodium (Na^+), and potassium (K^+) ions.

B. Four subtypes of calcium channels have been identified. Classic calcium entry blockers inhibit almost exclusively L-type channels that are prominent in heart and vascular tissue, but do not contribute to synaptic stimulus-secretion coupling characteristic of T, N, and P channels.

II. PHARMACOLOGIC EFFECTS

A. Based on the known effects of Ca^{2+} transport on the action potential, it is predictable that calcium entry blockers will produce decreased myocardial contractility, decreased heart rate, decreased rate of conduction of cardiac impulses through the atrioventricular node, and vascular smooth muscle relaxation with associated vasodilation and decreases in blood pressure.

B. These drugs are similar in antihypertensive efficacy but differ in their effects on the atrioventricular node and degree of peripheral vasodilation (Table 18-1).

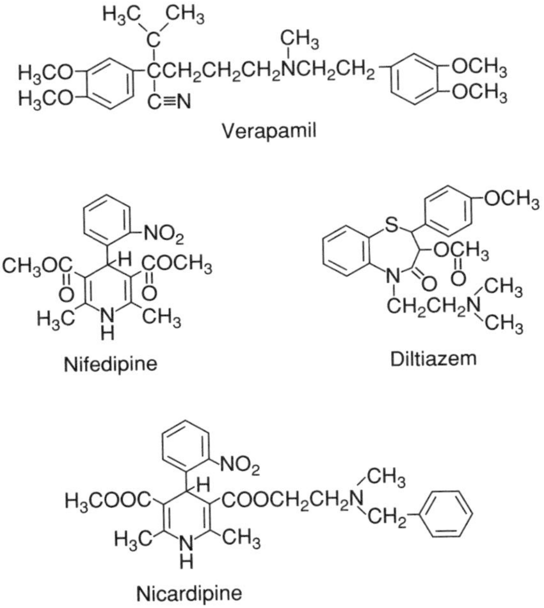

FIGURE 18–1. Calcium entry blockers.

III. CLINICAL USES (Table 18-2)

A. Calcium entry blockers are particularly useful in the treatment of **essential hypertension** and management of **supraventricular cardiac tachydysrhythmias.**
   1. **Essential Hypertension**
      a. Drugs with more specific vasodilating actions and less negative inotropic effects may be preferable in patients with congestive heart failure related to chronic essential hypertension.
      b. The antihypertensive efficacy of calcium entry blockers directly parallels the pretreatment blood pressure, with little or no effect on normotensive subjects.
   2. **Supraventricular Cardiac Tachydysrhythmias**
      a. Verapamil, 75 to 150 $\mu g \cdot kg^{-1}$ IV (5 to 10 mg IV for an adult) infused over 3 to 5 minutes, is effective in terminating paroxysmal supraventricular tachy-

Table 18–1
Comparative Effects of Calcium Entry Blockers

	Verapamil	Nifedipine	Diltiazem	Nicardipine
Blood pressure	−	−	−	−
Heart rate	−	+/NC	−	+/NC
Nodal conduction	−	NC	−	NC
Myocardial contractility	−	NC	−	NC
Peripheral vasodilation	−	−	−	−

− indicates decrease, + indicates increase, NC indicates no change.

Table 18–2
Clinical Uses of Calcium Entry Blockers

Essential hypertension

Supraventricular cardiac tachydysrhythmias

Coronary artery vasospasm

Exercise-induced angina pectoris

Cerebral artery vasospasm

Cerebral protection (?)

Myocardial protection

---

cardia by delaying conduction of cardiac impulses through the atrioventricular node.

   b. Depending on conduction through the accessory pathway, verapamil may or may not be beneficial in the management of patients with preexcitation syndromes, such as Wolff-Parkinson-White syndrome.

3. Coronary Artery Vasospasm. Verapamil (administered intravenously) and nifedipine (administered orally or sublingually) are equally effective in the treatment of coronary artery vasospasm (angina pectoris at rest in association with S-T changes on the electrocardiogram [ECG]).

4. Exercise-Induced Angina Pectoris

   a. Improvement in the balance of oxygen supply and demand is the presumed mechanism for the effectiveness of calcium entry blockers in the treatment of angina pectoris owing to coronary atherosclerosis.

   b. The beneficial effect of nifedipine in the treatment of exercise-induced angina pectoris appears to be due principally to its peripheral vasodilator action rather than to an effect on the coronary arteries.

5. Cerebral Artery Vasospasm

   a. The initial event in the development of vasospasm (common 4 to 14 days after subarachnoid hemorrhage) may be an intracellular influx of Ca^{2+} that causes contraction of smooth muscle cells in large cerebral arteries, leading to ischemic neurologic deficits.

   b. **Nimodipine** is a lipid-soluble analogue of nifedipine that gains entrance into the central nervous system and selectively blocks the influx of extracellular Ca^{2+}.

6. **Cerebral Protection.** The theoretical basis (unproven in humans) for considering calcium entry blockers for cerebral protection is the observation that lack of oxygen interferes with the maintenance of the normal Ca^{2+} gradient across cell membranes, leading to increases in the intraneuronal concentration of this ion.

7. **Myocardial Protection**

    a. Calcium entry blockers may exert a protective effect during global myocardial ischemia associated with cardiopulmonary bypass by suppressing energy-dependent Ca^{2+}-mediated myocardial activity.

    b. The combination of blockade of slow channels with a calcium entry blocker and of fast channels with K^+ may result in greater decreases in myocardial oxygen consumption than either intervention alone.

IV. DRUG INTERACTIONS (Table 18-3)

A. The known pharmacologic effects of calcium entry blockers on cardiac, skeletal, and vascular smooth muscle, as well as on the conduction velocity of cardiac impulses, make drug interactions possible. Nevertheless, therapy with calcium entry blockers can be continued until the time of surgery without risk of significant drug interactions, especially with respect to conduction of cardiac impulses.

Table 18–3
Drug Interactions and Calcium Entry Blockers

Anesthetic drugs
Neuromuscular blocking drugs
Local anesthetics
Potassium-containing solutions
Dantrolene
Platelet function (interfering with calcium-mediated functions)
Digoxin (plasma concentration may be increased)

1. **Anesthetic Drugs**
   a. Myocardial depression and peripheral vasodilation produced by volatile anesthetics may be exaggerated by similar actions of calcium entry blockers (volatile anesthetics may interfere with Ca^{2+} movement across cell membranes or at the sinoatrial node [halothane]).
   b. Despite these theoretical concerns, there is evidence that patients being treated with calcium entry blockers do not experience unacceptable additive depressant effects when anesthetic drugs are administered (the possible exception being patients with preexisting left ventricular dysfunction).
   c. The chronic combined administration of calcium entry blockers and beta-adrenergic antagonists to patients, without preoperative evidence of cardiac conduction abnormalities, is not associated with cardiac conduction abnormalities in the perioperative period.
2. **Neuromuscular Blocking Drugs**
   a. Calcium entry blockers **potentiate** the effects of depolarizing and nondepolarizing neuromuscular blocking drugs (resembling the potentiation produced by mycin antibiotics).
   b. **Antagonism** of neuromuscular blockade may be impaired because of diminished presynaptic release of acetylcholine in the presence of a calcium entry blocker.
3. **Local Anesthetics.** Verapamil has potent local anesthetic activity which may increase the risk of local anesthetic toxicity when regional anesthesia is administered to patients being treated with this drug.
4. **Potassium-Containing Solutions**
   a. Calcium entry blockers slow the inward movement of K^+, and hyperkalemia may occur after exogenous potassium infusion (whole blood) to patients treated with calcium entry blockers.
   b. In animals, pretreatment with verapamil does not alter increases in plasma potassium concentration following the administration of **succinylcholine.**
5. **Dantrolene**
   a. The administration of dantrolene following treatment with a calcium entry blocker has been associated with myocardial depression and hyperkalemia.

(text continues on page 286)

Table 18-4
Characteristics of Calcium Entry Blockers

	Verapamil	Nifedipine	Diltiazem	Nicardipine	Nimodipine
Dosage					
Oral	80-160 mg every 8 hours	10-20 mg every 8 hours	60-90 mg every 8 hours	20 mg every 8 hours	240 mg every 24 hours
Intravenous	75-150 µg·kg⁻¹	5-15 µg·kg⁻¹	75-150 µg·kg⁻¹		
Absorption (%)					
Oral	>90	>90	>90		
Bioavailability	10-20	65-70	40	30	5-10
Onset of Effect (min)					
Oral	<30	<20	30	20-60	30-90
Sublingual		3			
Intravenous	1-3	1-3	1-3		

First-Pass Hepatic Extraction after Oral Administration (%)	75-90	40-60	70-80	20-40	90
Protein Binding (%)	90	90	70-80	98	99
Clearance Mechanisms					
Renal (%)	70	80	35	55	20
Hepatic (%)	15	<15	60	45	80
Active Metabolites	Yes	No	Yes		
Therapeutic Plasma Concentration (ng·ml⁻¹)	50-250	10-100	100-250	5-100	10-30
Elimination Half-Time	6-12	2-5	3-5	3-5	2

(b)

(Data from Reves JG, Kissin I, Lell WA, Tosone S. Calcium entry blockers: Uses and implications for anesthesiologists. Anesthesiology 1982;57:504-18 and Durand P-G, Lehat JJ, Foex P. Calcium-channel blockers and anaesthesia. Can J Anaesth 1991;38:75-89.)

b. Verapamil does not influence the ability of known triggering agents to evoke malignant hyperthermia in susceptible animals.

V. VERAPAMIL

A. Verapamil is a synthetic derivative of papaverine that is supplied as a racemic mixture.

   1. The dextro isomer is devoid of activity at slow calcium channels (L channels), but instead acts on fast sodium channels, which accounts for the local anesthetic effects of verapamil.

   2. The levo isomer is specific for slow calcium channels, and the predominance of this action accounts for the classification of verapamil as a calcium entry blocker.

B. Cardiovascular Effects

   1. Verapamil produces direct depressant effects on the sinoatrial node and delays antegrade transmission of cardiac impulses through the atrioventricular node.

   2. Negative inotropic effects of verapamil are not prominent, except in patients with preexisting left ventricular dysfunction.

   3. Verapamil possesses mild vasodilating properties (less than those of nifedipine), making this drug useful in the treatment of angina pectoris and essential hypertension.

C. Pharmacokinetics (Table 18-4)

   1. Oral verapamil is almost completely absorbed, but extensive hepatic first-pass metabolism limits its bioavailability to 10% to 20%.

   2. Demethylated metabolites of verapamil predominate (nearly complete hepatic metabolism occurs), with norverapamil possessing sufficient activity to contribute to the cardiac antidysrhythmic properties of the parent drug.

VI. NIFEDIPINE

A. Nifedipine has greater coronary and peripheral arterial vasodilator properties than verapamil.

   1. There is minimal effect on venous capacitance vessels.

   2. Unlike verapamil, nifedipine has little or no direct depressant effect on sinoatrial or atrioventricular nodal activity.

   3. Peripheral vasodilation and resultant decrease in

blood pressure produced by nifedepine activate baro-receptors leading to increased peripheral sympathetic nervous system activity, most often manifesting as tachycardia (counters the direct negative inotropic, chronotropic, and dromotropic effects of nifedipine).

B. Nifedipine is most often used to treat patients with angina pectoris, especially that due to coronary artery vasospasm.

C. Pharmacokinetics (Table 18–4)

  1. Hepatic metabolism is nearly complete with elimination of inactive metabolites in the urine.

  2. Abrupt discontinuation of nifedipine has been associated with coronary artery vasospasm.

VII. DILTIAZEM

A. Diltiazem has cardiovascular effects and clinical uses (treatment of angina pectoris) similar to those of verapamil.

B. Diltiazem exerts minimal cardiodepressant effects and is unlikely to interact with beta-antagonists to decrease myocardial contractility.

Chapter

19

Drugs Used in Treatment of Psychiatric Disease

About 20% of prescriptions written in the United States are for drugs intended to alter mood or behavior (Table 19-1). (Updated and revised from Stoelting RK. Drugs used in treatment of psychiatric disease. In: Pharmacology and Physiology in Anesthesia Practice. 2nd ed. Philadelphia, JB Lippincott, 1991;365-83.) Each class of drugs is administered for management of specific psychiatric disorders (Table 19-2).

I. PHENOTHIAZINES AND THIOXANTHENES

A. Phenothiazines and thioxanthenes have a high therapeutic index and a relatively flat dose-response curve, accounting for the remarkable safety of these drugs over a wide dose range.
   1. Depression of ventilation and physical dependence do not occur.
   2. In addition to their use in the treatment of psychiatric disease, phenothiazines and thioxanthenes possess other clinically useful properties, including **antiemetic** and **antihistamine effects** and **potentiation of analgesics.**
B. Mechanism of Action
   1. Phenothiazines and thioxanthenes most likely produce their antipsychotic actions by **antagonism of dopamine** as a neurotransmitter in the central nervous system.
   2. **Extrapyramidal side effects** and **antiemetic effects** of these drugs presumably reflect interference with the normal actions of dopamine (basal ganglia, limbic portions of the forebrain, chemoreceptor trigger zone).

Table 19–1
Classification of Drugs Useful in the Treatment of Psychiatric Disease

Phenothiazines
Chlorpromazine
Thioridazine
Fluphenazine
Perphenazine
Trifluoperazine

Thioxanthenes
Chlorprothixene
Thiothixene

Butyrophenones
Droperidol
Haloperidol

Lithium

Tricyclic Antidepressants
Amitriptyline
Clomipramine
Doxepin
Imipramine
Trimipramine
Amoxamine
Desipramine
Nortriptyline
Protriptyline

Tetracyclic Antidepressants
Maprotiline

Nontricyclic Antidepressant Drugs
Fluoxetine
Bupropion
Trazodone

Monoamine Oxidase Inhibitors
Phenelzine
Tranylcypromine
Pargyline
Isocarboxazid

Table 19–2
Clinical Uses of Drugs Used to Treat Psychiatric Disorders

Class	Disorder
Antipsychotics	Schizophrenia
Phenothiazines	
Thioxanthenes	
Butyrophenones	
Antipsychotics	Mania
Lithium	
Tricyclic antidepressants	Depression
Tetracyclic antidepressants	
Nontricyclic antidepressants	
Monoamine oxidase inhibitors	

    C. Metabolism of phenothiazines and thioxanthenes is principally by oxidation in the liver to inactive metabolites.

    D. Side Effects (Table 19-3)

      1. Cardiovascular Effects

        a. Tolerance to the hypotensive effects develops after several weeks, although some element of orthostatic hypotension may persist.

        b. A cardiac antidysrhythmic effect of chlorpromazine may reflect the potent local anesthetic activity of this drug.

      2. Neuroleptic malignant syndrome occurs in 0.5% to 1% of all patients treated with antipsychotic drugs and the mortality rate is 20% to 30% (ventilatory failure, cardiac failure and/or cardiac dysrhythmias, renal failure, thromboembolism).

        a. This syndrome typically develops over 24 to 72 hours in young males and is characterized by evidence of autonomic nervous system dysfunction (Table 19-4).

        b. This syndrome is distinguished from malignant hyperthermia by the fact that nondepolarizing neuromuscular blocking drugs produce flaccid paralysis in the presence of neuroleptic malignant syndrome, but not in the presence of malignant hyperthermia.

        c. The cause of neuroleptic malignant syndrome is unknown and, therefore, treatment is symptomatic (dopamine agonists may be beneficial).

Table 19–3
Side Effects of Phenothiazines and Thioxanthenes

Cardiovascular Effects
   Hypotension (depression of vasomotor reflexes, peripheral alpha-
   adrenergic blockade, direct relaxant effect on vascular smooth
   muscle, direct cardiac depression)
   Blunt pressor effects of epinephrine (alpha-adrenergic blockade)

Extrapyramidal Effects
   Acute dystonic reactions (initiation of therapy)
   Tardive dyskinesia (treatment longer than 1 year)

Endocrine Changes
   Stimulation of prolactin secretion (galactorrhea and gynecomastia)

Neuroleptic Malignant Syndrome

Obstructive Jaundice

Antiemetic Effects

Anticholinergic Effects

Sedation

Hypothermia

Drug Interactions
   Opioids (enhanced ventilatory depressant and miotic effects)
   Alcohol (effects enhanced)

Table 19–4
Manifestations of Neuroleptic Malignant Syndrome

Hyperthermia (mimics malignant hyperthermia)

Generalized hypertonicity of skeletal muscles (may be so severe as
to require skeletal muscle paralysis and mechanical ventilation of
the lungs)

Labile blood pressure

Tachycardia

Cardiac dysrhythmias

Fluctuating levels of consciousness

E. Clozapine is unique among antipsychotic drugs in that it rarely evokes extrapyramidal side effects. Sedation, seizures, and risk of agranulocytosis (necessitating weekly white blood cell counts) limit the usefulness of this drug.

II. BUTYROPHENONES

A. Butyrophenones (droperidol and haloperidol) are useful for **decreasing anxiety** accompanying psychoses (less effective against situational anxiety such as that present in the preoperative period), providing an **antiemetic effect,** and producing **neuroleptanalgesia.**

B. Mechanism of Action

1. Butyrophenones act at postsynaptic receptor sites to decrease the neurotransmitter function of dopamine in various areas of the central nervous system.

2. The short elimination half-time of droperidol (metabolized in the liver) is not consistent with the prolonged central nervous system effects of this drug (may reflect slow dissociation of droperidol from receptors or retention of droperidol in the brain).

C. Clinical Uses

1. Neuroleptanalgesia

a. Droperidol, combined with fentanyl in a 50:1 ratio (Innovar), produces a cataleptic state in which analgesia is intense (neuroleptanalgesia).

b. Disadvantages of neuroleptanalgesia are prolonged central nervous system depression and failure to depress sympathetic nervous system responses predictably to painful stimulation.

2. Antiemetic

a. Droperidol, administered intravenously (7.5 to 20 $\mu g \cdot kg^{-1}$), is a powerful antiemetic as a result of inhibition of dopaminergic receptors in the chemoreceptor trigger zone of the medulla.

b. Sedation and delayed discharge time may accompany the prophylactic administration of droperidol for its antiemetic effect.

c. Labyrinthine-induced vomiting (motion sickness) is not influenced by droperidol.

3. Decrease in shivering, as associated with deliberate hypothermia

D. Side Effects (Table 19-5)

1. Diphenhydramine, administered intravenously, is an effective treatment for droperidol-induced extrapyramidal reactions.

Table 19–5
Side Effects of Droperidol

Extrapyramidal reactions (avoid this drug in patients being
treated for Parkinson's disease)

Preoperative Medication Effects
Dysphoria (overwhelming fear of surgery)
Akathisia (restlessness in the legs)
Depression of carotid body drive to ventilation (dopamine acts as
an inhibitory neurotransmitter at the carotid body)

Central Nervous System Effects
Cerebral blood flow decreased more than cerebral metabolic
oxygen requirements (could be undesirable in patients with
cerebral vascular disease)

Cardiovascular Effects
Hypotension (acts on central nervous system and may cause
peripheral alpha-adrenergic blockade)
Hypertension (reflects stimulation of catecholamine release in
patients with pheochromocytoma)

---

2. Droperidol is a **cardiac antidysrhythmic** (may reflect alpha-adrenergic antagonist effects) and protects
against epinephrine-induced dysrhythmias.
3. Large doses of droperidol (0.2 to 0.6 mg·kg^{-1} IV)
depress conduction of cardiac impulses along accessory pathways responsible for tachydysrhythmias that
occur in patients with Wolff-Parkinson-White syndrome.
4. **Acute laryngeal dystonic reactions** (laryngospasm) represent extrapyramidal reactions that may
result in life-threatening upper airway obstruction
(treated with intravenous administration of diphenhydramine).
5. Haloperidol-induced torsades de pointes ventricular
trachycardia has been described.

III. LITHIUM

A. Lithium is used for treatment of mania and for the prevention of recurrent attacks of manic-depressive illness.
B. **Mechanism of Action**
1. At the cellular level, lithium ions act as imperfect

Table 19–6
Side Effects of Lithium

Peripheral edema

Benign diffuse thyroid enlargement

Hypothyroidism (lithium inhibits release of thyroid hormones)

Polydipsia and polyuria (may reflect inhibition of the action of antidiuretic hormone on renal adenylate cyclase)

Depression of T waves on the electrocardiogram

Leukocytosis

Sedation (? decreased anesthetic requirements)

Potentiation of neuromuscular blocking drugs

substitutes for sodium ions (Na^+) with respect to maintaining transmembrane potentials.
2. Lithium-induced decreases in the availability of cyclic adenosine monophosphate (AMP) result in decreased responses of receptors to neurotransmitters.

C. **Pharmacokinetics**
   1. Lithium is almost completely absorbed from the gastrointestinal tract and slowly enters the central nervous system.
   2. Approximately 95% of a single dose of lithium is eliminated in the urine.
      a. Reabsorption of lithium back into the circulation can be produced by diuretics (thiazide, furosemide) that cause increased renal elimination of Na^+.
      b. Sodium loading minimally enhances lithium excretion.

D. **Side Effects** (Table 19-6)

E. **Toxicity**
   1. The therapeutic range for lithium is narrow, with plasma concentrations lower than 0.8 mEq·L^{-1} often being ineffective, and levels higher than 1.5 mEq·L^{-1} possibly producing toxicity (Table 19-7).
   2. It is not uncommon for elderly patients who excrete lithium slowly to become confused, even in the presence of therapeutic plasma concentrations of this ion.
   3. Even short-term administration of a thiazide diuretic (also low-sodium diets) can quickly cause lithium toxicity.

Table 19-7
Manifestations of Lithium Toxicity

Toxic Effect	Plasma Lithium Concentration ($\mu Mol \cdot L^{-1}$)	Manifestations
Mild	1.0–1.5	Sedation Nausea and vomiting Skeletal muscle weakness Widening of the QRS complex on the electrocardiogram
Moderate	1.6–2.5	Confusion Unsteady gait Tremor Dysarthria Muscle fasciculations
Severe	>2.5	Coma Generalized fasciculations Seizures Extrapyramidal symptoms Impaired renal function Atrioventricular heart block Cardiac dysrhythmias Hypotension

(Adapted from Price LH, Heninger GR. Lithium in the treatment of mood disorders. N Engl J Med 1994;331:591–8.)

4. **Treatment** of lithium toxicity is supportive. If renal function is adequate, excretion of lithium can be modestly accelerated by osmotic diuresis and intravenous administration of saline.

IV. TRICYCLIC ANTIDEPRESSANTS AND RELATED DRUGS (Fig. 19-1)

A. Clinical Uses
1. **Alleviation of mental depression**
2. **Treatment of chronic pain** presumably reflects a link between serotonin and nociception and the ability of tricyclic antidepressants to block the uptake of this neurotransmitter.

B. Mechanism of Action
1. Tricyclic antidepressants potentiate the actions of bio-

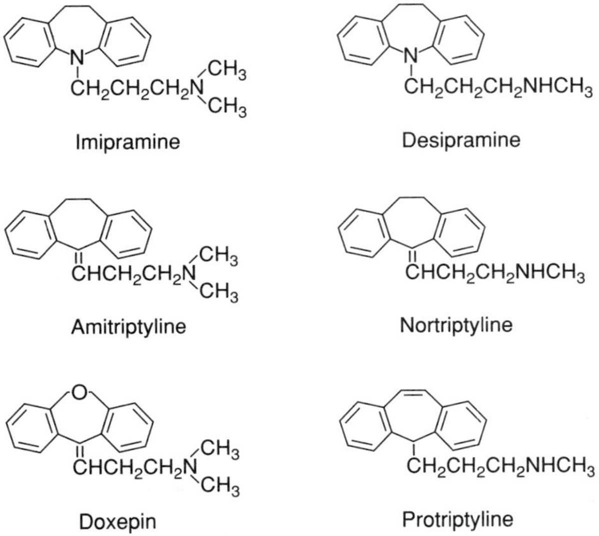

FIGURE 19–1. Tricyclic antidepressants.

genic amines (especially norepinephrine and/or serotonin) in the central nervous system by interfering
with the uptake (reuptake) of these amines into postganglionic sympathetic nervous system nerve endings.

2. Despite the prompt onset of inhibition of uptake, the
development of a therapeutic antidepressant effect
is inexplicably delayed for 2 to 3 weeks (suggests
antidepressant effects are not totally due to an accumulation of biogenic amines in the brain).

C. **Pharmacokinetics**

1. Tricyclic antidepressants are efficiently absorbed from
the gastrointestinal tract after oral administration, reflecting their high lipid solubility.

2. Tricyclic antidepressants are strongly bound to
plasma and tissue proteins which, in combination
with their high lipid solubility, results in a large volume of distribution (long elimination half-time makes
once-daily dosing intervals effective).

D. **Metabolism**

1. Tricyclic antidepressants undergo extensive hepatic

metabolism, often to active metabolites (imipramine to desipramine and nortriptyline).
   2. There is a wide variation in the rate of metabolism between patients.
E. Side Effects (Tables 19-8 and 19-9)
   1. Previous suggestions that tricyclic antidepressants increase the risk of cardiac dysrhythmias, myocardial depression, and sudden death have not been substantiated in the absence of drug overdose.
   2. Electrocardiographic effects of tricyclic antidepressants are probably benign and disappear with continued use.
   3. Phenylephrine in a decreased dose is recommended if a sympathomimetic is to be administered to a patient being treated with a tricyclic antidepressant (see Section VI D).
F. Tolerance
   1. Tolerance to anticholinergic effects (dry mouth, blurred vision, tachycardia) and orthostatic hypotension develops during chronic therapy with tricyclic antidepressants.
   2. Abrupt discontinuation of high doses of tricyclic antidepressants may be associated with a **mild withdrawal syndrome** (malaise, chills, coryza, skeletal muscle aching).
G. Toxicity
   1. Tricyclic antidepressant overdose probably represents the **most common life-threatening form of drug ingestion.**
   2. Progression from alert to life-threatening symptoms may be rapid, with intractable myocardial depression or ventricular cardiac dysrhythmias being the most frequent terminal event (Table 19-10).
   3. Plasma concentrations of tricyclic antidepressants do not allow prediction of the likely occurrence of seizures or cardiac dysrhythmias.
   4. The risk of life-threatening cardiac dysrhythmias persists for up to 10 days (comatose phase of tricyclic antidepressant overdose lasts 24 to 72 hours).
   5. Treatment of a life-threatening overdose of a tricyclic antidepressant is directed toward management of the central nervous system depression and cardiac toxicity (Table 19-11).
   a. Gastric lavage may be useful in early treatment

(text continues on page 300)

Table 19-8
Comparative Pharmacology of Antidepressant Drugs

	Anticholinergic Effect	Sedation	Orbostatic Hypotension	Time to Reach Steady State (days)	Special Considerations
Amitriptyline	++++	++++	++	4–10	Lower clearance of nortriptyline in elderly
Clomipramine	+++	+++	++	7–14	
Doxepin	++	+++	++	2–8	H-1 and H-2 antagonists
Imipramine	++	++	+++	2–5	
Trimipramine	++	+++	++	2–6	
Amoxamine	+++	++	+	2–7	Extrapyramidal effects, renal failure
Desipramine	+	+	+	2–11	
Nortriptyline	++	++	+	4–19	
Protriptyline	+++	+	+	14–19	
Maprotiline	++	++	+	6–10	Seizures
Fluoxetine	+	+/0	+		
Bupropion	0	0/+	0/+	1.5–5	Seizures
Trazodone	+	++	++	3–7	

0, none; +, slight; ++, moderate; +++, high; ++++ very high
(Adapted from Braverman B, O'Connor C, Barkin R. Pharmacology and anesthetic implication of antidepressants. In: Pharmacology and Physiology in Anesthetic Practices Updates 1993;1:1–15.)

Table 19–9
Side Effects of Tricyclic Antidepressants

Anticholinergic Effects (select desipramine when tachycardia
would be undesirable)

Cardiovascular Effects
Orthostatic hypotension
Depression of conduction of cardiac impulses (prolongation of P-R
interval and widening of the QRS complex on the
electrocardiogram)
Direct cardiac depressant effects (quinidine-like effects)

Central Nervous System Effects
Sedation (greatest with amitriptyline and doxepin)
Evidence of seizure activity on the electroencephalogram
(children may be especially vulnerable to seizure-inducing effects
of tricyclic antidepressants)

Drug Interactions
Sympathomimetics (hypertensive response to indirect-acting drugs
or epinephrine in local anesthetic solutions is enhanced,
reflecting increased availability of neurotransmitters)
Inhaled anesthetics (incidence of cardiac dysrhythmias may be
increased, especially if pancuronium is also administered or
exogenous epinephrine is injected)
Anticholinergics (possibility of enhanced central nervous system
effects)
Antihypertensives (may enhance rebound hypertension associated
with the abrupt withdrawal of clonidine)
Opioids (enhanced analgesic and ventilatory depressant effects)

Table 19–10
Features of Tricyclic Antidepressant Overdose

Prominent anticholinergic effects (mydriasis, flushed dry skin,
urinary retention, tachycardia)

Agitation and seizures followed by coma

Hypoventilation

Hypotension

Hypothermia

Widening of the QRS complex on the electrocardiogram (if longer
than 100 msec, there is an increased likelihood of seizures and
ventricular cardiac dysrhythmias)

Table 19–11
Pharmacologic Treatment of Tricyclic Antidepressant Overdose

Symptom	Treatment
Seizures	Diazepam Sodium bicarbonate Phenytoin
Ventricular cardiac dysrhythmias	Sodium bicarbonate Lidocaine Phenytoin
Heart block	Isoproterenol
Hypotension	Crystalloid or colloid solution Sodium bicarbonate Sympathomimetics Inotropes

(Data from Frommer DA, Kulig KW, Mark JA, Rumack B: Tricyclic antidepressant overdose. JAMA 1987;257:521–6; with permission.)

(assuming a cuffed tracheal tube is in place), whereas hemodialysis or drug-induced diuresis is not effective (reflects avid protein binding of tricyclic antidepressants).

  b. Coma usually resolves within 24 hours but is frequently severe enough to require upper airway protection with a cuffed tracheal tube.

  c. Acidosis associated with seizure activity may abruptly increase unbound tricyclic antidepressant plasma concentrations and predispose the patient to cardiac dysrhythmias (alkalinization of the plasma [pH higher than 7.45], either by intravenous administration of sodium bicarbonate or deliberate hyperventilation of the lungs, can temporarily reverse drug-induced cardiac toxicity).

V. NONTRICYCLIC ANTIDEPRESSANT DRUGS include fluoxetine, bupropion and trazodone.

  A. These drugs are no more effective than standard tricyclic antidepressant drugs, but do lack significant anticholinergic activity and exhibit minimal cardiovascular effects.

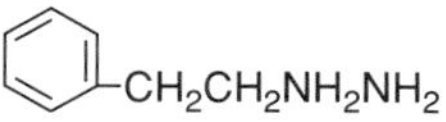

Phenelzine

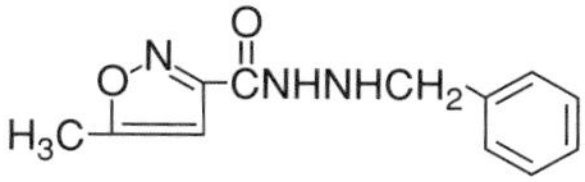

Isocarboxazid

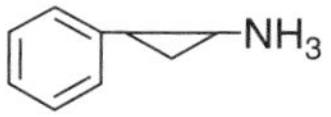

Tranylcypromine

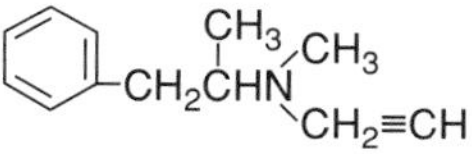

Selegiline

FIGURE 19–2. Monoamine oxidase inhibitors.

B. Mechanism of Action

1. Fluoxetine is a selective inhibitor of neuronal serotonin uptake.
2. Bupropion has an uncertain mechanism of action, although it does have some effect against the uptake of dopamine.
3. Trazodone seems to enhance neurotransmission through the serotonin system, the integrity of which appears to maintain an antidepressant response.

VI. MONOAMINE OXIDASE INHIBITORS (MAOIs)

A. MAOIs constitute a heterogenous group of drugs that have in common the ability to prevent oxidative deamination of naturally occurring monoamines in the central and peripheral autonomic nervous systems (Fig. 19-2).
   1. Clinically used MAOIs are classified as hydrazine or nonhydrazine derivatives, with a further subdivision based on the presence or absence of selectivity for the A or B form of the enzyme (Table 19-12).
   2. These drugs are administered only by the oral route.

B. Clinical Uses

1. The use of MAOIs is limited by serious drug interactions and hepatotoxicity.
2. MAOIs are used clinically not only for treatment of mental depression, but also of obsessive-compulsive disorders, eating disorders, chronic pain syndromes, and migraine headache.

C. Mechanism of Action

1. MAOIs form a stable and irreversible complex with monoamine oxidase enzyme, which is the principal

Table 19–12
Drug Selectivity for Monoamine Oxidase (MAO) Enzymes

	MAO-A	MAO-B
Hydrazine Compound		
Phenelzine	+	+
Isocarboxazid	+	+
Nonhydrazine Compound		
Tranylcypromine	+	+
Pargyline	?	+

(Data from Michaels I, Sevrins M, Shier, NQ, Barash PG. Anesthesia for cardiac surgery in patients receiving monoamine oxidase inhibitors. Anesth Analg 1984;63:1041–4; with permission.)

intraneuronal enzyme responsible for the oxidative deamination of amine neurotransmitters (dopamine, norepinephrine, epinephrine, serotonin).

  a. As a result, there is accumulation of amine neurotransmitters in the brain within a few hours, but as with tricyclic antidepressants, the therapeutic effects of MAOIs are delayed several days beyond the early increase in brain neurotransmitters.

  b. It seems likely that the initial increase in brain neurotransmitters produced by MAOIs activates a feedback loop that leads to decreased synthesis of these amines and delayed antidepressant effects.

  c. Chronic MAOI therapy is associated with a decrease in the responsiveness of alpha, beta, and serotonergic receptors manifesting as a general reduction in sympathetic nervous system activity.

  2. Two forms of monoamine oxidase enzyme have been defined on the basis of substrate preference (substrate specificity is concentration-dependent and may be overcome with high doses) (Table 19–12).

  a. MAO-A enzyme preferentially deaminates serotonin, dopamine, and norepinephrine, and its inhibition is clinically relevant.

  b. MAO-B enzyme preferentially deaminates phenylethamine and tyramine.

  3. Hypotensive effects of MAOIs (pargyline) are attributed to accumulation of a false neurotransmitter, **octapamine,** in postganglionic sympathetic nervous sys-

Table 19–13
Side Effects of Monoamine Oxidase Inhibitors

Sedation

Blurred vision and dryness of the mouth

Orthostatic hypotension (false neurotransmitter)

Hypertensive crises
  Sympathomimetics (greater incidence with indirect- than with
    direct-acting drugs)
  Tyramine in food (cheese, chicken liver, chocolate, wine)

Hyperthermia (meperidine, but not morphine or fentanyl, impairs
  neuronal uptake of serotonin)

Inhibition of hepatic enzymes (exaggerated depressant effects
  produced by opioids and barbiturates, possibly succinylcholine)

Increased anesthetic requirements (animal data)

Hepatotoxicity (hydrazine-containing compounds)

Peripheral neuropathy (may be related to pyridoxine deficiency)

tem nerve endings (release of which evokes less
intense vasoconstriction than norepinephrine).
  D. Side Effects (Table 19-13)
    1. A common recommendation in the past has been to
      discontinue MAOI therapy for a period of 14 to 21
      days before elective surgery.
        a. Adherence to this approach may place patients at
          risk for psychiatric complications, including sui-
          cide.
        b. There is growing appreciation that anesthesia can
          be safely administered to most patients in the pres-
          ence of chronic use of MAOIs (incidence of side
          effects is probably lower than previously sug-
          gested) (Table 19-14).
        c. Cell membrane receptor studies have shown that
          chronic treatment (longer than 14 to 21 days) with
          MAOIs or tricyclic antidepressant drugs results in
          physiologic adaptations (down-regulation) that de-
          crease the likelihood of adverse drug interactions
          (exaggerated blood pressure response to sympa-
          thomimetics).
        d. If hypotension occurs in a patient receiving an
          MAOI, direct-acting sympathomimetics, such as
          phenylephrine, in decreased doses are recom-
          mended.

Table 19–14
Guidelines for the Perioperative Management of Patients Treated with Monoamine Oxidase Inhibitors

Avoidance of meperidine (related opioids, such as fentanyl, sufentanil, and alfentanil, should be selected with caution)

Anticipation of possible prolonged response to muscle relaxants dependent on hydrolysis by plasma cholinesterase

Cautious use of sympathomimetics (titrate to effect, using decreased doses of direct-acting drugs)

Regional anesthesia when possible (avoid epinephrine in local anesthetic solution)

Postoperative pain management utilizing regional anesthesia or morphine

     e. For individuals receiving chronic (longer than 6 weeks) MAOI or tricyclic antidepressant therapy, administration of indirect or direct-acting sympathomimetic drugs is acceptable, although a high index of awareness of the potential risk of abnormal hemodynamic responses is indicated.

     f. Hypertensive crisis following ingestion of tyramine-containing foods is treated with a peripheral vasodilator (nitroprusside) or an alpha-adrenergic antagonist (phentolamine).

     g. Treatment of postoperative pain in patients receiving MAOIs should include a decreased dose of an opioid (about one fourth the usual dose) other than meperidine.

    2. Unlike tricyclic antidepressants, MAOIs do not produce seizure-like activity on the electroencephalogram or evoke cardiac dysrhythmias.

    3. Overdose with MAOIs is reflected by signs of excessive sympathetic nervous system activity (tachycardia, hyperthermia, mydriasis); seizures and coma (treatment is supportive, plus gastric lavage).

VII. DISULFIRAM

    A. Disulfiram inhibits acetaldehyde dehydrogenase activity necessary for the oxidation of acetaldehyde, which results from breakdown of alcohol by alcohol dehydrogenase.

    B. Ingestion of alcohol in the presence of disulfiram results in the accumulation of acetaldehyde, causing flushing,

vertigo, nausea, hyperventilation, tachycardia, and diaphoresis.

1. Sedation is predictable following waning of symptoms.
2. Severe reactions are infrequent but include hypoventilation, hypotension, cardiac dysrhythmias, cardiac
failure, syncope, and seizures.

C. **Management of anesthesia** in patients being treated
with disulfiram should include consideration of the potential presence of disulfiram-induced sedation (decreases
anesthetic drug requirements) and hepatoxicity (may
warrant preoperative liver function tests).

1. Unexplained hypotension during anesthesia that responds to ephedrine could reflect inadequate stores
of norepinephrine owing to disulfiram-induced inhibition of dopamine beta-hydroxylase (enzyme necessary
for the synthesis of norepinephrine).
2. Use of regional anesthesia may be influenced by reports of polyneuropathy occasionally occurring in patients treated with disulfiram.
3. Alcohol-containing solutions, such as used for skin
cleansing, should be avoided in these patients.

Prostaglandins are among the most prevalent of the naturally occurring, physiologically active endogenous substances (autacoids) having been detected in almost every tissue and body fluid. (Updated and revised from Stoelting RK. Prostaglandins. In: Physiology and Pharmacology in Anesthetic Practice. 2nd ed. Philadelphia, JB Lippincott, 1991;384–91.)

I. NOMENCLATURE AND STRUCTURE ACTIVITY RELATIONSHIPS

A. The generic term **eicosanoids** refers to the 20-carbon, hairpin-shaped fatty acid chain that includes a cyclopentane ring, characteristic of prostaglandins (Fig. 20–1).
B. The structure of prostaglandins is depicted by their generic designation (Table 20–1).

II. SYNTHESIS

A. Prostaglandins are derived principally from the polyunsaturated 20-carbon essential fatty acid, **arachidonic acid,** which is a ubiquitous component of cell membranes.
   1. Arachidonic acid is released from cell membranes by the action of phospholipase enzyme.
   2. Once released, arachidonic acid becomes available as a substrate for production of prostaglandins, via either the **cyclooxygenase** (widely distributed microsomal enzymes) or **lipoxygenase** (enzymes located principally in platelets, vascular endothelium, lungs, leukocytes) pathway (Fig. 20–2).

III. MECHANISM OF ACTION

A. In many tissues, prostaglandins act on specific receptors to stimulate synthesis of cyclic adenosine monophosphate (cyclic AMP).
B. Stimulation of smooth muscle by prostaglandins appears

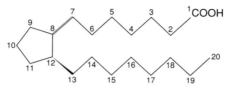

FIGURE 20–1. A 20-carbon, hairpin-shaped fatty acid chain is characteristic of prostaglandins.

Table 20–1
Nomenclature of Prostaglandins

	Notation	*Significance*
First two letters	PG	Prostaglandin
Third letter	PGE PGF	Indicates structures of the cyclopentane ring
Subscript after third letter	PGE_1 PGE_2	Indicates number of double bonds
Alpha or beta following the subscript	PGF_{2a}	Orientation of the hydroxyl group at the number 9 carbon

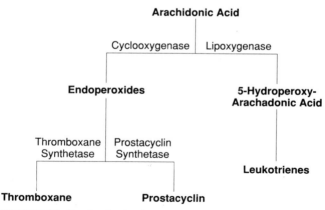

FIGURE 20–2. Synthesis of prostaglandins from arachidonic acid occurs via a cyclooxygenase pathway and a lipooxygenase pathway.

to be associated with the depolarization of cellular membranes and the release of calcium ions (Ca^{2+}).

IV. METABOLISM

A. Metabolism of prostaglandins to inactive substances is rapid, and is often confined to the site of their release.

B. The unique position of the pulmonary circulation between the venous and arterial circulation allows the lungs to act as a filter of many of the prostaglandins, thus protecting the cardiovascular system and other organs from prolonged effects due to recirculation of these substances.

V. EFFECTS ON ORGAN SYSTEMS (Table 20-2)

A. Hematologic System

1. Normal platelet function and hemostasis are likely to be strictly regulated by prostaglandins, as emphasized by the ability of nonsteroidal antiinflammatory drugs to interfere with normal platelet aggregation.

2. A normal thromboxane-to-prostacyclin ratio is important in maintaining the role of platelets in coagulation.

   a. An imbalance in the ratio of thromboxane (vasoconstriction) to prostacyclin (vasodilation) could lead to platelet aggregation and vasoconstriction in the arterial circulation or thromboembolism in the venous circulation.

   b. Bleeding disorders are likely in the presence of thromboxane depletion or excess prostacyclin.

3. **Iloprost** is a prostacyclin analogue that is a potent inhibitor of platelet aggregation.

B. Cardiovascular System

1. **Prostacyclin** is not inactivated in the lungs and, when administered intravenously, it causes a decrease in blood pressure resulting from a decrease in systemic vascular resistance (vasodilation occurs in several vascular beds, including coronary, renal, mesenteric, and skeletal muscle).

2. Alprostadil (PGE_1) is a potent relaxant of smooth muscle of the ductus arteriosus (used in neonates with ductus-dependent congenital heart disease [pulmonary atresia] to maintain patency of the ductus arteriosus until surgery can be performed). When used to produce controlled hypotension, PGE_1 decreases

Table 20–2
Comparative Effects of Prostaglandins

	Platelet Aggregation	Systemic Vascular Resistance	Airway Resistance	Uterine Muscle Tone
Thromboxane	↑	↑	↑	
Prostacyclin	↓	↓	↓	
Iloprost	↓	↓	↓	
Alprostadil (PGE$_1$)	↓	↓	↑	
Carboprost				↑
Dinoprost (PGF$_{2a}$)		↑/↓	↑	↑
Dinoprostone (PGE$_2$)				↑

↑, increased; ↓, decreased

blood pressure principally by relaxing vascular smooth muscle of resistance vessels.

C. Pulmonary Circulation

1. Pulmonary vasoconstriction may be related to increased circulatory concentrations of thromboxane, PGE_2, and PGE_{2a}.
2. Protamine-induced production of the prostaglandin vasoconstrictor, thromboxane, may manifest clinically as pulmonary hypertension and bronchoconstriction.

D. Lungs

1. The lungs are a major site of prostaglandin synthesis (producing bronchodilation or bronchoconstriction).
2. An imbalance between the production of thromboxane and prostacyclin in the lungs might contribute to symptoms of bronchial asthma.
3. **Leukotrienes** are several thousand times more potent than histamine as constrictors of bronchial smooth muscle.
   a. A predominant role of leukotrienes in asthma-induced bronchoconstriction is evidenced by the ineffectiveness of antihistamines in some patients.
   b. The relatively slow metabolism of leukotrienes in the lungs contributes to long-lasting bronchoconstriction.

E. Kidneys

1. The kidneys are a major site of prostaglandin synthesis, and intrarenal release of prostaglandins may be an important mechanism for regulating renal blood flow and glomerular filtration rate. The impact of prostaglandins on renal function appears to depend on the underlying physiological state of the kidneys.
2. The antihypertensive effect of normally functioning kidneys may be related to their capacity to synthesize and release into the circulation PGE_2 or prostacyclin, which causes diuresis, natriuresis, and a decrease in blood pressure.
3. Renal vasodilation produced by PGE_2 or prostacyclin may offset renal vasoconstriction produced by events such as drug-induced increases in sympathetic nervous system activity.
4. Inhibition of cyclooxygenase enzyme by aspirin or nonsteroidal antiinflammatory drugs may interfere with normal renal prostaglandin protective mechanisms and accentuate catecholamine-induced renal vasoconstriction (see Chapter 11).

F. Gastrointestinal Tract. Certain prostaglandins inhibit

gastric acid secretion evoked by histamine or gastrin. Miso-prostol is an analogue of PGE_1 that is effective in the healing of gastric or duodenal ulcers as associated with administration of nonsteroidal antiinflammatory drugs (not as effective as H-2 receptor antagonists, and it has more side effects).

G. **Uterus**
   1. The nongravid and gravid uterus are contracted by PGE_2 and PGF_{2a}, leading to the speculation that these prostaglandins are important in the initiation and main-tenance of labor (used to induce labor or cause abor-tion).
   2. Increased synthesis of prostaglandins in the endome-trium is speculated to be a possible cause of dysmenor-rhea (aspirin relieves pain of dysemenorrhea).
   3. **Carboprost** is a synthetic analogue of naturally oc-curring PGF_{2a}, administered to produce induction of elective abortion (nausea, vomiting, and an increase in body temperature [which must be differentiated from endometritis] may occur).
   4. **Dinoprost (PGF_{2a})** is administered intra-amniotically to induce uterine contractions for elective abortion (bronchospasm and seizures are possible side effects in predisposed patients).
   5. **Dinoprostone (PGE_2)** is administered most often as a vaginal suppository to induce elective abortion (side effects include tachycardia, tachypnea, hyperthermia, and sepsis).

H. **Immune System**
   1. Prostaglandins, such as prostacyclin, contribute to the signs and symptoms of inflammation, accentuating the pain and edema produced by bradykinin.
   2. Prostaglandins may suppress the release of chemical mediators from mast cells or decrease antibody re-sponses, possibly enhancing acceptance of tissue transplants.

21

Histamine and Histamine Receptor Antagonists

Histamine is a naturally occurring endogenous substance (autacoid) that produces intense physiologic effects when released locally or into the circulation (Fig. 21–1). (Updated and revised from Stoelting RK. Histamine and histamine receptor antagonists. In: Pharmacology and Physiology in Anesthetic Practice. 2nd ed. Philadelphia, JB Lippincott, 1991;393–406.)

I. HISTAMINE

A. Histamine is present in mast cells (skin, lungs, gastrointestinal tract) and basophils (circulation).

B. **Synthesis**
1. Synthesis of histamine in tissues is by decarboxylation of histadine.
2. Histamine is stored in vesicles in a complex with heparin to be released subsequently in response to antigen-antibody reactions or stimuli, such as drugs.
3. Histamine does not easily cross the blood–brain barrier, and central nervous system effects are usually not evident.

C. **Metabolism** of histamine is by methylation (histamine-N-methyltransferase) or deamination (histaminase) to inactive metabolites.

D. **Receptors**
1. Effects of histamine are mediated via histamine receptors that are classified as H-1, H-2, and H-3 (Table 21–1).
    a. Histamine causes vascular endothelium to release nitric oxide which stimulates guanylate cyclase and

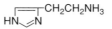

FIGURE 21–1.   Histamine.

increases levels of cyclic guanosine monophosphate (cyclic GMP) in vascular smooth muscle, causing vasodilation.
   b. The gene encoding the H-1 receptor has been cloned.
2. H-1 receptors mediate histamine-induced contraction of smooth muscle in the gastrointestinal tract and bronchi and cause pruritus and sneezing by sensory nerve stimulation.
3. H-2 receptors mediate histamine-induced secretion of gastric hydrogen ions (H^+) and are responsible for

Table 21–1
Effects Mediated by Activation of Histamine Receptors

	Receptor Subtype Activated
Increased intracellular cyclic guanosine monophosphate	H-1
Mediation of release of prostacyclin	H-1
Slowed conduction of cardiac impulses through the atrioventricular node	H-1
Coronary artery vasoconstriction	H-1
Bronchoconstriction	H-1
Increased intracellular cyclic adenosine monophosphate	H-2
Central nervous system stimulation	H-2
Cardiac dysrhythmias	H-2
Increased myocardial contractility	H-2
Increased heart rate	H-2
Coronary artery vasodilation	H-2
Bronchodilation	H-2
Increased secretion of acidic gastric fluid	H-2
Increased capillary permeability	H-1, H-2
Peripheral vascular vasodilation	H-1, H-2
Inhibited synthesis and release of histamine	H-3

Table 21–2
Effects of Histamine on Organ Systems

Cardiovascular System
>   Dilatation of arterioles and capillaries
>>   Flushing (blush area)
>>   Decreased peripheral vascular resistance
>>   Decreased blood pressure (prevented by pretreatment with
>>   combination of H-1 and H-2 receptor antagonists)
>>   Increased capillary permeability
>
>   Positive inotropic effect (involving direct effects, as well as the
>   ability of histamine to evoke the release of catecholamines from
>   the adrenal medulla)
>   Positive chronotropic effect
>   Cardiac dysrhythmias

Airways
>   Bronchoconstriction (accentuated in patients with obstructive
>   airway disease)
>   Bronchodilation

Gastric Hydrogen Ion Secretion (direct stimulant effect on
parietal cells)

Allergic Reactions (histamine only one of several chemical
mediators released)

---

cardiac and central nervous system effects of histamine.

4. **H-3 receptors** most likely function as autoreceptors
to inhibit the synthesis and release of histamine.

E. **Effects on Organ Systems** (Table 21–2)

II. HISTAMINE RECEPTOR ANTAGONISTS

A. Depending on what responses to histamine are inhibited,
drugs are classified as H-1 or H-2 receptor antagonists
(Table 21–3).
1. Histamine receptor antagonists produce a competitive
and reversible interaction.
2. H-1 and H-2 receptor antagonists do not inhibit release
of histamine, but rather attach to receptors and prevent
responses mediated by histamine.
a. Blood pressure decreases following drug-induced
histamine release are prevented by prior administration of H-1 and H-2 receptor antagonists (block-

Table 21-3
Classification of Histamine Receptor Antagonists

	Sedative Effects	Anticholinergic Activity	Antiemetic Effects	Duration of Action (h)	Adult Oral Dose (mg)
H-1 Antagonists					
First Generation					
Diphenhydramine	+++	+++	++	3–6	50
Pyrilamine	+	0	0	3–6	25–50
Chlorpheniramine	+	+	0	4–12	2–4
Brompheniramine	+	+	0	4–12	4–8
Promethazine	++	+++	+++	4–24	25–50
Second Generation					
Terfenadine	0	0	0	6–12	60
Astemizole	0	0	0	12–24	10
Loratidine	0	0	0	12–24	10
H-2 Antagonists					
Cimetidine	+*	0	0	5–7	300
Ranitidine	0	0	0	8–12	150
Famotidine	0	0	0	12	20–40
Nizatidine	0	0	0	8–12	150

0, none; +, mild; ++, moderate; +++, marked.
*Manifested as confusion and agitation.
(Adapted from Simons FER, Simons KJ. The pharmacology and use of H1-receptor antagonist drugs. N Engl J Med 1994;330:1663–70.)

ade of either receptor alone does not completely prevent the subsequent blood pressure-lowering effects of histamine).

   b. Responses to histamine-releasing drugs are better controlled by histamine receptor antagonists than are allergic responses (presumably chemical mediators in addition to histamine are involved in allergic responses).

B. H-1 receptor antagonists are among the most widely used medications in the world (Fig. 21-2).

   1. First generation H-1 receptor antagonists are relatively sedating (and inexpensive), whereas second generation antagonists are relatively nonsedating (Table 21-3).

   2. H-1 receptor antagonists are highly selective for H-1 receptors, having little effect on H-2 and H-3 receptors.

   3. Pharmacokinetics of H-1 receptor antagonists are characterized by reliable absorption from the gastrointestinal tract and extensive metabolism in the liver such that little, if any drug, is excreted unchanged in the urine.

   4. Side Effects (Table 21-2)

   5. Acute overdose with an H-1 receptor antagonist, particularly if it occurs in small children, can produce a flushed face, fever, mydriasis, and central nervous system excitation culminating in seizures.

   6. Clinical Uses (Table 21-4)

C. H-2 Receptor Antagonists (Fig. 21-3)

   1. Despite the presence of H-2 receptors throughout the body, inhibition of histamine binding to receptors on gastric parietal cells is the major beneficial clinical effect of H-2 receptor antagonists (Table 21-3).

   2. Cimetidine is a selective and competitive H-2 receptor antagonist that blocks histamine-induced secretion of H^+ by gastric parietal cells (no significant effect on gastric emptying time, lower esophageal sphincter tone, or pancreatic secretions).

   a. Pharmacokinetics of cimetidine are characterized by prompt absorption from the small intestine, followed by renal excretion of 50% to 70% of the unchanged drug (elimination half-time is doubled in anephric patients) (Table 21-5).

   b. Clinical Uses (Table 21-6)

   c. Side Effects (Table 21-7)

   3. Ranitidine is a selective and competitive H-2 receptor antagonist that has the same clinical uses as cimetidine

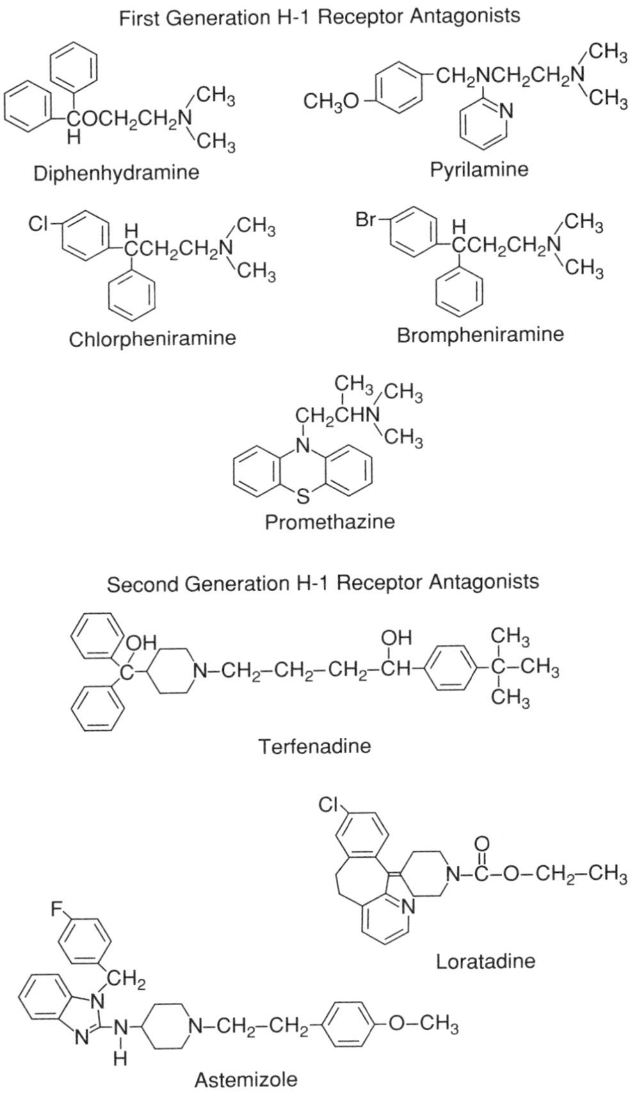

FIGURE 21–2. First generation H-1 receptor antagonists and second generation H-1 receptor antagonists.

Table 21–4
Clinical Uses of H-1 Receptor Antagonists

Symptomatic treatment of allergic rhinoconjunctivitis (sneezing, rhinorrhea, conjunctivitis)

Prophylaxis and treatment of motion sickness

Allergic dermatitis (pruritus, urticaria)

Insomnia

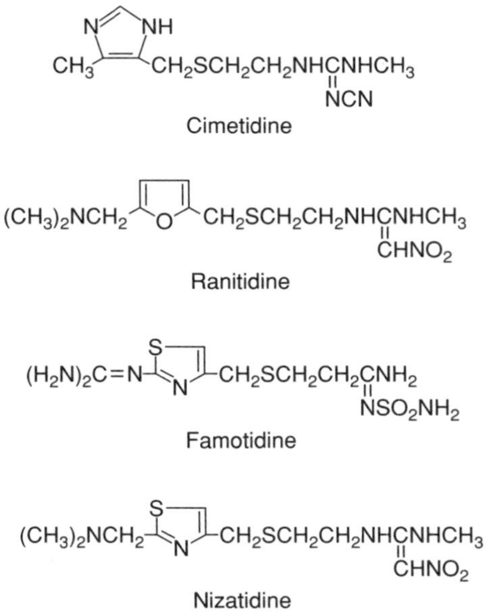

Cimetidine

Ranitidine

Famotidine

Nizatidine

FIGURE 21–3. H-2 receptor antagonists.

but is five to eight times more potent in antagonizing H^+ secretion by gastric parietal cells (inhibition lasts 8 to 12 hours).

  a. **Pharmacokinetics** are characterized by a more significant hepatic first-pass effect than for cimetidine and renal excretion of about 50% of the drug in an unchanged form (elimination half-time is pro-

(text continues on page 321)

Table 21-5
Pharmacokinetics of H-2 Receptor Antagonists

	Cimetidine	Ranitidine	Famotidine	Nizatidine
Absorption				
Bioavailability (%)	60	50	43	98
Time to peak plasma concentration (h)	1–2	1–3	1–3.5	1–3
Volume of distribution (L·kg[21])	0.8–1.2	1.2–1.9	1.1–1.4	1.2–1.6
Protein binding (%)	13–26	15	16	26–35
Clearance (ml·min[21])	450–650	568–709	417–483	667–850
Hepatic clearance (%)				
Oral	60	73	50–80	22
Intravenous	25–40	30	25–30	25
Renal clearance (%)				
Oral	40	27	25–30	57–65
Intravenous	50–80	50	65–80	75
Elimination half-time (h)	1.5–2.3	1.6–2.4	2.5–4	1.1–1.6

(Adapted from Feldman M, Burton ME. Histamine-2 receptor antagonists. N Engl J Med 1990;1672–80.)

Table 21–6
Clinical Uses of Cimetidine

Treatment of duodenal ulcer disease

Preoperative increase in gastric fluid pH (3 to 4 mg·kg^{-1} orally, 1.5 to 2 hours before induction of anesthesia; no effect on pH of gastric fluid already in stomach)

Preoperative preparation of patients with history of allergy (combined with an H-1 receptor antagonist and corticosteroid)

Prophylaxis against blood pressure effects of drug-induced histamine release (must be combined with an H-1 receptor antagonist)

Table 21–7
Side Effects of Cimetidine

Cardiovascular changes following intravenous injection
   Hypotension (peripheral vasodilation)
   Bradycardia
   Heart block

Increased airway resistance (loss of H-2 receptor–mediated bronchodilation)

Central nervous system dysfunction (most likely with high plasma concentrations associated with renal dysfunction)
   Confusion
   Hallucinations
   Seizures
   Coma

Gastric achlorhydria (weakens gastric barrier to bacteria) and predisposition to systemic infection and overgrowth of *Candida albicans*

Pulmonary infections (inhaled secretions; more likely if acid-killing effect of gastric secretions on bacteria is altered)

Mild increases in serum transaminase enzymes

Transient increases in serum creatinine (reversible interstitial nephritis)

Neutropenia and thrombocytopenia

Gynecomastia (antiandrogen effect)

Slowed metabolism of drugs (propranolol, diazepam, lidocaine, phenytoin, tricyclic antidepressants) that normally undergo high hepatic extraction (reflecting drug-induced decreases in hepatic blood flow and inhibition of hepatic mixed function P-450 oxidase system)

longed in the elderly and in the presence of renal dysfunction [decrease dose by half]) (Table 21–5).

   b. Side effects are less likely to follow administration of ranitidine than of cimetidine (central nervous system dysfunction and slowed rate of hepatic metabolism of drugs are unlikely).

  4. Famotidine is a potent (40-mg dose is equivalent to 150 mg of ranitidine), highly selective H-2 receptor antagonist.

   a. Inhibition of gastric H^+ secretion lasts for 12 hours.

   b. Effects on hepatic blood flow are negligible, and this drug has almost no adverse hemodynamic effects.

III. OMEPRAZOLE

A. Omeprazole blocks gastric acid secretion by selective inhibition of the H^+-K^+-ATPase proton pump (final common step in acid secretion) in the parietal cell membrane.

B. Virtual anacidity can be achieved for sustained periods (superior to H-2 receptor antagonists for the treatment of gastric ulcer disease).

C. Clinical Uses

  1. Omeprazole is superior to H-2 receptor antagonists for the treatment of reflux esophagitis and is the best drug available for patients with the Zollinger-Ellison syndrome.

  2. Duodenal and, possibly, gastric ulcers heal more rapidly with omeprazole than with H-2 receptor antagonist therapy (yet it has no clear superiority, as H-2 receptor antagonists are eventually effective in 90% of patients).

IV. CROMOLYN

A. Cromolyn inhibits antigen-induced release of histamine and other autacoids, including leukotrienes, from pulmonary mast cells (release of histamine from basophils is not altered).

B. Administration is by inhalation and excretion of unchanged drug in the urine and bile is in approximately equal amounts.

C. The principal use of cromolyn is in the prophylactic treatment of bronchial asthma (no value if administered after the onset of bronchoconstriction).

Chapter

22

Renin, Plasma Kinins, and Serotonin

Renin, plasma kinins, and serotonin are endogenous vasoactive substances (autacoids) with important and widespread physiologic effects. (Updated and revised from Stoelting RK. Renin, plasma kinins, and serotonin. In: Pharmacology and Physiology in Anesthetic Practice. 2nd ed. Philadelphia, JB Lippincott, 1991:407–14.)

I. **RENIN** is a proleolytic enzyme that is synthesized and stored by juxtaglomerular cells present in the walls of renal afferent arterioles as they enter the glomeruli (Table 22-1).
   A. **Formation of Angiotensins** (Fig. 22-1)
      1. **Converting enzyme,** which is present in highest concentrations in the lungs (an estimated 20% to 40% of angiotensin I is converted to angiotensin II during a single pulmonary circulation), is also responsible for the breakdown of plasma kinins, creating a situation in which the most potent endogenous vasoconstrictor (angiotensin II) and vasodilator (bradykinin) are cleared by the same enzyme.
      2. **The renin-angiotensin-aldosterone system** is important in maintaining blood pressure and intravascular fluid volume during sodium deprivation or in the presence of hypovolemia (no active role in the sodium-repleted patient).
   B. **Effects on Organ Systems**
      1. Vasoconstriction and stimulation of the synthesis and secretion of aldosterone (retention of sodium and water and loss of potassium and hydrogen) by the adrenal cortex are the principal physiologic effects of angiotensin II.
      2. Effects of angiotensin are most likely mediated through specific receptors.

322

Table 22–1
Stimuli for the Release of Renin

Decrease in Renal Perfusion Pressure
   Hemorrhage
   Dehydration
   Chronic sodium depletion
   Renal artery stenosis

Sympathetic Nervous System Stimulation
   Activation of beta-adrenergic receptors

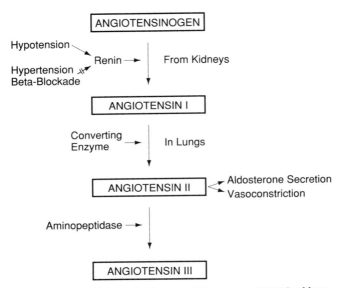

FIGURE 22–1.   Schematic diagram of the renin-angiotensin-aldosterone system.

Table 22–2
Physiologic Effects of Angiotensin II

Cardiovascular Effects

Vasoconstriction of precapillary arterioles (greatest in skin, splanchnic vasculature, and kidneys) and, to a lesser extent, postcapillary venules; 40 times more potent than norepinephrine

Decreased cardiac output

Decreased intravascular fluid volume

Central Nervous System

Enhanced central outflow of sympathetic nervous system impulses (hypertension)

Enhanced release of adrenocorticotrophic hormone

Peripheral Autonomic Nervous System

Enhanced responsiveness of the innervated organ to norepinephrine

Stimulation of the release of catecholamines from the adrenal medulla

Adrenal Cortex

Synthesis and secretion of aldosterone

    C. Cardiovascular Effects (Table 22-2)
    D. Central Nervous System (Table 22-2)
    E. Peripheral Autonomic Nervous System (Table 22-2)
    F. Adrenal Cortex (Table 22-2)
    G. Factors that Alter Plasma Renin Activity (Table 22-3)
    H. Exogenous infusion of angiotensin II produces intense vasoconstriction (more potent than that produced by norepinephrine) that may increase blood pressure to dangerous levels and produce myocardial ischemia.
    I. Antagonists of the Renin-Angiotensin-Aldosterone System (Table 22-3).

  II. PLASMA KININS (kallidin, bradykinin) are the most potent endogenous vasodilators known (about 10 times more potent than histamine).

 III. SEROTONIN (5-hydroxytryptamine [5HT]) is an endogenous vasoactive substance that also serves as an inhibitory neurotransmitter in the central nervous system.

Table 22–3
Factors that Alter Plasma Renin Activity

Increased Plasma Renin Activity
   Positive end-expiratory pressure
   Nitroprusside-induced hypotension (may contribute to
      tachyphylaxis)
   Volatile anesthetics and sodium depletion
   Activation of the sympathetic nervous system (cardiopulmonary
      bypass)

Decreased Plasma Renin Activity
   Beta-adrenergic blockade
   Blockade of receptors responsive to angiotensin II (saralasin)
   Inhibition of converting enzyme (captopril)

No Change in Plasma Renin Activity
   Trimethaphan-induced hypotension (blockade of sympathetic
      nervous system ganglia)
   Volatile anesthetics in the presence of sodium repletion

A. **Mechanism of Action**
   1. Receptors specific for serotonin are confirmed by the
      effectiveness of serotonin antagonists (methysergide,
      cyproheptadine, and kentanserin antagonize the ef-
      fects of serotonin on peripheral tissues, but not in the
      central nervous system).
   2. Serotonin receptors and alpha receptors have many
      overlapping functions.
   3. All serotonin receptors seem to be involved in the
      state characterized as anxiety.
B. **Synthesis and Metabolism**
   1. Serotonin is synthesized in cells from tryptophan (car-
      cinoid tumors that synthesize serotonin may divert so
      much tryptophan from protein synthesis to production
      of serotonin that hypoalbuminemia and pellegra re-
      sult).
   2. Serotonin undergoes oxidative deamination by mono-
      amine oxidase, ultimately resulting in the formation
      of **5-hydroxyindolacetic acid.**
C. **Effects on Organ Systems** (Table 22–4)
D. **Antagonists**
   1. **Tricyclic antidepressants** inhibit the uptake of sero-
      tonin back into tryptaminergic nerve endings, similar
      to the effect exerted on catecholamines.
   2. **Methysergide** is a congener of lysergic acid (lacks

Table 22—4
Effects of Serotonin on Organ Systems

Vasoconstriction (splanchnic, renal, cerebral circulation)

Vasodilation (skeletal muscles, skin)

Bronchoconstriction (especially in patients with bronchial asthma)

Increased activity of the gastrointestinal tract

significant central nervous system effects) that inhibits peripheral vasoconstriction evoked by serotonin.

   a. Uses of this drug include prophylaxis against development of migraine and other vascular headaches.

   b. Methysergide is useful in treating malabsorption and diarrhea in patients with carcinoid syndrome.

3. **Cyproheptadine** is able to block receptors for both histamine and serotonin and, in addition, this drug possesses weak anticholinergic activity and mild central nervous system depressant properties.

   a. This drug is useful in the treatment of intestinal hypermotility associated with carcinoid syndrome and in the postgastrectomy dumping syndrome.

   b. Side effects of cyproheptadine include sedation and dry mouth.

4. **Ketanserin** selectively antagonizes the effects of serotonin at peripheral 5-HT$_2$ receptors (also acts at alpha-1, histamine-1, and dopamine receptors), thus attenuating serotonin-induced vasoconstriction, bronchoconstriction, and platelet aggregation.

   a. This drug is useful in the treatment of patients with carcinoid.

   b. Antihypertensive effects of this drug may reflect alpha-1 antagonist actions unrelated to actions at serotonin receptors.

5. Highly selective 5-HT$_3$ receptor antagonists (ondansetron, granisetron) have revolutionized the management of chemotherapy-induced vomiting.

Chapter

23

Hormones as Drugs

Preparations that contain active hormones secreted endogenously by endocrine glands may be administered as drugs most often as replacement therapy to provide a physiologic effect. (Updated and revised from Stoelting RK. Hormones as drugs. In: Pharmacology and Physiology in Anesthetic Practice. 2nd ed. Philadelphia, JB Lippincott, 1991;415–35.) Recombinant deoxyribonucleic acid (DNA) technology permits the production of pure hormones devoid of allergenic properties.

I. ANTERIOR PITUITARY HORMONES (Table 23-1)

A. Perioperative replacement of anterior pituitary hormones may be necessary for patients receiving exogenous hormones because of prior hypophysectomy.

B. Cortisol must be provided continuously, whereas thyroid hormone has such a long elimination half-time that it can be omitted for several days without adverse effects.

C. The loss of other anterior pituitary hormones does not have immediate implications.

II. THYROID GLAND HORMONES (Fig. 23-1)

A. Evidence for the effectiveness of thyroid hormone replacement (levothyroxine, liothyronine) in the treatment of hypothyroidism is found in the return of the plasma concentration of thyroid stimulating hormone (TSH) to normal levels.

B. Certain carcinomas of the thyroid gland, particularly papillary tumors, may remain sensitive to TSH.

III. DRUGS THAT INHIBIT THYROID HORMONE SYNTHESIS (Table 23-2)

A. Iodide is particularly useful in the treatment of hyperthyroidism prior to elective thyroidectomy (often combined with propranolol).

B. Iatrogenic hypothyroidism must be considered preoper-

Table 23–1
Anterior Pituitary Hormones

Growth hormone (used to treat hypopituitary dwarfism)

Prolactin

Gonadotropins (used to treat infertility and cryptorchism)
    Luteinizing hormone
    Follicle-stimulating hormone

Adrenocorticotrophic hormone (ACTH) (used as a diagnostic aid in patients with suspected adrenal insufficiency and administered therapeutically to evoke the release of cortisol)

Thyroid stimulating hormone

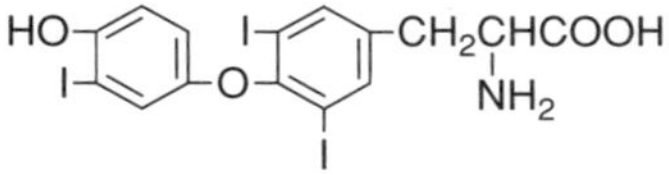

Triiodothyronine (T_3)

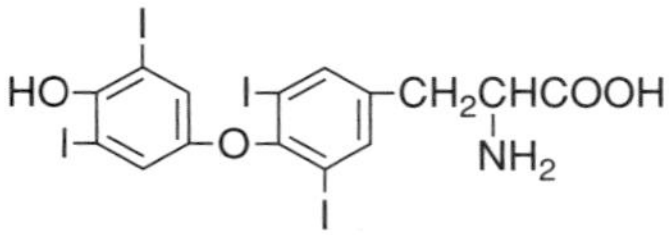

Thyroxine (tetraiodothyronine, T_4)

FIGURE 23–1.   Thyroid gland hormones.

Table 23–2
Drugs that Inhibit Thyroid Hormone Synthesis

Antithyroid drugs (block hormone synthesis)
    Propylthiouracil
    Methimazole

Inhibitors of iodine transport mechanisms (inhibit uptake of iodide ions by the thyroid gland)
    Thiocyanate
    Perchlorate

Iodide (high doses inhibit release of thyroid hormone within 24 hours)

Radioactive iodine (trapped by thyroid gland with subsequent emission of destructive beta rays)

atively in a patient who has previously been treated with radioactive iodine (^{131}D).

1. The principal indication for ^{131}I treatment is hyperthyroidism in elderly patients and in patients with heart disease.
2. Most thyroid carcinomas, except for follicular carcinoma, accumulate little radioactive iodine.

IV. OVARIAN HORMONES

A. **Estrogens** are effective in treating unpleasant side effects of menopause (viewed simplistically as an endocrine-deficiency state) and, in combination with progestins, are an effective oral contraceptive (Fig. 23–2).
   1. The presence of receptors for estrogen increases the likelihood of a palliative response to estrogen therapy in women with metastatic breast cancer.
   2. **Nausea** is the most frequent unpleasant symptom associated with the use of estrogen.
   3. **Antiestrogens** (clomiphene, tamoxifen) bind to estrogen receptors, resulting in increased secretion of gonadotropins and enhanced fertility.

B. **Progesterone**
   1. Orally active derivatives of progesterone are designated **progestins** (often combined with estrogens as oral contraceptives).
   2. Dysfunctional uterine bleeding can be treated with small doses of progestin with the goal being induction of progesterone-withdrawal bleeding.

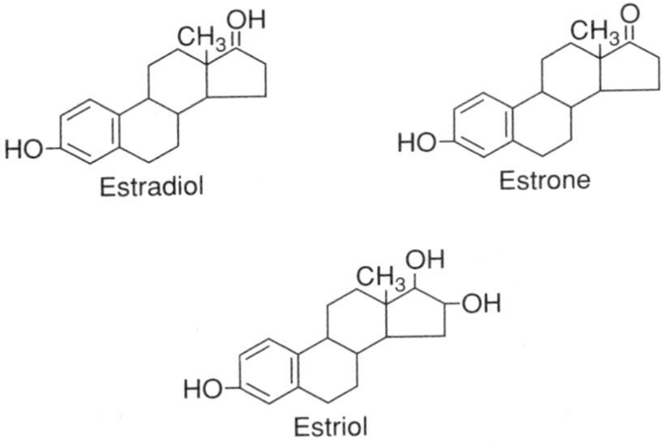

Estradiol

Estrone

Estriol

FIGURE 23–2. Estrogens.

Table 23–3
Side Effects of Oral Contraceptives

Thrombophlebitis and thromboembolism
  Increased blood concentrations of clotting factors
  Increased platelet aggregation

Nausea and vomiting

Weight gain

Hypertension (water and sodium retention)

Myocardial infarction

Stroke

Altered glucose tolerance curve (in patients with preclinical diabetes mellitus)

Cholelithiasis

Mental depression and fatigue

---

3. Mifepristone inhibits the action of progesterone (antiprogestins) and is effective in abortion induction, contraception, and the treatment of patients with cancer and Cushing's syndrome.

C. **Oral Contraceptives**
  1. The combination of estrogen and progestin inhibits ovulation, presumably by preventing release of follicle-stimulating hormone by estrogen and luteinizing hormone by progesterone.
  2. **Side effects** of oral contraceptives are believed to be most often due to estrogens (Table 23-3).

V. ANDROGENS

A. Androgens are most often administered to males to stimulate the development and maintenance of secondary sexual characteristics (Fig. 23-3).
  1. Androgens enhance erythropoiesis and may be useful in the treatment of aplastic and hemolytic anemia.
  2. The efficacy of anabolic steroids to improve athletic performance is not documented and is condemned on ethical grounds.

B. **Side Effects**
  1. Dose-related **cholestatic hepatitis** and jaundice are particularly likely to accompany androgen therapy for palliation in neoplastic disease.
  2. Retention of sodium and water is also likely to accom-

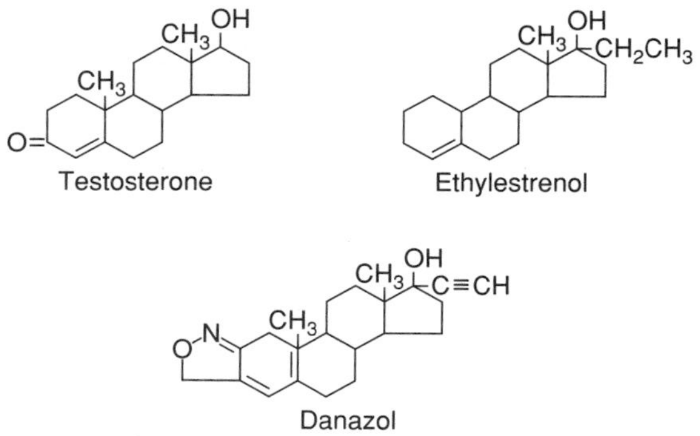

FIGURE 23–3. Androgens.

pany palliative treatment of cancer with high doses of androgens.

C. Danazol has low androgenic activity and is the preferred androgen for treatment of hereditary angioedema (stimulates production of deficient plasma protein factors).

D. Finasteride is a 5-alpha-reductase inhibitor (selectively blocks dihydrotestosterone production and androgen action in the prostate and skin) that is potentially useful in treating benign prostatic hyperplasia, male pattern baldness, hirsutism, and possibly, acne.

VI. CORTICOSTEROIDS

A. The actions of corticosteroids are classified according to their **glucocorticoid effects** (antiinflammatory response) and their **mineralocorticoid effects** (distal renal tubular reabsorption of sodium in exchange for potassium ions) (Table 23–4).

B. Structure Activity Relationships

1. All corticosteroids are constructed on the same primary molecular framework, designated as the **steroid nucleus** (Fig. 23–4).

2. Introduction of a double bond (prednisolone and prednisone) results in synthetic corticosteroids with more potent antiinflammatory effects than the two closely related natural hormones, cortisol (hydrocortisone) and cortisone.

Table 23-4
Comparative Pharmacology of Endogenous and Synthetic Corticosteroids

	Antiinflammatory Potency	Sodium-Retaining Potency	Equivalent Dose (mg)	Elimination Half-Time (b)	Duration of Action (b)	Route of Administration
Cortisol	1	1	20	1.5–3	8–12	Oral, IV, IM, IA
Cortisone	0.8	0.8	25	0.5	8–36	Oral, IM
Prednisolone	4	0.8	5	2–4	12–36	Oral, IV, IM, IA
Prednisone	4	0.8	5	3–4	18–36	Oral
Methylprednisolone	5	0.5	4	2–4	12–36	Oral, IV, IM, IA
Betamethasone	25	0	0.75	5	36–54	Oral, IV, IM, IA
Dexamethasone	25	0	0.75	3.5–5	36–54	Oral, IV, IM, IA
Triamcinolone	5	0	4	3.5	12–36	Oral, IM, IA
Fludrocortisone	10	125	—	—	24	Oral

IV, intravenous; IM, intramuscular; IA, intraarticular

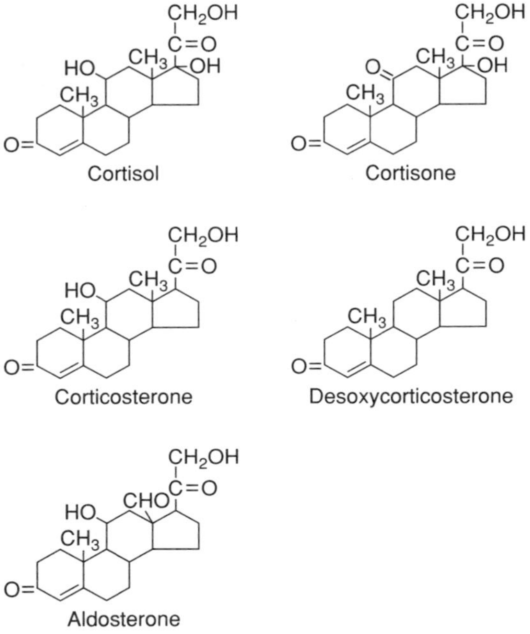

FIGURE 23–4. Endogenous corticosteroids.

    3. Mineralocorticoid effects and the rate of hepatic metabolism of these synthetic drugs are less than those of the natural hormones.

C. Pharmacokinetics (Table 23–1)

    1. Corticosteroids are promptly absorbed after oral, topical, or aerosol administration.

    2. After release, cortisone is converted to cortisol in the liver.

D. Synthetic Corticosteroids (Table 23–4; Fig. 23–5)

    1. Prednisolone is an analogue of cortisol that is useful for its antiinflammatory effects and is acceptable for sole replacement therapy in adrenocortical insufficiency because of the presence of glucocorticoid and mineralocorticoid effects.

    2. Prednisone is an analogue of cortisone that is rapidly converted to prednisolone after its absorption.

    3. Methylprednisolone is the methyl derivative of

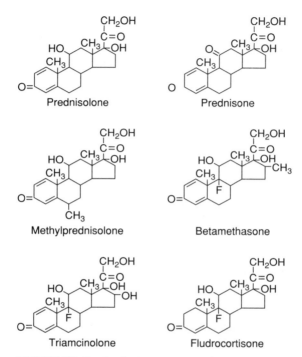

FIGURE 23–5.   Synthetic corticosteroids.

prednisolone. When administered **intraarticularly,** it has a prolonged effect; when administered **intravenously,** it produces an intense antiinflammatory effect.

4. **Betamethasone** is a fluorinated derivative of prednisolone that lacks the mineralocorticoid effects of cortisol and is thus unacceptable for sole replacement therapy in adrenocortical insufficiency.

5. **Dexamethasone** is a fluorinated derivative of prednisolone that is commonly chosen to treat certain types of cerebral edema.

6. **Triamcinolone** is a fluorinated derivative of prednisolone (less mineralocorticoid effect than prednisolone) that produces prolonged therapeutic effects

Table 23–5
Clinical Uses of Steroids

Replacement therapy for deficiency states

Antiinflammatory effect (palliative)

Cerebral edema (global ischemic injury)

Acute laryngotracheobronchitis (croup)

Aspiration pneumonitis (empiric)

Lumbar disc disease

Organ transplantation (often in combination with cyclosporine)

Asthma

Rheumatoid arthritis

Collagen diseases

Ocular inflammation (uveitis and iritis)

Cutaneous disorders

Postintubation laryngeal edema (unproven efficacy)

Ulcerative colitis

Myasthenia gravis

Hypercalcemia

Cardiac arrest (value for global cerebral ischemia is unproven)

when injected intraarticularly. It is commonly selected for epidural injections in the treatment of lumbar disc disease.

a. Epidural injection of triamcinolone, 80 mg, as administered to treat low back pain, may result in suppression of the hypothalamic-pituitary-adrenal axis (decreased release of cortisol in response to stress) for nearly 2 months (effect is more severe if midazolam is administered for sedation during the epidural injection).

b. For these reasons, it may be reasonable to provide supplemental cortisol for patients undergoing surgery who have received epidural steroids in the previous 1 to 3 months.

E. Clinical Uses (Table 23-5)

1. With the exception of treatment of deficiency states, the administration of corticosteroids for treatment of disease states is palliative or empirical.

2. Prednisolone or prednisone is recommended when an antiinflammatory effect is desired, as the low min-

Table 23–6
Side Effects of Cyclosporine

Nephrotoxicity

Hypertension

Limb paresthesias

Headache, confusion, and somnolence

Seizures

Cholestasis

Allergic reactions

eralocorticoid potency of these drugs limits sodium and water retention when large doses are administered to produce the desired glucocorticoid effect.

3. For treatment of lumbar disc disease, a common regimen is epidural injection of 25 to 50 mg of triamcinolone or 40 to 80 mg of methylprednisolone with 5 ml of lidocaine at the interspace corresponding to the distribution of pain.

4. **Cyclosporine** selectively inhibits helper T-lymphocyte–mediated immune responses and, in combination with corticosteroids, has greatly increased the success of organ transplantation.

   a. Cyclosporine must be administered before T-lymphocyte cells undergo proliferation as a result of exposure to specific antigens presented by organ transplantation.

   b. Serious side effects may accompany administration of cyclosporine, emphasizing the need to monitor blood concentrations and decrease the dose accordingly to minimize adverse effects (Table 23-6).

F. **Side Effects** (Table 23-7)

1. Corticosteroid therapy, including epidural steroid injection for treatment of back pain, may result in suppression of the hypothalamic-pituitary-adrenal axis with the result that release of cortisol in response to stress, such as that produced by surgery, is blunted or does not occur (see Section VI, D6).

2. The larger the dose and the more prolonged the therapy, the greater is the likelihood of suppression.

3. **Corticosteroid supplementation** is increased whenever the patient being treated for chronic hypo-

Table 23–7
Side Effects of Chronic Corticosteroid Therapy

Suppression of the hypothalamic-pituitary-adrenal axis (dose and
  duration of therapy necessary to produce this effect are unknown)

Electrolyte and metabolic changes
  Hypokalemic metabolic alkalosis
  Edema and weight gain
  Hyperglycemia
  Redistribution of body fat (buffalo hump, moon facies)

Osteoporosis

Peptic ulcer disease

Skeletal muscle myopathy

Central nervous system dysfunction
  Neuroses and psychoses
  Cataracts

Peripheral blood changes
  Lymphocytopenia

Inhibition of normal skeletal growth

adrenocorticism undergoes a surgical procedure
(based on concern that these patients may be susceptible to cardiovascular collapse because they cannot
release additional endogenous cortisol in response
to the stress of surgery).

4. **Corticosteroid supplementation** is controversial
in the management of the patient who may manifest
suppression of the hypothalamic-pituitary-adrenal
axis because of current or previous administration
of corticosteroids for treatment of a disease unrelated
to pituitary or adrenocortical dysfunction (Table
23–8).

Table 23–8
Corticosteroid Supplementation

Daily maintenance dose of corticosteroid with the preoperative
  medication (no evidence to support the need to increase dose
  preoperatively)

Cortisol, 25 mg IV, at the induction of anesthesia

Cortisol, 100 mg continuously IV, during the following 24 hours
  (200 mg per 24 hours in presence of burns or sepsis)

      5. Endogenous cortisol production during stress introduced by major surgery or extensive burns does not exceed 150 mg daily.

G. Inhibitors of Corticosteroid Synthesis

   1. Metyrapone decreases cortisol secretion by inhibition of the 11-beta-hydroxylation reaction (used to treat excessive adrenocortical function that results from adrenal neoplasms).

   2. Aminoglutethimide inhibits the conversion of cholesterol to 20-alpha-hydroxycholesterol, thereby interrupting production of both cortisol and aldosterone.

VII. POSTERIOR PITUITARY HORMONES

A. Antidiuretic hormone (ADH) is secreted by the posterior pituitary and acts on the renal collecting ducts to increase permeability of cell membranes to water (water is passively reabsorbed from renal collecting ducts into extracellular fluid).

   1. Diabetes insipidus is due to inadequate secretion of ADH and manifests as polyuria and hypernatremia.

      a. Head trauma and surgery in the region of the pituitary are recognized causes of diabetes insipidus.

      b. The oral hypoglycemic drug **chlorpropamide** sensitizes renal tubules to the effects of low circulating concentrations of ADH (probably reflects inhibition of prostaglandin synthesis), accounting for its beneficial effects in patients with diabetes insipidus (hypoglycemia is a risk associated with this drug).

   2. Nephrogenic diabetes insipidus results from an inability of the renal tubules to respond to endogenous ADH or exogenous preparations (desmopressin, lypressin).

   3. Inappropriate and excessive secretion of ADH results in retention of water and dilutional hyponatremia (demeclocycline promotes diuresis by antagonizing the effects of ADH on renal tubules) (Table 23–9).

   4. Vasopressin is the exogenous preparation of ADH.

      a. Clinical uses of vasopressin include treatment of ADH-sensitive diabetes insipidus, evaluation of the urine-concentrating abilities of the kidneys (as

Table 23–9
Causes of Excessive Secretion of Antidiuretic Hormone

Head injury
Intracranial tumors
Meningitis
Pulmonary infections
Oat cell carcinoma

following administration of a fluorinated volatile anesthetic), and management of uncontrolled hemorrhage from esophageal varices (selective arterial administration a consideration).

  b. Side effects of vasopressin, even in small doses, may include coronary artery vasoconstriction and myocardial ischemia.

 5. Desmopressin is a synthetic analogue of ADH that is the drug of choice in the treatment of diabetes insipidus owing to inadequate ADH production by the posterior pituitary (administered intranasally).

B. Oxytocin is the second principal hormone secreted by the posterior pituitary, producing selective stimulation of uterine smooth muscle.

 1. Clinical uses of oxytocin are to induce labor at term and to counter uterine hypotonicity and decrease hemorrhage in the postpartum or postabortion period.

 2. Side Effects

  a. High doses of oxytocin produce a direct relaxant effect on vascular smooth muscle that manifests as hypotension and flushing (may be exaggerated in the presence of hypovolemia or when compensatory reflex responses are blunted by general anesthesia).

  b. Modern oxytocin preparations are not contaminated with ergot alkaloids, thus removing the risk of exaggerated vasoconstriction when administered in the presence of a sympathomimetic drug.

VIII. ERGOT DERIVATIVES

A. Ergonovine and its semisynthetic derivative, methylergonovine, produce a uterotonic action.

 1. Intravenous injection of these drugs has been associated with intense vasoconstriction (hypertension, seizures) and may produce additive effects when used with sympathomimetics, such as ephedrine and phenylephrine.

2. These drugs should be used with caution, if at all, in patients with pregnancy-induced hypertension, essential hypertension, cardiac disease, or atherosclerotic peripheral vascular disease.

B. Ergotamine may be effective in relieving migraine headaches.

IX. CHYMOPAPAIN

A. Chymopapain is a proteolytic enzyme that dissolves the proteoglycan portion of the nucleus pulposus but does not affect collagenous components **(chemonucleolysis).**

B. Injection of chymopapain into the intervertebral space has been associated with life-threatening allergic reactions.

1. Preoperative administration of a corticosteroid plus an H-1 and H-2 receptor antagonist may decrease the incidence and severity of allergic reactions.

2. Known allergy to papaya is a contraindication to injection of chymopapain.

Chapter

24

Insulin and Oral Hypoglycemics

Insulin, administered exogenously, is the only effective treatment for Type 1 diabetes mellitus, whereas oral hypoglycemics may serve as an alternative therapy for patients with Type II diabetes mellitus. (Updated and revised from Stoelting RK. Insulin and oral hypoglycemics. In: Pharmacology and Physiology in Anesthetic Practice. 2nd ed. Philadelphia, JB Lippincott, 1991;436–44.)

I. INSULIN

A. The two most important effects of insulin are to facilitate transport of glucose across cell membranes and to enhance phosphorylation of glucose within cells.

B. Structure Activity Relationships. Insulin consists of two chains of amino acids joined by three disulfide bonds.

C. Pharmacokinetics

1. Despite rapid clearance of insulin from the plasma following intravenous injection (elimination half-time of 5 to 10 minutes) there is a **sustained pharmacologic effect** (30 to 60 minutes) because insulin is tightly bound to tissue receptors.

2. Insulin is secreted into the portal venous system at a daily rate of approximately 40 units (basal state 1 unit·h^{-1} and increases promptly in response to food intake).

3. Despite extensive hepatic first-pass metabolism, the presence of renal dysfunction prolongs the disappearance rate of circulating insulin to a greater extent than does hepatic disease.

4. The sympathetic and parasympathetic nervous system innervates the insulin-producing islet cells (alpha stimulates and beta or parasympathetic inhibits).

Table 24-1
Classification of Insulin Preparations

| | Hours after Subcutaneous Administration* | | | | |
	Onset	Peak	Duration	Modifier	Source
Fast-acting					
Regular	0.5–1	2–4	6–8	None	B,P,H
Semilente	1–3	5–10	16	Zinc	B,P
Intermediate-acting					
Isophane (NPH)	2–4	6–12	18–26	Protamine	B,P,H
Lente	2–4	6–12	18–26	Zinc	B,P,H
Long-acting					
Protamine zinc	4–8	14–24	28–36	Protamine	B,P
Ultralente	4–8	14–24	28–36	Zinc	B,P

*Approximate.
B, bovine; P, porcine; H, human (Humulin), NPH, neutral (N) solution, protamine (P), with origin in Hagedorn's laboratory (H).

D. Receptors for insulin in cell membrane surfaces become fully saturated with low circulating concentrations of insulin (1 to 2 units·h^{-1}, administered continuously as an intravenous infusion).

E. Preparations

1. Insulin preparations differ in their concentration (U-100 = 100 units·ml^{-1}), time to onset, duration of action, purity, and species of origin.

   a. The potency of insulin is 22 to 26 units for every 1 mg of hormone produced by the pancreas.

   b. A total daily exogenous dose of insulin for treatment of diabetes mellitus is usually in the range of 20 to 60 units (may be acutely increased by sepsis or trauma).

2. **Human insulins** are produced by processes (recombinant deoxyribonucleic acid technology) designed to synthesize insulin identical to that produced by the human pancreas.

3. **Classification** (Table 24-1)

   a. **Regular insulin** is the only insulin preparation that can be administered intravenously as well as subcutaneously (in the perioperative period, it is adminis-

Table 24–2
Side Effects of Exogenous Insulin Administration

Hypoglycemia (especially in the absence of carbohydrate intake in the preoperative period)

Allergic Reactions
  Local (erythematous indurated area)
  Systemic (antibodies to insulin or protamine)

Lipodystrophy

Insulin Resistance (greater than 100 units daily)
  Acute (associated with trauma or infection and presence of increased circulating concentrations of cortisol)
  Chronic (associated with circulating antibodies against insulin)

Drug Interactions
  Countering hypoglycemic action of insulin (glucagon, adrenocorticotrophic hormone, estrogens)
  Inhibiting secretion of insulin (epinephrine)
  Potentiating effects of insulin (monoamine oxidase inhibitors)

(text continues on page 346)

Table 24-3
Classification and Pharmacokinetics of Sulfonylurea Oral Hypoglycemics

	Relative Potency	Average Dose (mg)	Doses per Day	Duration of Action* (h)	Elimination Half-Time* (h)
First Generation					
Tolbutamide	1	1500	2–3	6–10	4–8
Acetohexamide	2.5	1000	2	12–18	1.3–6
Tolazamide	5	250	1–2	16–24	4.7–8
Chlorpropamide	6	250	1	24–72	30–36
Second Generation					
Glyburide	150	7.5	1–2	18–24	4.6–12
Glipizide	100	10	1–2	16–24	4–7

*Approximate

Table 24-4
Side Effects of Sulfonylurea Oral Hypoglycemics

	Overall Incidence of Side Effects (%)	Incidence of Hypoglycemia (%)	Antidiuretic	Diuretic
Tolbutamide	3	<1	Yes	Yes
Acetohexamide	4	1	No	Yes
Tolazamide	4	1	No	Yes
Chlorpropamide	9	4–6	Yes	No
Glyburide	7	4–6	No	Yes
Glipizide	6	2–4	No	Yes

tered as a single injection [1 to 5 units IV] or as a continuous infusion [0.5 to 2 units·h^{-1}]).

   b. The plasma insulin level required for 50% of maximum oxidation of glucose is 5 μmol·L^{-1} (administration of 7 units IV achieves a peak plasma concentration of about 1000 μmol·L^{-1}).

   c. **Isophane insulin** (NPH) is conjugated with protamine (0.005 mg·unit^{-1}) to delay its absorption from its subcutaneous injection site.

   d. **Lente insulin** is a mixture of 30% semilente insulin (prompt onset) and 70% ultralente insulin (extended duration), and can be used interchangeably with NPH.

4. **Side Effects** (Table 24-2)

   a. General anesthesia and treatment with beta antagonists may mask the symptoms of hypoglycemia (tachycardia, diaphoresis, hypertension), or the symptoms may be confused with responses to painful stimulation in a lightly anesthetized patient.

   b. Rebound hyperglycemia caused by sympathetic nervous system activity in response to hypoglycemia **(Somogyi effect)** may mask the correct diagnosis of hypoglycemia.

   c. Treatment of hypoglycemia is with 50 to 100 ml of 50% glucose, administered intravenously.

II. ORAL HYPOGLYCEMICS (Table 24-3)

A. It is estimated that 5% to 10% of patients who at first achieve satisfactory glycemic control with oral hypoglycemics experience secondary failure each year.

B. **Mechanism of Action**

1. Sulfonylureas increase islet beta cell sensitivity to glucose so more insulin is released.

2. These drugs are ineffective in the absence of endogenous insulin production.

C. **Pharmacokinetics** (Table 24-3)

D. **Side Effects** (Table 24-4)

1. **Tolbutamide** is the shortest acting and least potent sulfonylurea and is extensively metabolized in the liver.

2. **Acetohexamide** is converted to an active metabolite that is dependent on renal excretion (not recommended for patients with renal disease).

3. **Chlorpropamide** is unique in being associated with

reactions similar to those produced by disulfiram (facial flushing after ingestion of alcohol) and with the inappropriate secretion of antidiuretic hormone (hyponatremia may be severe).

4. **Glipizide** undergoes rapid clearance from the plasma which minimizes the potential for long-lasting hypoglycemia.

Chapter

25
Diuretics

Diuretics are classified according to (1) the mechanism by which they alter the excretion of solute and (2) their site of action on renal tubules (Tables 25-1 and 25-2). (Updated and revised from Stoelting RK. Diuretics. In: Pharmacology and Physiology in Anesthetic Practice. 2nd ed. Philadelphia, JB Lippincott, 1991;445-54.)

I. THIAZIDE DIURETICS

A. Thiazide diuretics are administered orally to **treat essential hypertension,** often as the initial sole therapy or in combination with a more potent antihypertensive drug, and to **mobilize edema fluid** associated with renal, hepatic, or cardiac dysfunction.

B. **Mechanism of Action**
1. Thiazide diuretics produce diuresis by inhibiting reabsorption of sodium (Na^+) and chloride (Cl^-) ions at various sites in the renal tubules (Table 25-2).
2. The result is a marked increase in the urinary excretion of Na^+, Cl^-, bicarbonate (HCO_3^-) and potassium (K^+) ions (Table 25-3).

C. **Antihypertensive Effect**
1. The acute antihypertensive effect of thiazide diuretics is due to a decrease in extracellular fluid volume and, often, a decrease in cardiac output.
2. The sustained antihypertensive effect of thiazide diuretics is due to peripheral vasodilation.

D. **Side Effects** (Table 25-4)
1. The increased possibility of **digitalis toxicity** and **potentiation of nondepolarizing neuromuscular blocking drugs** should be considered.
2. The presence of **orthostatic hypotension** may reflect diuretic-induced hypovolemia (increased hematocrit and blood urea nitrogen concentration).

II. LOOP DIURETICS (Tables 25-2 and 25-3)

A. **Pharmacokinetics**
1. **Ethacrynic acid** is excreted by the kidneys as unchanged drug.

Table 25–1
Classification of Diuretics

Thiazide Diuretics
  Chlorothiazide
  Hydrochlorothiazide
  Benzthiazide
  Cyclothiazide

Loop Diuretics
  Ethacrynic Acid
  Furosemide

Osmotic Diuretics
  Mannitol
  Urea

Potassium-sparing Diuretics
  Triamterene
  Amiloride

Aldosterone Antagonists
  Spironolactone

Carbonic Anhydrase Inhibitors
  Acetazolamide

---

  2. **Furosemide** (0.1 to 1 mg·kg^{-1} IV) is extensively bound to proteins.
     a. Glomerular filtration and renal tubular secretion account for approximately 50% of furosemide excretion.
     b. About one third of a dose of furosemide is metabolized or excreted unchanged in the bile.
  B. **Clinical Uses** (Table 25-5)
  C. **Side Effects** (Table 25-4 and Section I, D1-2)
     1. Administration of furosemide in the presence of oliguria due to hypovolemia can further exaggerate hypovolemia and aggravate renal ischemic changes that result from poor renal blood flow.
     2. Continued urine output in the presence of furosemide cannot be considered evidence of adequate intravascular fluid volume, cardiac output, and renal blood flow.
     3. Furosemide may enhance the **nephrotoxic potential** of aminoglycoside antibiotics and can cause deafness,

(text continues on page 353)

Table 25-2
Sites of Action of Diuretics

	Thiazide Diuretics	Loop Diuretics	Osmotic Diuretics	Potassium-Sparing Diuretics	Aldosterone Antagonists	Carbonic Anhydrase Inhibitors
Early proximal convoluted tubule			+			
Proximal convoluted tubule	+	+				+++
Medullary portion of ascending loop of Henle		+++	+++			
Cortical portion of ascending loop of Henle	+++	+	+			
Distal convoluted tubule	+	+	+	+++		+
Collecting duct					+++	

+, minor site of action; +++, major site of action
(Adapted from Merin RG, Bastron RD. Diuretics. In: Smith NT, Miller RD, Corbascio AN, eds. Drug Interactions in Anesthesia. Philadelphia: Lea and Febiger 1986; 206–24; with permission.)

Table 25-3
Effects of Diuretics on Urine Composition

	Volume (ml·min^{2l})	pH	Sodium (mEq·L^{2l})	Potassium (mEq·L^{2l})	Chloride (mEq·L^{2l})	Bicarbonate (mEq·L^{2l})
No drug	1	6.4	50	15	60	1
Thiazide diuretics	13	7.4	150	25	150	25
Loop diuretics	8	6.0	140	25	155	1
Osmotic diuretics	10	6.5	90	15	110	4
Potassium-sparing diuretics	3	7.2	130	10	120	15
Carbonic anhydrase inhibitors	3	8.2	70	60	15	120

(Adapted from Tonnesen AS. Clinical pharmacology and use of diuretics. In: Hershey SG, Bamforth BJ, Zander H, eds. Review Courses in Anesthesiology. Philadelphia: JB Lippincott Co. 1983; 217–26; with permission.)

Table 25-4
Side Effects of Diuretics

	Hypokalemic, Hypochloremic, Metabolic Alkalosis	Hyperkalemia	Hyperglycemia	Hyperuricemia	Hyponatremia
Thiazide diuretics	Yes	No	Yes	Yes	Yes
Loop diuretics	Yes	No	Minimal	Minimal	Yes
Potassium-sparing diuretics	No	Yes	Minimal		Minimal
Aldosterone antagonists	No	Yes	No	No	Yes

Table 25–5
Clinical Uses of Loop Diuretics

Mobilization of edema fluid (associated peripheral vasodilation contributes to value in treatment of pulmonary edema)

Treatment of increased intracranial pressure (response not influenced by alterations in the blood–brain barrier)

Differential diagnosis of acute oliguria
  Excessive antidiuretic hormone effect (offset with furosemide, 0.1 mg·kg^{-1} IV)
  Acute renal failure (controversial)

---

    especially with prolonged high plasma concentrations.

   4. Plasma concentrations of **lithium** may be increased acutely by the intravenous administration of furosemide in the perioperative period (reflects decreased lithium clearance in the presence of diuretic-induced decreases in Na$^+$ reabsorption).

   5. Patients who are allergic to drugs containing a sulfonamide nucleus (sulfonamide antibiotics or thiazide diuretics) may be at increased risk for developing allergic reactions when treated with furosemide.

III. OSMOTIC DIURETICS

  A. Mannitol is an inert six-carbon sugar that is most frequently administered intravenously, as it is not absorbed from the gastrointestinal tract.

  B. Mechanism of Action (Table 25–3)

   1. Mannitol increases the osmolarity of renal tubular fluid (completely filtered at the glomeruli and none reabsorbed) which prevents reabsorption of water.

     a. As a result of this osmotic effect on the renal tubular fluid, there is an osmotic diuretic effect with urinary excretion of water, Na$^+$, Cl$^-$, and HCO$_3^-$ (Table 25–3).

     b. Urinary pH is not altered by mannitol-induced osmotic diuresis.

   2. In addition to renal tubular effects, intravenous administration of mannitol also increases plasma osmolarity, thus drawing fluid from intracellular to extracellular spaces (acute expansion of intravascular fluid volume may have detrimental effects in patients with poor myocardial function).

Table 25–6
Clinical Uses of Mannitol

Prophylaxis against acute renal failure
    Cardiovascular surgery
    Extensive trauma
    Surgery in presence of jaundice
    Hemolytic transfusion reactions (unproven)

Treatment of increased intracranial pressure (0.25 to 1 $g \cdot kg^{-1}$ IV)

Differential diagnosis of acute oliguria (diuresis does not occur when oliguria is due to decreased glomerular filtration rate or impaired renal tubular function)

Reduction of intraocular pressure (glycerin administered orally does not cause diuresis and is an alternative to mannitol)

    C. Clinical Uses (Table 25-6)
    D. Side Effects
        1. Pulmonary edema is a risk in selected patients owing to acute mannitol-induced increases in intravascular fluid volume.
        2. Hypovolemia may follow excessive secretion of water and Na^+.
        3. Diuresis secondary to mannitol does not alter the elimination rate of long-acting nondepolarizing neuromuscular blocking drugs (predictable because clearance of these drugs depends on glomerular filtration, which is not altered by mannitol).
        4. If the blood–brain barrier is not intact, mannitol may enter the brain and draw fluid with it, producing **rebound intracranial hypertension.**
        5. The brain eventually adapts to sustained increases in plasma osmolarity such that the chronic use of mannitol is likely to become less effective in lowering intracranial pressure.
        6. Venous thrombosis is not likely to occur after intravenous administration of mannitol, and tissue necrosis is unlikely if extravasation occurs.
    E. Urea is an effective osmotic diuretic but, compared to mannitol, produces a greater degree of rebound increase in intracranial pressure and incidence of venous thrombosis.

IV. POTASSIUM-SPARING DIURETICS

    A. Diuresis produced by diuretics, such as triamterene and

Table 25–7
Clinical Uses of Acetazolamide

Reduction of intraocular pressure (carbonic anhydrase inhibition decreases formation of aqueous humor)

Petit mal and grand mal epilepsy (inhibits seizure activity by producing metabolic acidosis)

Familial periodic paralysis (metabolic acidosis increases potassium concentration in skeletal muscles)

Stimulate ventilation in patients with metabolic alkalosis

amiloride, is characterized by inhibition of K^+ secretion into the distal renal tubules (Tables 25–2 and 25–3).

B. **Clinical Uses.** The greatest value of potassium-sparing diuretics is in their combination with thiazide diuretics to offset their opposite effects on urinary excretion of K^+.

C. **Side Effects** (Table 25–4)

V. ALDOSTERONE ANTAGONISTS

A. **Spironolactone** is the prototype of drugs that act as competitive antagonists at receptor sites on collecting ducts that otherwise respond to aldosterone (Table 25–2).

B. **Clinical Uses.** Spironolactone is often prescribed for fluid overload owing to cirrhosis of the liver on the assumption that decreased hepatic function and metabolism lead to increased plasma concentrations of aldosterone.

C. **Side Effects** (Table 25–4)

VI. CARBONIC ANHYDRASE INHIBITORS

A. Acetazolamide is a sulfonamide drug that produces non-competitive inhibition of carbonic anhydrase enzyme, particularly in the proximal renal tubules (Table 25–3).

1. Excretion of hydrogen ions is decreased and loss of HCO_3^- is increased.

2. The net effect of these changes is excretion of an alkaline urine in the presence of **hyperchloremic metabolic acidosis.**

B. **Clinical Uses** (Table 25–7)

26

Gastric Antacids, Stimulants, and Antiemetics

Selected patients may benefit from treatment with gastric antacids, stimulants, and antiemetics. (Updated and revised from Stoelting RK. Gastric antacids, stimulants, and antiemetics. In: Pharmacology and Physiology in Anesthetic Practice. 2nd ed. Philadelphia, JB Lippincott, 1991;455-65.)

I. GASTRIC ANTACIDS

A. Gastric antacids are drugs that neutralize or remove acid from gastric contents (aluminum, calcium, and magnesium salts react with hydrochloric acid to form less acidic salts).

B. Side Effects

1. In the presence of renal failure, all antacids except aluminum compounds can cause **metabolic alkalosis.**

2. **Alkalinization of the urine** may alter renal elimination of drugs and predispose patients to urinary tract infections and, if chronic, to urolithiasis.

C. Drug Interactions

1. The rate of absorption of salicylates, indomethacin, and naproxen is increased when gastric fluid pH is increased.

2. Absorption of cimetidine, tetracyclines, and digoxin may be decreased.

D. Commercial Preparations (Table 26-1)

E. Antacid Selection

1. There is considerable variation in the acid-neutralizing effects of different antacids (Table 26-2).

2. There is no evidence that mixtures of antacids have greater beneficial effects than those provided by an individual antacid.

Table 26–1
Commercial Preparations of Antacids

Aluminum hydroxide

Sucralfate (complex of sulfated sucrose and aluminum hydroxide)

Calcium carbonate (milk-alkali syndrome is a rare complication of chronic administration manifesting as hypercalcemic alkalosis, nausea, and occasionally, renal failure)

Magnesium oxide

Sodium bicarbonate

F. Preoperative Administration of Antacids

1. Despite the ability of antacids to increase gastric fluid pH and theoretically decrease the risk associated with aspiration, it has not been documented that routine use of antacids in the preoperative period is efficacious.

   a. The duration of antacid action is highly dependent on gastric emptying time (opioids slow gastric motility and prolong the pH-elevating effects of antacids).

   b. Repeated administration of antacids, such as to the parturient who has also received opioids, can result in a greatly increased gastric fluid volume (more

Table 26–2
Contents (mg per 5 ml) of Particulate Antacids

	Aluminum Hydroxide	Magnesium Hydroxide	Calcium Carbonate	Sodium
Aludrox	307	103		1.1
Amphojel	320			6.9
Di-Gel	282	85		10.6
Gelusil	200	200		0.7
Maalox	225	200		1.35
Mylanta	200	200		0.68
Riopan	480			0.3
Tums			500	<3
WinGel	180	160		<2.5

logical to administer an antacid as a single dose approximately 30 minutes before the induction of anesthesia).

G. **Particulate antacids** may cause a foreign body reaction if inhaled into the lungs during aspiration of gastric contents.

H. **Nonparticulate antacids,** such as sodium citrate, are less likely to cause a foreign body reaction if aspirated into the lungs, and their mixing with gastric fluid is more complete and rapid (15 to 30 minutes) than is that of particulate antacids.

II. GASTROINTESTINAL PROKINETICS

A. **Metoclopramide** (methoxychloroprocainamide) is a dopamine antagonist that is structurally similar to procainamide but lacks local anesthetic activity.

   1. **Mechanism of Action**

      a. Metoclopramide produces selective cholinergic stimulation of the gastrointestinal tract (increased motility and relaxation of the pylorus following administration of 10 to 20 mg IV).

      b. Atropine opposes metoclopramide-induced increases in lower esophageal sphincter tone and gastrointestinal hypermotility.

   2. **Pharmacokinetics**

      a. Metoclopramide is rapidly absorbed after oral administration and crosses the placenta.

      b. Impairment of renal function prolongs the elimination half-time of metoclopramide and necessitates a decrease in dosage.

   3. **Clinical Uses** (Table 26–3)

   4. **Side Effects** (Table 26–4)

Table 26–3
Clinical Uses of Metoclopramide

Preoperative reduction of gastric fluid volume (10 to 20 mg IV over 3 to 5 minutes, administered 15 to 30 minutes before induction of anesthesia in selected adult patients)

Treatment of gastroparesis

Production of an antiemetic effect (antagonism of dopamine receptors in the chemoreceptor trigger zone and reversal of gastric stasis, as produced by opioids)

Table 26–4
Side Effects of Metoclopramide

Extrapyramidal reactions (1 in 500 patients)

Sedation (not observed following a single dose)

Galactorrhea

Enhanced central nervous system depressant effects of antidepressant drugs

Inhibitory effect (*in vitro*) on plasma cholinesterase activity

Increased intraluminal pressures in presence of intestinal obstruction

---

  B. Cisapride stimulates gastric emptying by enhancing the release of acetylcholine from nerve endings in the myenteric plexus in the wall of the gastrointestinal tract (lacks dopamine antagonist effects).
    1. Opioid-induced gastric stasis, which may be an important cause of postoperative nausea and vomiting, is reversed by cisapride.
    2. Cisapride increases lower esophageal sphincter pressure.

III. ANTIEMETICS (see Chapters 19 and 21)

  A. Antiemetic drugs have potential undesirable side effects (sedation, dysphoria, extrapyramidal reactions).
    1. Antiemetic prophylaxis may be justified in subpopulations of patients who are at greater risk for developing postoperative nausea and vomiting (Table 26–5).
    2. No currently available antiemetic drug will antagonize all receptor sites involved in the emetic response (Table 26–6, see also Fig. 41–11).

Table 26–5
Subpopulations of patients at Greatest Risk for Developing Postoperative Nausea and Vomiting

History of motion sickness

History of previous postoperative emesis

Laparoscopic gynecologic procedures

Extracorporeal shock wave lithotripsy

Strabismus surgery

Table 26-6
Receptor Site Affinity of Antiemetic Drugs

	Dopamine-2	Muscarinic/Cholinergic	Histamine	Serotonin
Phenothiazines				
Chlorpromazine	++++	++	++++	+
Fluphenazine	++++	+	++	0
Prochlorperazine	++++			
Butyrophenones				
Haloperidol	++++	0	++	0
Droperidol	++++	0	+	+
Domperidone	++++			
Antihistamines				
Diphenhydramine	+	++	++++	0
Promethazine	++	++	++++	0
Anticholinergics				
Scopolamine	+	++++	+	0
Benzamides				
Metoclopramide	+++	0	+	++
Antiserotonins				
Ondansetron				+++
Granisetron				++++
Tricyclic antidepressants				
Amitriptyline	+++	+++	++++	0
Nortriptyline	++	++	+++	0

0, no activity; +, minimal activity; ++, moderate activity; +++, marked activity; ++++, very high activity.
(Adapted from Watcha MF, White PF. Postoperative nausea and vomiting: Its etiology, treatment and prevention. Anesthesiology 1992;77:162–84.)

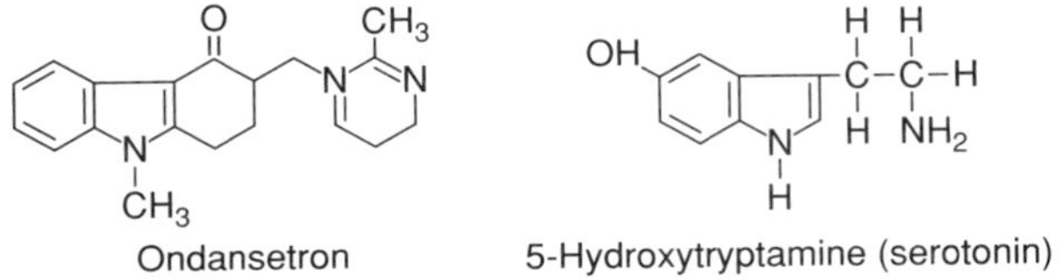

Ondansetron   5-Hydroxytryptamine (serotonin)

FIGURE 26–1. Chemical structure of ondansetron and 5-hydroxytryptamine.

3. Antiemetic drugs may be more effective when used in combinations designed to block several different receptors (limited by sedation).

B. Domperidone is a dopamine receptor antagonist that does not easily cross the blood–brain barrier.

1. Restriction of antidopaminergic activity to peripheral sites allows domperidone to influence the chemoreceptor trigger zone (outside the blood–brain barrier) without affecting the basal ganglia (extrapyramidal reactions do not occur).

2. Domperidone is not useful for treatment of postoperative nausea and vomiting or that induced by opioids.

C. Ondansetron

1. Ondansetron is structurally related to serotonin and produces selective 5-hydroxytryptamine subtype 3 (5-HT$_3$) receptor antagonism (Fig. 26–1).

2. **Side Effects**

a. Headache, diarrhea, and transient increases in liver transaminase enzymes have been described in patients treated with ondansetron.

b. Side effects commonly observed with other antiemetics (hypotension, sedation, restlessness, dry mouth, dysphoria, extrapyramidal symptoms) do not occur with ondansetron as it does not alter dopamine, histamine, adrenergic, or cholinergic receptor activity.

c. Antagonism of 5-HT$_3$ receptors may have a mood-elevating effect.

3. **Clinical Uses** (Table 26–7)

4. When nausea and vomiting do occur in patients treated with ondansetron, the symptoms are often mild compared with those in patients treated with other antiemetics.

5. **Granisetron** is a 5-HT$_3$ receptor antagonist that produces a long-lasting (24 hours) antiemetic effect follow-

Table 26-7
Clinical Uses of Ondansetron

Prevention of nausea and vomiting produced by cancer
  chemotherapy
Prophylaxis against postoperative nausea and vomiting (4 to 8 mg IV
  just before induction of anesthesia in an adult patient is more
  effective than droperidol or metoclopramide)
Treatment of postoperative nausea and vomiting

ing a single dose ($40\ \mu g \cdot kg^{-1}$ IV at the time of anesthetic
induction).

D. Diphenidol acts on the vestibular apparatus and may be
  a useful antiemetic for nausea and vomiting associated
  with irradiation, chemotherapeutic drugs, and general anesthesia.

27

Anticoagulants

Anticoagulants are drugs that delay or prevent the clotting of blood by exerting direct or indirect actions on the coagulation system. (Updated and revised from Stoelting RK. Anticoagulants. In: Pharmacology and Physiology in Anesthetic Practice. 2nd ed. Philadelphia, JB Lippincott, 1991;466–76.)

I. **HEPARIN** is a negatively charged mucopolysaccharide organic acid that is present endogenously in high concentrations in the liver and granules of mast cells and basophils.

   A. **Commercial Preparations**
      1. A **unit of heparin** is defined as the volume of heparin solution that will prevent 1 ml of citrated sheep blood from clotting for 1 hour following the addition of 0.2 ml of 1:100 calcium chloride.
      2. Because the potency of different commercial preparations of heparin may vary greatly, the heparin dose is prescribed in units.

   B. **Clinical Uses**
      1. Commercially prepared solutions of heparin are used exclusively to produce an anticoagulant effect, as during specific operative procedures.
      2. Low-dose heparin is efficacious as primary prophylaxis against postoperative deep vein thrombosis and pulmonary embolism.
      3. Continuous intravenous infusion of a solution containing a small amount of heparin is commonly used to maintain patency of intravascular catheters.

   C. **Mechanism of Action**
      1. Heparin binds with antithrombin III, resulting in a 1000-fold increase in its activity as an inhibitor of thrombin (without thrombin, the coagulation cascade is inhibited at several points, and clot formation is suppressed).

2. In addition to its anticoagulant effects, heparin inhibits platelet function and increases the permeability of vessel walls.

D. Route of Administration
1. The recommended route of administration for heparin in ambulatory patients is subcutaneous (intramuscular injection may cause hematoma formation).
2. Administration of high doses of heparin is accomplished by intermittent or continuous intravenous infusion.
3. Heparin is a poorly lipid-soluble, high-molecular-weight substance that cannot easily cross lipid barriers (blood–brain barrier, placenta, gastrointestinal tract).

E. Duration of action of heparin is largely determined by the dose administered and body temperature.

F. Clearance of heparin is principally by metabolism in the liver by the enzyme heparinase to inactive metabolites that are eliminated by the kidneys.

G. Laboratory Evaluation of Coagulation
1. **Partial thromboplastin time (PTT)** is maintained approximately twice the patient's predrug value of 30 to 35 seconds.
2. **Activated coagulation time (ACT)** during cardiopulmonary bypass is commonly maintained longer than 300 seconds (normal is 90 to 120 seconds).

H. Side Effects (Table 27-1)

I. Protamine
1. Protamine is a positively charged alkaline molecule that combines with negatively charged acidic heparin to form a stable complex that is devoid of anticoagulant activity (specific antagonist of heparin's anticoagulant effects).
2. **Side Effects** (Table 27-2)
3. The protamine-heparin complex is removed by the reticuloendothelial system.

II. ORAL ANTICOAGULANTS (Table 27-3)

A. Clinical Uses
1. Among the coumarin derivatives, warfarin is the most widely used drug.
2. Oral anticoagulants, in combination with dipyridamole, are commonly used to decrease the incidence of thromboembolism associated with prosthetic heart valves and atrial fibrillation.

Table 27–1
Side Effects of Heparin

Hemorrhage (intraocular, intracranial)

Allergic reactions

Thrombocytopenia

Platelet count <100,000 cells·mm^{-3} (occurs in 30% to 40% of patients and is usually transient; probably reflects drug-induced platelet aggregation)

Platelet count <50,000 cells·mm^{-3} (occurs in 0.5% to 6% of patients and is often associated with resistance to heparin and the occurrence of thrombotic events; probably reflects drug-induced platelet antibodies)

Altered protein binding (displacement of alkaline drugs)

Cardiovascular changes (large IV doses administered rapidly may decrease systemic vascular resistance)

Decreased antithrombin III concentrations (fresh frozen plasma restores the levels to normal and promotes the anticoagulant effects of heparin)

B. Mechanism of Action
   1. The anticoagulant effect of coumarin derivatives reflects competitive inhibition of vitamin K, which is required for the formation of gamma carboxyglutamic acid in the liver.
   2. This amino acid is necessary for the normal synthesis of vitamin K–dependent clotting factors (factors II, VII, IX, and X).
C. Distribution and Clearance
   1. Warfarin is rapidly and completely absorbed within 1 hour after oral ingestion (crosses the placenta).

Table 27–2
Side Effects of Protamine

Hypotension (rapid intravenous injection is most likely to evoke release of histamine in the lungs)

Pulmonary hypertension (complement activation and thromboxane release)

Allergic reactions (at-risk patients may be those treated with protamine-containing insulin preparations or those allergic to fish)

Table 27-3
Comparative Pharmacology of Oral Anticoagulants

	Time to Peak Effect (h)	Duration After Discontinuation (days)	Initial Adult Dose (mg)	Maintenance Adult Dose (mg)
Warfarin	36–72	2–5	15, first day 10, second day 10, third day	2.5–10
Dicumarol	36–48	2–6	200–300, first day	25–200
Phenindione	18–24	1–2	300, first day 200, second day	25–200

2. Extensive protein binding contributes to a prolonged elimination half-time.

D. Laboratory Evaluation of Anticoagulation

1. Treatment with oral anticoagulants is best guided by the prothrombin time (PT) (sensitive to factors II, VII, and X), which is typically maintained at approximately twice the normal baseline of 12 to 15 seconds.

2. An excessively prolonged PT (longer than 30 seconds) is not readily shortened by omitting a dose (in contrast to the rapid and predictable response that occurs with the omission of a single dose of heparin).

E. Management Prior to Elective Surgery

1. Relatively minor surgical procedures can be performed safely in patients receiving oral anticoagulants

2. For major surgery, discontinuation of oral anticoagulants 1 to 3 days preoperatively is recommended to permit the PT to return to within 20% of the normal range.

3. In emergency situations, intravenous administration of vitamin K, fresh whole blood, or fresh frozen plasma may be necessary to abruptly counter the effects of oral anticoagulants.

4. Vitamin K, 1 to 5 mg IV administered to adults, will usually return the PT to a normal range within 4 to 24 hours.

F. Drug Interactions

1. It is hazardous to administer any drug containing aspirin during oral anticoagulant therapy.
   a. Even a single 325-mg tablet of aspirin can impair platelet aggregation.
   b. Acetaminophen and sodium salicylate lack effects on platelets and therefore do not interact adversely when administered for antipyresis to patients being treated with oral anticoagulants.

2. Phenylbutazone impairs platelet aggregation, displaces warfarin from albumin, and inhibits the metabolism of warfarin.

G. Side Effects (Table 27-4)

Table 27-4
Side Effects of Oral Anticoagulant Therapy

Hemorrhage (gastrointestinal, intracranial)

Compression neuropathy

Teratogenic effects

III. ANTITHROMBOTIC DRUGS

A. Antithrombotic drugs (aspirin, dipyridamole, dextran) suppress platelet function and are used primarily for treatment of arterial thrombotic disease.

B. Heparin and oral anticoagulants suppress function or synthesis of clotting factors and are used to control venous thromboembolic disorders.

IV. THROMBOLYTIC DRUGS

A. Thrombolytic therapy (streptokinase, recombinant tissue plasminogen activator, urokinase), when initiated soon after an acute myocardial infarction, preserves left ventricular function and reduces mortality.

1. These drugs promote the dissolution of thrombi by stimulating the conversion of endogenous plasminogen to plasmin.

2. **Plasmin** is a proteolytic enzyme that hydrolyzes fibrin.

B. **Side Effects**

1. Spontaneous bleeding (especially intracranial hemorrhage) is the principal risk of thrombolytic therapy.

2. Bleeding is particularly likely in patients who have recently undergone surgery or invasive diagnostic procedures, emphasizing the fact that these drugs do not distinguish between the fibrin of a thrombus and the fibrin of a hemostatic plug.

3. Fever is common in treated patients, and allergic reactions may occur.

4. Steptokinase is less expensive than recombinant tissue plasminogen activator, but is more likely to cause hypotension and allergic reactions.

V. APROTININ

A. Aprotinin is a serine protease inhibitor that is isolated from bovine lung.

B. **Mechanism of Action**

1. High-dose aprotinin (2 million kallikrein inhibitor units [KIU]) inhibits fibrinolytic activity by virtue of its ability to inhibit proteases, such as trypsin, plasmin, and plasma and tissue kallikrein.

2. High-dose aprotinin may partially inhibit the intrinsic coagulation pathway while leaving the extrinsic pathway intact.

3. Low-dose aprotinin (1 million KIU) produces plasma

Table 27–5
Clinical Uses of Aprotinin

Acute pancreatitis

Shock syndromes

Hyperfibrinolytic hemorrhage

Decrease in intraoperative blood loss
  Repeat cardiac surgery requiring cardiopulmonary bypass
  Primary cardiac surgery in presence of a coagulopathy
  Total hip replacement

concentrations that are adequate to inhibit plasmin alone.

C. Clinical Uses (Table 27-5)

D. Side Effects

1. Aprotinin may alter whole blood clotting time in the presence of heparin (patients may require additional heparin, even in the presence of an ACT that appears to represent adequate anticoagulation).

   a. In patients being treated with aprotinin, additional heparin should be administered, either in a fixed dose or according to a dosage regimen based on body weight and duration of cardiopulmonary bypass.

   b. Alternatively, heparin can be administered on the basis of heparin levels measured by a method, such as protamine titration, that is not affected by aprotinin.

2. The activated PTT is significantly prolonged by aprotinin.

Chapter

28

Antibiotics

The therapeutic value and associated dangers of antibiotics are particularly relevant to the care of patients in the perioperative period and those in the intensive care unit who are at high risk for hospital-acquired infections. (Updated and revised from Stoelting RK. Antibiotics. In: Pharmacology and Physiology in Anesthetic Practice. 2nd ed. Philadelphia, JB Lippincott, 1991;477–503.) In seriously ill patients or patients with decreased immune defense mechanisms, selection of bactericidal rather than bacteriostatic antibiotics is often recommended (Table 28-1). Narrow-spectrum antibiotics should be considered, before broad-spectrum or combination antibiotic therapy is prescribed, to preserve normal bacterial flora of the patient (Table 28-2).

I. PROPHYLACTIC ANTIBIOTICS

    A. Prophylactic antibiotics are indicated for most of the commonly performed surgical procedures (Table 28-3).

    B. Cephalosporins are the antibiotics of choice for surgical procedures in which skin flora and the normal flora of the gastrointestinal and genitourinary tracts are the most likely pathogens.

    C. Timing of antibiotic administration must coincide with bacterial innoculation.

        1. Prolongation of prophylactic antibiotic therapy beyond the first postoperative day provides no additional protection.

        2. Pseudomembranous colitis is the most frequent complication of prophylactic antibiotics.

II. PENICILLINS

    A. The bactericidal action of penicillins reflects the ability of these antibiotics to interfere with the synthesis of peptidoglycan, which is an essential component of the cell walls of susceptible bacteria.

    B. Benzylpenicillin is the drug of choice for treat-

Table 28–1
Examples of Bactericidal and Bacteriostatic Antibiotics

Bactericidal	Bacteriostatic
Penicillins	Tetracyclines
Cephalosporins	Chloramphenicol
Aminoglycosides	Erythromycin
Colistin	Clindamycin
Vancomycin	Sulfonamides
Co-trimoxazole	

ing pneumococcal, streptococcal, meningococcal, and clostridial infections.

1. Most staphylococcal infections (60% to 80%) are caused by bacteria that produce penicillinase (an enzyme that hydrolyzes the beta-lactam ring of penicillin), and thus are resistant to treatment with most penicillins.
2. Transient bacteremia occurs in most patients undergoing dental extractions, emphasizing the importance of prophylactic penicillin in patients with congenital or acquired heart disease who undergo dental procedures.
3. **Route of Administration**
   a. Potassium salts of penicillin are most commonly administered intravenously, with 1.7 mEq of potassium being present in every 1 million units of

Table 28–2
Examples of Narrow-Spectrum and Broad-Spectrum Antibiotics

Narrow-Spectrum	Broad-Spectrum
Benzylpenicillin	Ampicillin
Erythromycin	Cephalosporins
Clindamycin	Aminoglycosides
	Tetracyclines
	Fluoroquinolones
	Azithromycin

Table 28–3
Examples of Surgical Procedures for Which a Benefit May Be Derived from Prophylactic Antibiotics

Gynecologic Surgery
    Cesarean section
    Hysterectomy—abdominal or vaginal

Orthopedic Surgery
    Arthroplasty of joints, including replacement
    Open reduction of fractures

General Surgery
    Cholecystectomy
    Colon surgery
    Appendectomy
    Gastric resection
    Penetrating abdominal trauma

Urologic Surgery

Surgery on Nose, Mouth, and Pharynx
    Tonsillectomy
    Incisions through oral or pharyngeal mucosa

Cardiothoracic and Vascular Surgery
    Coronary artery bypass graft
    Valve annuloplasty or replacement
    Pacemaker insertion
    Thoracotomy
    Peripheral vascular surgery (possible exception, carotid endarterectomy)

Neurosurgical Procedures
    Shunt procedures
    Craniotomy

---

      penicillin (may cause hyperkalemia in patients who are in renal failure).

    b. Penicillin is a potent convulsant when administered into the intrathecal space.

4. Excretion of penicillin is principally by renal tubular secretion.

5. Duration of action of penicillin is pronged by simultaneous administration of probenecid, which blocks renal tubular secretion of this antibiotic.

III. PENICILLINASE-RESISTANT PENICILLINS (methicillin, oxacillin, cloxacillin, nafcillin) are indicated for the treatment of infections caused by staphylococci that produce this enzyme.

IV. BROAD-SPECTRUM ANTIBIOTICS (ampicillin, carbenicillin) are bactericidal against gram-positive and gram-negative bacteria that do not produce penicillinase (therefore, they are ineffective in treating most staphylococcal infections).

V. ALLERGY TO PENICILLINS

    A. Allergic reactions (most often rash, rarely hypotension, bronchospasm, and laryngeal edema) occur in 1% to 10% of patients treated with penicillins, making these antibiotics the most allergenic of all drugs (penicillin accounts for 75% of fatal anaphylactic reactions).

    B. Patients allergic to penicillin are three to four times more likely to experience allergic reactions to other drugs unrelated to antibiotics.

    C. Cross-Reactivity

        1. The presence of a common nucleus (beta-lactam ring) in penicillins and cephalosporins means there is potential cross-reactivity between these antibiotics (it is estimated that 1.1% to 1.7% of patients who are allergic to penicillin are also allergic to cephalosporins).

        2. Cephalosporins are often selected for administration to patients with a history of cutaneous reaction following treatment with penicillins.

        3. Cephalosporins cannot be administered safely to patients with a history of an immediate or accelerated reaction (hypotension, bronchospasm, angioedema) to any of the penicillins.

VI. CEPHALOSPORINS

    A. Bacteria can produce cephalosporinases (beta-lactamases) that disrupt the beta-lactam ring structure of cephalosporins and thus inhibit their antibacterial activity.

        1. These drugs depend on renal excretion, emphasiz-

Table 28–4
Classification of Cephalosporins

First Generation
   Cefazolin
   Cephalexin
   Cephalothin

Second Generation
   Cefamandole
   Cefoxitin

Third Generation
   Cefotaxime
   Cefoperazone
   Ceftriaxone

ing the need to decrease the dose in the presence of renal dysfunction.

   2. Allergy to cephalosporins, as with penicillins, is the most common adverse response associated with administration of these antibiotics (occurs in less than 2% of patients, an incidence that is much less than that associated with penicillins).

B. Classification (Table 28–4)

VII. AMINOGLYCOSIDES

A. Aminoglycosides (streptomycin, gentamicin, tobramycin, amikacin, kanamycin, neomycin) are poorly lipid-soluble drugs that are rapidly bactericidal for aerobic gram-negative bacteria because of their ability to inhibit protein synthesis in bacterial ribosomes.

B. Route of Administration
   1. Poor lipid solubility results in poor absorption after oral administration and limited entrance into the central nervous system (intrathecal administration may be necessary).
   2. Rapid systemic absorption occurs after intramuscular injection.

C. Excretion of aminoglycosides is almost exclusively by glomerular filtration.

D. Side Effects (Table 28–5)
   1. Reappearance of neuromuscular blockade is a possibility if aminoglycosides are administered systemi-

Table 28–5
Side Effects of Aminoglycosides

Ototoxicity (vestibular and/or auditory dysfunction)

Nephrotoxicity (acute tubular necrosis)

Skeletal muscle weakness (decreased prejunctional release of acetylcholine and reduced postsynaptic sensitivity to the neurotransmitter)

Potentiation of nondepolarizing neuromuscular blocking drugs (penicillins, cephalosporins, tetracyclines, and erythromycin are devoid of effects at the neuromuscular junction)

cally in the early postoperative period to a patient who has been judged to have adequately recovered from neuromuscular blocking drugs administered during anesthesia.

2. Oral neomycin, which is used to decrease the bacterial population of the gastrointestinal tract prior to abdominal surgery, is unlikely to produce effects at the neuromuscular junction because this antibiotic is not absorbed into the systemic circulation.

VIII. VANCOMYCIN

A. Vancomycin is the only clinically effective treatment of methicillin-resistant staphylococcal infection.

1. Patients who are allergic to penicillins or cephalosporin antibiotics are likely to be treated with vancomycin when a staphylococcal infection is present.

2. Vancomycin is a useful antibiotic, especially in cardiac, orthopedic, and neurosurgical procedures involving implantation of a foreign body.

B. **Side Effects**

1. Accidental rapid intravenous infusion (recommended infusion time is 30 to 60 minutes) of vancomycin has been associated with profound hypotension and even cardiac arrest.

2. Hypotension is typically accompanied by signs of histamine release, often characterized by intense facial and truncal erythema (**"red-man syndrome"**).

3. Vancomycin can produce allergic reactions, presumably mediated by IgG and complement, which

are characterized by hypotension, erythema, and occasionally, bronchospasm.

4. Arterial hypoxemia may accompany the administration of vancomycin.

IX. TETRACYCLINES possess a wide range of antibiotic activity against gram-positive and gram-negative bacteria (myocoplasma, chlamydia, Rickettsia).

X. ERYTHROMYCIN is administered orally and is effective against *Haemophilus influenzae, Neisseria gonorrhoeae,* mycoplasma, streptococcal infections (pharyngitis), and pneumococcal pneumonia.

XI. CLINDAMYCIN resembles erythromycin in antibacterial activity except that it is more active against many anaerobic bacteria.

XII. POLYMYXIN AND COLISTIN are effective against gram-negative bacteria, including *Escherichia coli,* Klebsiella, and *Pseudomoras aeruginosa* (urinary tract infections).

XIII. FLUOROQUINOLONE ANTIBIOTICS (norfloxacin, aprofloxacin, ofloxacin) are bactericidal against most gram-positive and gram-negative bacteria.

XIV. AZITHROMYCIN is an azalide, belonging to a subclass of macrolide antibiotics that is distributed in tissues with resulting high concentrations in cells (phagocytes and fibroblasts) following oral administration. A total dose of 1.5 g (500 mg on day 1 and 250 mg on days 2–5) is effective against gram-positive and gram negative bacteria.

XV. BACITRACIN is effective typically against a variety of gram-positive bacteria.

XVI. SULFONAMIDES prevent normal use of para-aminobenzoic acid by bacteria to synthesize folic acid.

    A. Drug fever is a common side effect of sulfonamide treatment.

    B. Co-trimoxazole is a combination of trimethoprim

with sulfamethoxazole that results in synergistic antibacterial action (especially useful in treatment of urinary tract infections).

XVII. URINARY TRACT ANTISEPTICS (methenamine, nalidixic acid, nitrofurantoin, phenazopyridine) are concentrated in the renal tubules, making them effective for the treatment of infections in the kidney and bladder.

XVIII. DRUGS FOR TREATMENT OF TUBERCULOSIS

    A. Isoniazid is the primary drug for the chemotherapy of tuberculosis. It is used in combination with a second drug to offset the impact of resistance that commonly develops during therapy (alone, it is used for prophylaxis).

        1. Excretion is by metabolism (hepatic acetylation), with patients being categorized as rapid or slow acetylators (genetically determined).

        2. Side effects of isoniazid can be minimized by prophylactic therapy with pyridoxine (isoniazid increases excretion of this vitamin) (Table 28–6).

    B. Rifampin inhibits the growth of most gram-positive and gram-negative bacteria (used for prophylaxis against meningococcal disease).

        1. Rifampin is effective because of its ability to inhibit ribonucleic acid (RNA) synthesis in bacteria at concentrations below those that produce this effect in normal cells.

        2. Clearance of rifampin is by hepatic deacetylation, with the active metabolite entering the bile.

        3. Side effects of rifampin are infrequent but, with

Table 28–6
Side Effects of Isoniazid

Precipitation of seizures (especially in patients with a history of epilepsy)

Optic neuritis

Mental changes (euphoria, memory loss)

Excessive sedation (in slow acetylators)

Hepatotoxicity (reflected by liver transaminase levels)

Enhanced defluorination of volatile anesthetics

high doses, may include thrombocytopenia, anemia, hepatic dysfunction, and occasionally, hepatorenal syndrome.

   C. Ethambutol is tuberculostatic and is used in combination with isoniazid for the treatment of active tuberculosis.

   D. Multidrug-resistant tuberculosis is increasing in frequency and poses a unique threat to patients with decreased immune function.

      1. Excretion of ethambutol is highly dependent on renal function.

      2. Side effects of ethambutol include optic neuritis (dose-dependent) and decreased renal excretion of uric acid.

XIX. ANTIFUNGAL DRUGS

   A. Nystatin is a fungistatic and fungicidal antibiotic (used primarily to treat Candida infections) that lacks effects on bacteria (superinfections do not occur).

   B. Amphotericin B is the most effective antifungal drug for managing infections due to yeasts and fungi (cryptococcal infection of the lungs or meninges, histoplasmosis, coccidioidomycosis, blastomycosis, sporotrichosis, disseminated candidiasis).

      1. Oral absorption is poor, so the drug must be administered intravenously if therapeutic concentrations are to be achieved in infected tissues.

      2. Side Effects (Table 28–7)

   C. Glucytosine is converted to fluorouracil exclusively in fungal cells by the enzyme cytosine deaminase (se-

Table 28–7
Side Effects of Amphotericin B

Impaired renal function (monitoring of plasma creatinine concentrations recommended)
Hypokalemia
Hypomagnesemia
Fever, chills, dyspnea, and hypotension (during intravenous administration)
Allergic reactions
Seizures
Anemia and thrombocytopenia

lective effect avoids cytotoxicity of fluorouracil on normal cells).

1. Oral absorption is excellent, as is penetration into the cerebrospinal fluid and aqueous humor.
2. Renal excretion of unchanged drug is the principal route of elimination.
3. Hepatotoxicity may occur.

D. Griseofulvin

1. Mycotic diseases of the skin, hair, and nails respond to griseofulvin.
2. **Side effects** include headache, peripheral neuritis, fatigue, blurred vision, syncope, renal dysfunction, and hepatotoxicity.

XX. ANTIVIRAL DRUGS

A. Host cell surface receptors and enzymes that are unique for viruses provide a mechanism for the development of antiviral drugs with selective activity.

B. Idoxuridine

1. The antiviral activity of idoxuridine is mainly limited to DNA viruses; it is usually used for the topical treatment of herpes simplex keratitis lesions.
2. Rapid inactivation of nucleotidases precludes its administration by other than intravenous or topical routes.

C. Amantadine inhibits replication of influenza A virus and has prophylactic value (70% protection) when administered to persons who have had contact with an active case of the virus.

1. This drug also has therapeutic value in the treatment of patients with Parkinson's disease.
2. Amantadine accumulates in patients with impaired renal function, and excessive plasma concentrations are associated with central nervous system toxicity, including seizures and coma.

D. Vidarabine is effective in the treatment of herpes simplex encephalitis and keratoconjunctivitis (inhibits viral DNA polymerase).

E. Acyclovir, administered topically or orally, is effective in the initial and recurrent treatment of genital herpes.

F. Famciclovir and its active metabolite (penciclovir) are effective, when administered orally, in the treatment of acute, uncomplicated herpes zoster.

G. Zidovudine inhibits replication of some retroviruses

and is associated with a high incidence of granulocytopenia and anemia.

XXI. CYTOKINES

A. Cytokines are a group of polypeptides (synthesized in macrophages and monocytes) that includes the **interleukins** (IL 1-12), **tumor necrosis factor,** and **interferons.**

1. Interleukins control many aspects of immune and inflammatory responses (fever, myocardial depression, hypotension).

2. Tumor necrosis factor and IL-1 have been implicated as mediators of the sepsis syndrome and rheumatoid arthritis (a naturally occurring IL-1 receptor antagonist may have therapeutic value).

3. The principal cytokine released after surgery is IL-6.

4. Circulating concentrations of IL-6 are proportional to the severity of surgery (lower after laparoscopic cholecystectomy vs. laparotomy).

5. IL-6 stimulates protein synthesis in the liver (metabolic response) and plays an important role in inflammation.

Chapter

29

Chemotherapeutic Drugs

Effectiveness of chemotherapy requires that there be complete destruction (total cell-kill) of all cancer cells, because a single surviving clonogenic cell can give rise to sufficient progeny to ultimately kill the host. (Updated and revised from Stoelting RK. Chemotherapeutic drugs. In: Pharmacology and Physiology in Anesthetic Practice. 2nd ed. Philadelphia, JB Lippincott, 1991; 504–20.) The logical outgrowth of the recognition for the need of total cell-kill is the use of several chemotherapeutic drugs concurrently or in a planned sequence (allows administration of the largest possible doses of drugs, each working by different mechanisms and not sharing similar toxic effects). Often, **myelosuppression** is the dose-limiting factor for chemotherapeutic drugs.

I. CLASSIFICATION (Table 29-1)

A. Knowledge of drug-induced adverse effects and evaluation of appropriate laboratory tests (hemoglobin, platelet count, white blood cell count, coagulation profile, plasma electrolytes, liver and renal function tests, electrocardiogram, chest radiograph) may be useful in the preoperative evaluation of patients being treated with chemotherapeutic drugs.

1. Attention to asepsis is essential because immunosuppression makes these patients susceptible to iatrogenic infection.

2. A history of diarrhea may be associated with electrolyte disturbances and decreased intravascular fluid volume.

3. The response to inhaled and injected drugs may be altered by drug-induced cardiac, hepatic, or renal dysfunction.

4. The response to muscle relaxants may be prolonged by impaired renal function or drug-induced decreases in plasma cholinesterase activity.

Table 29–1
Classification of Chemotherapeutic Drugs and Associated Side Effects

	Immunosuppression	Thrombocytopenia	Leukopenia	Anemia	Cardiac Toxicity	Pulmonary Toxicity	Renal Toxicity	Hepatic Toxicity	Nervous System Toxicity	Stomatitis	Plasma Cholinesterase Inhibition
Alkylating Drugs											
Nitrogen Mustards											
Mechlorethamine	+	+++	+++			+			++		++
Cyclophosphamide	++++	+	++	+			+	+		+	++
Melphalan	+	++	++	++		+					+
Chlorambucil	+	++	++	++		+		+	+		+
Alkyl Sulfonates											
Busulfan	+	+++	+++	+++		++	++			+	+
Nitrosoureas											
Carmustine		++	++	++		+	+	+		++	
Lomustine		+++	+++	++				+		++	
Semustine		++	++	++				+		++	
Streptozocin		+	+	+			+++	+++			
Antimetabolites											
Folic Acid Analogues											
Methotrexate	+++	+++	+++	+++		+	++	+		+++	
Pyrimidine Analogues											
Fluorouracil	++++	+++	+++	+++					+	+++	
Cytarabine	+++	+++	+++			+		+		+	

Purine Analogues											
Mercaptopurine	+++	+++					++			++	+++
Azathioprine	++++	++++					++				
Thioguanine	+++	+					++		+++	+++	+++
Vinca Alkaloids											
Vinblastine	++	+		+			+			++	+
Vincristine	++	+		+			++		++	++	
Antibiotics											
Dactinomycin	++	+++	+++			+++	+++			+++	+++
Daunorubicin	+	+++	++			+++	++		+	+++	+++
Doxorubicin		+++	++			+++	++		+	+++	+++
Bleomycin		+	+		+++		+				+++
Plicamycin	+	+++++	++	+++	+++		++		++	++	+++
Mitomycin		+++	+++		+	+	++++		+	+	+++
Enzymes											
Asparaginase	++	+	+	+		+	+		+	+++	+
Synthetics											
Cisplatin	+	++	++			+	++	++++			
Hydroxyurea	++	+++	+++				++		+++		++
Procarbazine	+	++	+++				++		++		++
Mitotane											
Hormones											
Corticosteroids	+++	+++			+++						
Progestins											
Estrogens/Androgens											

+, minimal; ++, mild; +++, moderate; ++++, marked.

B. Alkylating Drugs (Table 29-1)

1. These chemotherapeutic drugs undergo electrophilic chemical reactions that result in formation of covalent linkages (alkylation) with various nucleophilic substances, principally deoxyribonucleic acid (DNA).

2. **Side Effects** (Table 29-1)

   a. Bone marrow suppression is the most important dose-limiting factor in the clinical use of alkylating drugs.

   b. All alkylating drugs are powerful central nervous system stimulants (nausea, vomiting, and seizures).

C. Antimetabolites (Table 29-1)

1. These drugs interact with specific enzymes, leading to inhibition of that enzyme and subsequent synthesis of an aberrant molecule that cannot function normally.

2. **Side Effects** (Table 29-1)

   a. The principal targets for the antimetabolite chemotherapeutic drugs are the proliferating bone marrow cells and gastrointestinal cells.

   b. Most of these drugs are also potent immunosuppressants.

D. Vinca Alkaloids (Table 29-1)

1. Vinca alkaloids bind with an essential protein component of microtubules, arresting cell division in metaphase.

2. **Clinical Uses**

   a. The most important clinical use of vinblastine is with bleomycin and cisplatin in the treatment of metastatic testicular tumors.

   b. Lymphomas, including Hodgkin's disease, are responsive to these drugs (rapid onset of vinca alkaloids often necessitates the concomitant administration of allopurinol to prevent the complications of hyperuricemia).

3. **Side effects** include myelosuppression, alopecia, skeletal muscle weakness, and peripheral neuropathy.

E. Antibiotics (Table 29-1)

1. **Daunorubicin and doxorubicin** may produce a unique dose-related cardiomyopathy (when doxorubicin is given by intermittent bolus injection, the risk of cardiac toxicity is probably less than 3% with a cumulative dose of less than 400 mg·m^2 of body surface area) (Table 29-2).

2. **Bleomycin** may produce dose-dependent **pulmonary toxicity** in 5% to 10% of treated patients (Table 29-3).

   a. Enhanced pulmonary toxicity in the presence of bleo-

Table 29–2
Anthracycline Antibiotics and Cardiomyopathy

Acute Cardiomyopathy
  Benign and transient, manifesting principally as changes on the electrocardiogram (nonspecific ST-T changes and decreased QRS voltage)

Rapidly Progressive Cardiomyopathy
  Insidious onset (dry, productive cough)
  Irreversible congestive heart failure
  High mortality

---

  mycin therapy and high concentrations of oxygen has not been a consistent observation.
  b. Replacement of fluids with colloids, rather than crystalloids, is intended to decrease the likelihood of pulmonary interstitial edema in bleomycin-treated patients undergoing surgery (accumulation of interstitial fluid may reflect impaired lymphatic function caused by bleomycin-induced fibrotic changes in the lung).
F. Enzymes (Table 29-1)
G. Synthetics (Table 29-1)
H. Hormones (Table 29-1)

Table 29–3
Bleomycin-Induced Pulmonary Toxicity

Mild Pulmonary Toxicity
  Exertional dyspnea and normal resting PaO_2 values

Severe Pulmonary Toxicity
  Interstitial pneumonitis and fibrosis
  Increased alveolar-to-arterial difference for oxygen
  Decreased pulmonary diffusion capacity

Chapter

30

Antiepileptic Drugs

The antiepileptic drug selected to treat epilepsy is determined by the characteristics of the seizure experienced by the patient (Table 30-1). (Updated and revised from Stoelting RK. Antiepileptic drugs. In: Pharmacology and Physiology in Anesthetic Practice. 2nd ed. Philadelphia, JB Lippincott, 1991;521-9.) The incidence of epilepsy (a collective term used to designate a group of chronic central nervous system disorders characterized by the sudden onset of disturbances of sensory, motor, autonomic, or psychic origin) is between 0.3% to 0.6% of the population. The disturbances associated with epilepsy are usually transient and are almost always associated with abnormal discharges on the electroencephalogram.

I. MECHANISM OF SEIZURE ACTIVITY

A. Seizure activity in most patients with epilepsy has a localized or focal origin, and the spread of seizure activity to neighboring cells is presumably restrained by normal inhibitory mechanisms.

B. If the spread of a seizure focus into areas of normal brain is sufficiently extensive, the entire brain is activated and a tonic-clonic seizure with unconsciousness ensues (if the spread is localized, the seizure produces signs and symptoms characteristic of the anatomic focus).

II. MECHANISM OF DRUG ACTION

A. Most antiepileptic drugs act by decreasing the spread of excitation from a seizure focus to normal neurons.

B. Complete drug-induced control of seizures can be achieved in up to 50% of patients treated with antiepileptic drugs (Table 30-2).

Table 30–1
Selection of Drug Based on Seizure Type

Seizure Type	Drug Therapy
Focal seizures	Phenytoin Phenobarbital Primidone Carbamazepine
Petit mal (absence) seizures	Ethosuximide Valproic acid Clonazepam
Grand mal (tonic-clonic) seizures	Phenytoin Phenobarbital Carbamazepine Valproic acid
Myoclonic seizures	Valproic acid Clonazepam Corticosteroids

III. PLASMA CONCENTRATIONS (Table 30-3)

IV. HYDANTOINS (Table 30-2)

A. **Phenytoin** is the prototype of hydantoins and is the drug administered for treatment of focal seizures and grand mal seizures.
  1. The antiepileptic activity of phenytoin is not accompanied by sedation.
  2. **Mechanism of Action**
     a. Phenytoin limits the development and spread of activity from a seizure focus by exerting a stabilizing effect on neuron cell membranes, especially in the cerebral cortex.
     b. This stabilizing effect is most likely a result of drug-induced alterations in the movement of ions (decreased flux of sodium ions during action potentials) across cell membranes.
  3. **Pharmacokinetics** (Table 30-3)
  4. **Side Effects** (Table 30-4)

V. BARBITURATES (Table 30-2)

A. **Phenobarbital** is effective in the suppression of grand mal epilepsy and focal epilepsy and is the drug used

Table 30–2
Antiepileptic Drugs

Hydantoins	Valproic acid
Phenytoin	Oxazolidinediones
Mephenytoin	Trimethadione
Phenacemide	Paramethadione
Barbiturates	Benzodiazepines
Phenobarbital	Clonazepam
Mephobarbital	Diazepam
Metharbital	Acetazolamide
Primidone	
Carbamazepine	
Succinimides	
Ethosuximide	
Methsuximide	
Phensuximide	

most frequently for prophylaxis against the recurrence of febrile seizures.

   1. Pharmacokinetics (Table 30-3)
   2. Side Effects (Table 30-5)

VI. PRIMIDONE is a deoxybarbiturate that is principally used in the treatment of focal epilepsy

   A. Pharmacokinetics (Table 30-3)
   B. Side effects of primidone include sedation, nystagmus, vertigo, nausea, and vomiting.

VII. CARBAMAZEPINE is useful in the treatment of psychomotor epilepsy and the management of patients with trigeminal and glossopharyngeal neuralgias.

   A. Pharmacokinetics (Table 30-3)
   B. Side effects of carbamazepine include sedation, vertigo, diplopia, nausea, vomiting, and ataxia. Less common toxic effects require monitoring of bone marrow, hepatic, and renal function in patients treated with this drug.

VIII. SUCCINIMIDES (Table 30-2)

   A. Ethosuximide has a characteristic effect on thalamocortical excitation which is presumed to be important in the etiology of petit mal epilepsy.

Table 30-3
Pharmacokinetics of Antiepileptic Drugs

	Plasma Therapeutic Concentration ($\mu g \cdot ml^{-1}$)	Protein Binding (%)	Volume of Distribution ($L \cdot kg^{-1}$)	Elimination Half-Time (b)	Clearance ($ml \cdot kg^{-1} \cdot min^{-1}$)	Site of Clearance and Percent
Phenytoin	10–20	90	0.64	24	Dose-dependent	Hepatic, 98%
Phenobarbital	10–20	40–60	0.8	90	0.09	Hepatic, 75% Renal, 25%
Primidone	5–10	20	0.8	8	0.78	Hepatic, 60% Renal, 40%
Carbamazepine	4–12	80	1.4	13–17	0.58	Hepatic, 98%
Ethosuximide	40–100	NS	0.72	60	0.26	Hepatic, 80% Renal, 20%
Valproic Acid	50–100	80–90	0.13	12	0.12	Hepatic, >70%
Clonazepam	0.02–0.08	50	3.2	24–36	0.92	Hepatic, 98%

NS, not significant.

Table 30–4
Side Effects of Phenytoin

Cerebellar-vestibular dysfunction (nystagmus, ataxis, diplopia, vertigo)

Peripheral neuropathy

Gingival hyperplasia

Allergic reactions

Megaloblastic anemia

Gastrointestinal irritation

Hyperglycemia

---

1. **Pharmacokinetics** (Table 30-3)
2. **Side effects** of ethosuximide include nausea, vomiting, sedation, headache, and hiccup.

IX. VALPROIC ACID

A. Valproic acid is a branched chain carboxylic acid that is effective in the treatment of petit mal epilepsy.
   1. **Pharmacokinetics** (Table 30-3)
   2. **Side Effects**
      a. Nausea and vomiting are uncommon, and sedation and ataxia are less frequent than after administration of other antiepileptic drugs.
      b. Valproic acid may affect platelet aggregation, so bleeding time is often determined prior to initiating therapy.
      c. The ketone test may show a false-positive result

Table 30–5
Side Effects of Phenobarbital

Sedation (tolerance develops with chronic therapy)

Possible hyperactivity in children and confusion in the elderly

Scarlatiniform rash

Megaloblastic anemia

Nystagmus and ataxia

Congenital malformations

Drug interactions (enzyme induction)

because valproic acid is partly eliminated as a
ketone-containing metabolite.
   d. Liver function is often monitored, as chronic therapy with valproic acid may produce hepatotoxicity.

X. OXAZOLIDINEDIONES (Table 30-2)

   A. Thalamic nuclei are particularly sensitive to these drugs,
which is consistent with the speculated importance of
the thalamocortical system in the etiology of petit mal
epilepsy.
   B. Pharmacokinetics
   1. Trimethadione is metabolized in the liver to an
active metabolite, dimethadione, which is responsible for its antiepileptic activity.
   2. Paramethadione undergoes demethylation in the
liver to an active metabolite that is responsible for
its antiepileptic activity.

XI. BENZODIAZEPINES (Table 30-2)

   A. Clonazepam is useful in the treatment of petit mal
epilepsy, as well as myoclonic seizures in children.
   1. Pharmacokinetics (Table 30-3)
   2. Side Effects (Table 30-6)
   B. Diazepam is effective in the treatment of status epilepticus and local anesthetic-induced seizures (0.1 mg·kg^{-1}
IV every 5 to 10 minutes until seizure activity has been
suppressed).

XII. ACETAZOLAMIDE is a carbonic anhydrase inhibitor that
may be effective in the treatment of petit mal epilepsy.

Table 30–6
Side Effects of Clonazepam

Sedation (tends to subside with chronic therapy)

Ataxia

Behavioral disturbances (hyperactivity, irritability)

Salivary and bronchial secretions

Status epilepticus with abrupt discontinuation

Chapter

31

Drugs Used for Treatment of Parkinson's Disease

The goal of treating Parkinson's disease is to enhance the inhibitory effect of dopamine (inhibitory neurotransmitter) or reduce the stimulating effect of acetylcholine (excitatory neurotransmitter) on the extrapyramidal system by the administration of centrally acting drugs. (Updated and revised from Stoelting RK. Drugs used for treatment of Parkinson's disease. In: Pharmacology and Physiology in Anesthetic Practice. 2nd ed. Philadelphia, JB Lippincott, 1991;530–5.) Regardless of the drug(s) selected, treatment of Parkinson's disease is always palliative, emphasizing that therapy does not halt progression of neuronal degeneration.

In patients with Parkinson's disease, the basal ganglia content of dopamine is only approximately 10% of normal. As a result, there is an excess of excitatory cholinergic activity manifesting as tremor, skeletal muscle rigidity, bradykinesia, and disturbances of posture. In addition to these classic peripheral manifestations, many afflicted patients become mentally depressed and some develop cognitive and mental deficits that may progress to delirium.

I. LEVODOPA

    A. Levodopa, as the immediate metabolic precursor of dopamine, acts by replenishing the depleted stores of dopamine in the basal ganglia.

        1. The usual daily maintenance dosage of levodopa is 3 to 8 g administered orally in at least four divided doses.

        2. Abrupt discontinuation of levodopa therapy may result in a precipitous return of symptoms of Parkinson's disease (levodopa should be continued throughout the perioperative period, being included in the preoperative medication).

B. **Metabolism**

1. Approximately 95% of orally administered levodopa is rapidly decarboxylated to dopamine by a hepatic first-pass effect, reflecting the activity of the enzyme dopa decarboxylase.

   a. The resulting dopamine cannot easily cross the blood–brain barrier to exert a beneficial therapeutic effect, whereas increased plasma concentrations of dopamine often lead to undesirable side effects (nausea, vomiting, cardiac dysrhythmias).

   b. Inhibition of the peripheral activity of dopa decarboxylase enzyme (see Section II) greatly increases the fraction of administered levodopa that remains available to cross the blood–brain barrier.

2. Most of the metabolites of levodopa (dopamine and its metabolite, homovanillac acid) are excreted by the kidneys.

3. Urinary metabolites of levodopa may cause a false-positive test result for ketoacidosis.

C. **Side Effects** (Table 31-1)

D. **Drug Interactions** (Table 31-2)

II. CARBIDOPA

A. Carbidopa inhibits the peripheral enzyme activity of dopa decarboxylase, which results in more levodopa being available to enter the central nervous system, where it is converted to dopamine.

1. Carbidopa does not cross the blood–brain barrier, so enzyme activity in the brain is not altered.

2. The combination of carbidopa with levodopa allows a decrease of up to 75% in the dose of levodopa while at the same time reducing the likelihood of dose-dependent side effects resulting from high plasma concentrations of dopamine.

B. Administered alone, carbidopa lacks pharmacologic activity.

III. AMANTADINE

A. Amantadine is an antiviral drug that produces symptomatic improvement in patients with Parkinson's disease, presumably by facilitating the release of dopamine from intact dopaminergic terminals (also delays uptake back into nerve endings and exerts anticholinergic effects).

Table 31–1
Side Effects of Dopamine

Gastrointestinal Dysfunction
Nausea and vomiting (dopamine-induced stimulation of the chemoreceptor trigger zone)

Abnormal Involuntary Movements
Faciolingual tics
Grimacing
Rocking movements
Irregular gasping breathing pattern (dyskinesia of the diaphragm)

Behavioral Disturbances
Confusion
Delirium

Cardiovascular Changes *(alpha and beta effects of dopamine)*
Cardiac dysrhythmias (propranolol an effective treatment)
Orthostatic hypotension

Endocrine Effects
Inhibition of prolactin secretion
Hypokalemia (associated with increased levels of aldosterone)

Decreased Anesthetic Requirements *(not a consistent finding)*

Table 31–2
Drug Interactions and Levodopa Treatment

Antagonists for Effects of Dopamine
Phenothiazines
Butyrophenones (droperidol may provoke severe skeletal muscle rigidity)
Metoclopramide

Inhibitors of Catecholamine Inactivation
Monoamine oxidase inhibitors (hypertension and hyperthermia)

Synergistic Actions
Anticholinergic drugs

Enhancement of Dopa-Decarboxylase Activity
Pyridoxine (present in multivitamin preparations)

   B. More than 90% of amantadine is excreted unchanged by the kidneys, necessitating dosage adjustments in patients with renal dysfunction.
   C. Side Effects (Table 31–3)

IV. BROMOCRIPTINE

   A. Bromocriptine is a direct-acting dopamine receptor agonist that is used most often to supplement treatment regimens that depend primarily on levodopa.
   B. Extensive hepatic first-pass metabolism occurs, and most of the metabolites are excreted in the bile.
   C. Less than 10% of bromocriptine is excreted unchanged or as inactive metabolites in the urine.

V. SELEGILINE

   A. Selegiline is a highly selective inhibitor of monoamine oxidase type B enzyme and is effective in the treatment of Parkinson's disease by virtue of its inhibition of the intercerebral metabolism of dopamine (maximizes the therapeutic efficacy of dopamine).
   B. Selegiline does not alter the peripheral metabolism of norepinephrine, which minimizes the likelihood of adverse responses during anesthesia in response to sympathomimetics.
   C. Dyskinesia is the most common side effect of treatment with selegiline.

VI. ANTICHOLINERGIC DRUGS

   A. Centrally acting anticholinergic drugs (benztropine, cycrimine, trihexyphenidyl) are presumed to blunt the effects of the excitatory neurotransmitter acetylcholine.

   B. Trihexyphenidyl is particularly useful in reducing the

Table 31–3
Side Effects of Amantadine

Difficulty concentrating
Enhancement of the effects of anticholinergic drugs
Livedo reticularis
Erythromelalgia

tremor and excess salivation associated with Parkinson's disease.

1. Side effects are less prominent than with atropine, but may include mydriasis, cycloplegia, dry mouth, tachycardia, sedation, and confusion.
2. The mydriatic effect of this drug could precipitate acute glaucoma in a susceptible patient.

32

Drugs Used to Treat Hyperlipoproteinemia

Elevation of blood cholesterol is a major risk factor for the development of atherosclerosis and, in particular for death from coronary artery disease and nonhemorrhagic stroke. (Updated and revised from Stoelting RK. Drugs used to treat hyperlipoproteinemia. In: Pharmacology and Physiology in Anesthetic Practice. 2nd ed. Philadelphia, JB Lippincott, 1991:536–40.) Because low-density lipoproteins (LDL) are the principal cholesterol-carrying lipoproteins in plasma, there is a predictable association between increases in the plasma concentrations of LDL cholesterol and accelerated atherogenesis (coronary artery disease). Removal of LDL cholesterol from the plasma occurs principally by attachment to LDL receptors on the surfaces of liver cells. Synthesis of these receptors is genetically determined, with one gene inherited from each patient (heterozygous in approximately 1 in 500 patients and plasma cholesterol levels are about twice the normal level). Decreasing risk factors, especially cessation of smoking and control of hypertension, in combination with efforts to lower plasma concentrations of cholesterol will decrease the risk of coronary artery disease. It is estimated that 15% to 20% of the population has hypercholesterolemia.

I. DRUGS THAT LOWER PLASMA CONCENTRATIONS OF CHOLESTEROL (Table 32–1)

A. Nicotinic Acid
1. Nicotinic acid is a water-soluble vitamin that lowers plasma concentrations of LDL cholesterol by 10% to 15%.
2. **Side Effects** (Table 32–2)

B. Clofibrate characteristically decreases plasma concentrations of triglycerides.

C. Cholestyramine is the chloride salt of an ion exchange resin that lowers LDL cholesterol levels and decreases mor-

Table 32–1
Drugs that Lower Plasma Concentrations of Cholesterol*

Nicotinic acid

Clofibrate

Gemfibrozil

Cholestyramine

Colestipol

Probucol

Lovastatin

Compactin

Dextrothyroxine

---

*Dietary regulation and weight reduction must continue during drug therapy.

---

bidity and mortality associated with coronary artery disease.
  1. **Side effects** include abdominal pain, constipation (offset with high fluid intake), and impairment of absorption of fat-soluble vitamins (hypoprothrombinemia).
  2. **Hyperchloremic acidosis** can occur because cholestyramine is a chloride form of an ion exchange resin.
  D. **Probucol** lowers LDL cholesterol levels and also provides a protective effect against atherogenesis by acting as an antioxidant (inhibition of LDL oxidation).
  E. **Lovastatin** is a fungal metabolite that acts as a specific and reversible inhibitor of the rate-limiting enzyme for the synthesis of cholesterol.

Table 32–2
Side Effects of Nicotinic Acid

Hepatic dysfunction

Hyperglycemia

Gout

Cutaneous flushing (prostaglandin release)

Pruritus

---

1. Inhibition of cholesterol synthesis in the liver triggers an increase in synthesis of hepatic LDL surface receptors, leading to an increase in hepatic uptake of cholesterol and a subsequent lowering of the plasma concentrations of LDL cholesterol.
2. **Pharmacokinetics.** Lovastatin undergoes extensive hepatic metabolism, and metabolites are excreted through the biliary tract.

33
Central Nervous System Stimulants and Muscle Relaxants

Drugs that stimulate the central nervous system as their primary action are classified as analeptics (convulsants) (Table 33-1). (Updated and revised from Stoelting RK. Central nervous system stimulants and muscle relaxants. In: Pharmacology and Physiology in Anesthetic Practice. 2nd ed. Philadelphia, JB Lippincott, 1991: 541-8.) Centrally acting muscle relaxants act in the central nervous system or directly on skeletal muscles to relieve spasticity (Table 33-1).

I. CENTRAL NERVOUS SYSTEM STIMULANTS

A. **Doxapram** is a centrally acting analeptic that selectively increases minute ventilation by activating the carotid bodies (stimulant effect on the medullary respiratory center is absent).

1. Doxapram, 1 mg·kg^{-1} IV, produces a transient increase in ventilation (due more to tidal volume than to breathing frequency) similar to that produced by a PaO$_2$ of 38 mmHg acting on the carotid bodies.

a. There is a large margin of safety, as the dose that stimulates ventilation is 20 to 40 times less than that which produces seizures.

b. Continuous infusion of doxapram (2 to 3 mg·min^{-1}), as required to produce a sustained effect on ventilation (single intravenous dose lasts 5 to 10 minutes), often results in evidence of subconvulsive central nervous system stimulation (hypertension, tachycardia, cardiac dysrhythmias, vomiting, increased body temperature).

Table 33–1
Classification of Centrally Acting Stimulants and Relaxants

Central Nervous System Stimulants
Doxapram
Methylphenidate
Methylxanthines
    Theophylline
    Theobromine
    Caffeine
Nicotine
Almitrine

Centrally Acting Muscle Relaxants
Mephenesin
Benzodiazepines
Baclofen
Cyclobenzaprine
Dantrolene

       c. Doxapram is extensively metabolized, with less than 5% of an intravenous dose being excreted unchanged in the urine.

    2. Clinical Uses (Table 33-2)

  B. Methylphenidate is useful in the treatment of hyperkinetic syndromes in children and may be effective in the treatment of narcolepsy, either alone or in combination with tricyclic antidepressants.

  C. Methylxanthines are represented by theophylline (see Chapter 12), theobromine, and caffeine.

    1. Clearance of methylxanthines is greatly prolonged in the neonate compared with that in the adult (important to consider when methylxanthines are used as analeptics to treat primary apnea of prematurity).

Table 33–2
Clinical Uses of Doxapram

Maintenance of ventilation during administration of supplemental oxygen to patients with chronic obstructive pulmonary disease (not indicated for drug-induced coma or acute exacerbation of chronic lung disease)

Arousal from residual effects of inhaled anesthetics (transient, nonspecific)

    2. Caffeine is present in a variety of beverages and non-prescription medications (common cold remedies, in an attempt to offset the sedating effects of antihistamines) (Table 33-3).
      a. Postdural puncture headache may respond to caffeine, 300 mg orally (presumably reflects a cerebral vasoconstrictor effect).
      b. Postoperative headache may reflect the effects of caffeine withdrawal in susceptible patients.
D. Nicotine is a highly addictive substance (withdrawal syndrome) that is readily absorbed (respiratory, buccal, skin) and undergoes extensive metabolism, principally in the liver, to **cotinine.**
    1. Effects on Organ Systems (Table 33-4)
    2. Overdose (fatal dose about 60 mg, one cigarette delivers up to 2.5 mg) from nicotine (vomiting, hypotension, intercostal muscle paralysis) requires supportive treatment.
E. Almitrine
    1. Almitrine is a peripheral chemoreceptor agonist that improves PaO_2 and decreases $PaCO_2$ in patients with chronic respiratory failure.
    2. It is presumed that this improvement in gas exchange is due to enhancement of hypoxic pulmonary vasoconstriction.

Table 33-3
Caffeine Content of Common Substances

	Caffeine (mg)
Coffee (150 ml)	66-142
Tea (150 ml)	15-47
Cocoa (150 ml)	13
Coca Cola (360 ml)	65
Pepsi-Cola (360 ml)	43
Dr. Pepper (360 ml)	61
Mountain Dew (360 ml)	55
Candy Bar (1.2 oz)	5
No-Doz	100

(Data from Bunker ML, McWilliams M. Caffeine content of common beverages. J Am Diet Assoc 1979;74:28-32; with permission.)

Table 33–4
Effects of Nicotine on Organ Systems

Central Nervous System
  Tremor
  Increased ventilation (carotid and aortic bodies)

Cardiovascular System
  Peripheral vasoconstriction
  Hypertension
  Tachycardia

Gastrointestinal Tract
  Vomiting and diarrhea

II. CENTRALLY ACTING MUSCLE RELAXANTS

A. **Baclofen** is an analogue of gamma-aminobutyric acid that may be administered for treatment of spasticity resulting from disease (multiple sclerosis) or injury of the spinal cord.

1. Use of baclofen is limited by its side effects (sedation, skeletal muscle weakness, confusion).

2. Sudden discontinuation of chronic baclofen therapy may result in tachycardia and both auditory and visual hallucinations.

B. **Dantrolene** produces skeletal muscle relaxation by a direct action on excitation-contraction coupling, presumably by decreasing the amount of calcium released from the sarcoplasmic reticulum (neuromuscular transmission and electrical properties of skeletal muscle membranes are not altered).

1. Therapeutic doses have little or no effect on cardiac and smooth muscles.

2. **Pharmacokinetics**

   a. Absorption of dantrolene from the gastrointestinal tract, as well as intravenous injection (may cause phlebitis owing to alkalinity of drug solution), provides sustained dose-related plasma concentrations of drug (Figs. 33–1 and 33–2).

   b. Diuresis may accompany intravenous administration of dantrolene, reflecting the addition of mannitol to the dantrolene powder to make the solution isotonic (urinary catheter may be recommended).

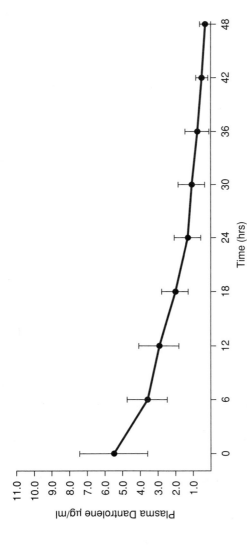

FIGURE 33–1. Plasma dantrolene concentrations following induction of anesthesia (time 0) and until 48 hours postoperatively in 10 malignant hyperthermia-susceptible patients. The total dose of dantrolene was 5 mg·kg⁻¹, administered orally in three or four divided doses, with the last dose given 4 hours before induction of anesthesia. All patients had plasma concentrations of dantrolene exceeding 2.8 μg·ml⁻¹ for at least 6 hours following induction of anesthesia. (From Allen GC, Cattrain CB, Peterson RG, Lakende M. Plasma levels of dantrolene following oral administration in malignant hyperthermia-susceptible patients. Anesthesiology 1988;67:900-4; with permission.)

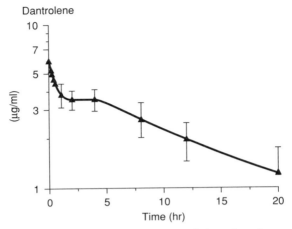

FIGURE 33–2. Plasma concentrations of dantrolene in venous blood following induction of anesthesia and administration of dantrolene, 2.4 mg·kg^{-1} IV, to 10 children. Mean ± SD. (From Lerman J, McLeod ME, Strong HA. Pharmacokinetics of intravenous dantrolene in children. Anesthesiology 1989;70:625–9; with permission.)

Table 33–5
Clinical Uses of Dantrolene

Skeletal muscle spasticity

Prophylaxis in patients susceptible to malignant hyperthermia*
    Dantrolene, 5 mg·kg^{-1} orally, in three or four divided doses every
    6 hours with the last dose 4 hours preoperatively
                                    or
    Dantrolene, 2.4 mg·kg^{-1} IV (over 10 to 30 minutes), just prior to
    induction of anesthesia

Treatment of malignant hyperthermia
    Dantrolene, 2 mg·kg^{-1} IV, until symptoms subside or a cumulative
    dose of 10 mg·kg^{-1} is reached

*Known triggering drugs must also be avoided.

Table 33–6
Side Effects of Dantrolene

Skeletal muscle weakness

Nausea

Diarrhea

Uterine atony

Hepatitis*

Pleural effusion*

*Occur only with chronic therapy.

    c. Dantrolene is metabolized in the liver, principally to 5-hydroxydantrolene (weakly active), and less than 1% of the drug appears unchanged in the urine.

    d. Blood levels of dantrolene of at least 2.8 $\mu g \cdot ml^{-1}$ are recommended when the drug is being administered for prophylaxis against or treatment of malignant hyperthermia.

3. Clinical Uses (Table 33–5)

4. Side Effects (Table 33–6)

Chapter

34
Vitamins

Vitamins are a group of structurally diverse organic substances that must be provided in the diet (supplemental vitamins being unnecessary in the presence of a balanced diet) for the subsequent synthesis of cofactors that are essential for various metabolic reactions. (Updated and revised from Stoelting RK. Vitamins. In: Pharmacology and Physiology in Anesthetic Practice. 2nd ed. Philadelphia, JB Lippincott, 1991:549–59.) Dietary vitamin supplements are medically indicated only for specific situations (Table 34–1).

Table 34–1
Medical Indications for Dietary Vitamin Supplements

Inadequate intake (socioeconomic conditions, self-imposed dieting)
Malabsorption (liver and biliary tract disease, diarrhea, alcoholism)
Increased needs (parturients, infants)
Antibiotic therapy (synthesis of vitamin K)
Hyperalimentation

I. WATER-SOLUBLE VITAMINS (Table 34-2)

II. FAT-SOLUBLE VITAMINS (Table 34-3)

A. Fat-soluble vitamins are metabolized slowly and excessive ingestion may produce toxic effects.

B. **Vitamin D,** despite its name, functions as a hormone.

C. **Vitamin K**
1. **Replacement therapy** is not effective when severe hepatocellular disease is responsible for decreased production of clotting factors.
2. **Phytonadione,** 10 to 20 mg orally, or administered intravenously at a rate of 1 mg·min^{-1} (associated risks of hypotension and bronchospasm), is usually adequate to reverse the effects of oral anticoagulants in adults.

(text continues on page 411)

Table 34–2
Classification of Water-Soluble Vitamins

	Causes of Deficiency	Symptoms of Deficiency	Treatment of Deficiency
Vitamin B Complex			
Thiamine (B_1)	Increased metabolic rate (hyperalimentation, parturients, lactation)	Beriberi Korsakoff's syndrome	Oral or intravenous supplementation
Riboflavin (B_2)		Pharyngitis Angular stomatitis Glossitis Peripheral neuropathy	Oral supplementation
Nicotinic acid (Niacin)	Tryptophan-deficient corn diets (alcoholism) Carcinoid syndrome	Pellagra	Supplementation of flour with nicotinic acid
Pyridoxine (B_6)	Alcoholism Isoniazid Hydralazine	Seizures Peripheral neuropathy Anemia	Oral supplementation

Pantothenic acid Biotin	Rarely occurs Hyperalimentation	Glossitis Anorexia Dermatitis	Oral or intravenous supplementation
Cyanocobalamin (B_{12})	Gastric achlorhydria Inadequate intrinsic factor Bacterial overgrowth Resection of the ileum Nitrous oxide (see Chapter 2)	Megaloblastic (pernicious) anemia Demyelination Psychosis (elderly patients)	Oral or intramuscular supplementation Folic acid
Folic acid	Alcoholism Methotrexate Phenytoin	Megaloblastic anemia	Oral supplementation
Ascorbic acid (vitamin C)	Alcoholism Hyperalimentation Sepsis	Scurvy	Oral supplementation

Table 34-3
Classification of Fat-Soluble Vitamins

	Causes of Deficiency	Symptoms of Deficiency	Treatment of Deficiency	Symptoms of Toxicity
Vitamin A	Diet inadequate in milk, fruits, vegetables	Night blindness Hyperkeratosis Urinary calculi Spontaneous abortion Respiratory infections	Dietary or oral supplements	Increased intracranial pressure Osteoblastic activity leading to hypercalcemia Hepatosplenomegaly
Vitamin D	Inadequate bile salts or sunlight Phenytoin	Hypocalcemia Rickets Osteomalacia		Hypercalcemia (polyuria, polydipsia, proteinuria) Skeletal muscle weakness)
Vitamin E (Tocopherol)	Only limited evidence exists that vitamin E is nutritionally significant or of any value in therapy as an antioxidant.			
Vitamin K	Inadequate bile salts Inadequate bacterial flora owing to antibiotics Liver disease Neonates Hyperalimentation	Decreased plasma concentrations of factors II, VII, IX, and X (prolonged prothrombin time) Ecchymoses Spontaneous bleeding	Vitamin K (phytonadione, menadione)	

    a. The oral and intramuscular routes of administration for phytonadione are less likely than the intravenous route to cause side effects and are thus preferred for nonemergency reversal of oral anticoagulants.

    b. Even large doses of phytonadione are ineffective against heparin-induced anticoagulation.

Chapter

35

Minerals

Many minerals function as essential constituents of enzymes and regulate a variety of physiologic functions (Table 35-1). (Updated and revised from Stoelting RK. Minerals. In: Pharmacology and Physiology in Anesthetic Practice. 2nd ed. Philadelphia, JB Lippincott, 1991:560-9.) In the absence of absorption abnormalities, severe mineral deficiency is unlikely because most minerals, with the exception of zinc, are present in foods. Nevertheless, iron deficiency is common, especially in infants and females consuming inadequate diets. Mineral deficiencies may develop during prolonged hyperalimentation.

I. **CALCIUM** is present in the body in greater amounts than any other mineral.
   A. The plasma concentration of calcium is maintained between 4.5 and 5.5 $mEq \cdot L^{-1}$ (8.5 to 10.5 $mg \cdot dl^{-1}$) by an endogenous control system that includes vitamin D, parathyroid hormone, and calcitonin.
      1. **Ionized calcium** represents about 45% of the total plasma concentration (normal plasma ionized calcium concentration is 2 to 2.5 $mEq \cdot L^{-1}$), and is responsible for the presence or absence of physiologic effects of calcium.
         a. Acidosis increases and alkalosis decreases the plasma ionized calcium concentration.
         b. Albumin in plasma binds nonionized calcium (hypocalcemia owing to hypoproteinemia is not accompanied by symptoms unless the plasma ionized fraction of calcium is also decreased).
      2. **Role of Calcium** (Table 35-2)
      3. **Cardiovascular Effects**
         a. Calcium chloride (7 $mg \cdot kg^{-1}$ IV) transiently increases myocardial contractility and cardiac output and decreases calculated systemic vascular resistance.
         b. Volatile anesthetics may induce myocardial de-

Table 35–1
Physiologic Functions of Minerals

Maintenance of osmotic pressure

Transport of oxygen

Skeletal muscle contraction

Integrity of the central nervous system

Growth and maintenance of tissues and bones

Hematopoiesis

        pression by inhibiting calcium uptake by the sarcoplasmic reticulum.

B. Hypocalcemia (plasma calcium concentration lower than 4.5 mEq·L^{-1})

    1. Causes (Table 35–3)

        a. Supplemental intravenous administration of calcium is indicated to prevent citrate-induced hypocalcemia in the neonate receiving stored blood.

        b. Hypothermia or severe liver dysfunction may interfere with the ability to metabolize citrate to bicarbonate.

    2. Symptoms (Table 35–4)

    3. Treatment of hypocalcemia is with intravenous administration of calcium chloride (27 mg·ml^{-1}), calcium gluconate (9 mg·ml^{-1}), or calcium gluceptate (23 mg·ml^{-1}).

        a. Administered intravenously over 5 to 15 minutes, equivalent doses of calcium chloride (3 to 6 mg·kg^{-1}) and calcium gluconate (7 to 14 mg·kg^{-1}) produce similar effects on the plasma concentrations of calcium.

Table 35–2
Role of Calcium

Neuromuscular transmission

Skeletal muscle contraction

Cardiac muscle contractility

Blood coagulation

Exocytosis

Component of bone

Table 35–3
Causes of Hypocalcemia

Hypoalbuminemia

Hypoparathyroidism

Acute pancreatitis

Vitamin D deficiency

Chronic renal failure associated with hyperphosphatemia

Malabsorption states

Citrate binding of calcium (unlikely in adults unless rate of whole blood infusion exceeds 50 ml·70 kg^{-1}·min^{-1})

       b. Hyperkalemia that is life-threatening is initially treated by intravenous administration of calcium (10 to 20 ml of a 10% calcium chloride solution restores myocardial contractility).

   C. Hypercalcemia (plasma calcium concentration higher than 5.5 mEq·L^{-1})

      1. Causes (Table 35-5)

      2. Symptoms (Table 35-6)

      3. Treatment

         a. Asymptomatic patients with mild hypercalcemia are managed with intravenous administration of saline and furosemide to speed the renal excretion of calcium.

         b. The drug of choice for the treatment of life-threatening hypercalcemia is a biophosphorate such as disodium etidronate, which administered intravenously binds to hydroxyapatite in bone and acts as

Table 35–4
Symptoms of Hypocalcemia

Tetany

Circumoral paresthesias

Increased neuromuscular excitability

Laryngospasm

Seizures

Hypotension

Prolonged Q-T interval on the electrocardiogram (not a consistent finding)

Table 35–5
Causes of Hypercalcemia

Tumors (secrete substances that stimulate resorption of bone)
Hyperparathyroidism (may manifest following renal transplantation)
Sarcoidosis

a potent inhibitor of osteoclastic activity (allows surgery to be performed under elective conditions rather than as an emergency in an unstable hypercalcemic patient).

D. Bone Composition
   1. Bone is composed of an organic matrix (collagen fibers, chondroitin sulfate) that is strengthened by deposits of calcium and phosphate (combination known as hydroxyapatites).
   2. Bone is continually being deposited by osteoblasts and is constantly being absorbed at sites where osteoclasts are active (parathyroid hormone controls osteoclast activity).
   3. **Exchangeable calcium** reflects the buffering mechanism of bone to keep the calcium concentration in the extracellular fluid from changing excessively in either direction (a single passage of blood through bone will remove almost all excess calcium).
   4. **Teeth** (Fig. 35-1)
      a. **Structure.** The outer surface of the tooth is covered by a protein (enamel) that is extremely hard and resistant to corrosive agents, such as acids or enzymes.
      b. **Dentition.** Deciduous teeth erupt between 7 and

Table 35–6
Symptoms of Hypercalcemia

Sedation
Vomiting
Cardiac conduction disturbances
   Prolonged P-R interval
   Wide QRS complex
   Shortened Q-T interval
Renal damage

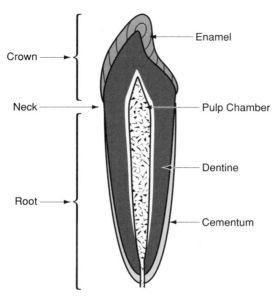

FIGURE 35–1. Schematic depiction of the functional parts of a tooth. (From Guyton AC. Textbook of Medical Physiology, 6th ed. Philadelphia: WB Saunders, 1986; with permission.)

> 24 months of age and remain in place until 6 to 13 years of age.
>
> **c. Dental caries** result from formation of acids by bacteria (which depend on carbohydrates for survival) that inhabit plaque.

II. PHOSPHATE

- **A.** Phosphate is important in energy metabolism and maintenance of acid-base balance (phosphate ions are the most abundant buffer ions in the distal renal tubules, allowing excretion of hydrogen ions).
  - **1.** Vitamin D stimulates the systemic absorption of phosphate from the gastrointestinal tract and reabsorption from the proximal renal tubules.
  - **2.** Parathyroid hormone facilitates renal excretion of phosphate.
- **B. Hypophosphatemia** (alcoholism, hyperalimentation)

Table 35–7
Causes of Hypomagnesemia

Alcoholism

Hyperalimentation

Malabsorption syndromes

Vomiting and diarrhea

Cardiopulmonary bypass (dilutional effects from pump-priming solutions)

is associated with skeletal muscle weakness, central nervous system dysfunction, and peripheral neuropathy.

III. **MAGNESIUM** is the fourth most plentiful cation in the body and the second most plentiful intracellular cation after potassium (about one-half of total body magnesium is present in bone).
   A. **Hypomagnesemia** (plasma magnesium concentration lower than 1.6 mEq·L^{-1}) may be the most common unrecognized electrolyte deficiency.
      1. **Causes** (Table 35-7)
         a. There is a strong correlation of hypomagnesemia with hypokalemia.
         b. A low serum magnesium concentration is almost always due to total body depletion of this cation.
      2. **Manifestations** (Table 35-8)
      3. **Treatment** of life-threatening hypomagnesemia is by infusion of magnesium, 10 to 20 mg·kg^{-1} IV, over 10 to 20 minutes.
   B. **Hypermagnesemia** (plasma concentration of magnesium higher than 2.6 mEq·L^{-1}) is most often due to

Table 35–8
Manifestations of Hypomagnesemia

Ventricular cardiac dysrhythmias

Neuromuscular symptoms (resembling those associated with hypocalcemia)

Seizures

Coma

Potentiation of nondepolarizing muscle relaxants

administration of magnesium to parturients to treat pregnancy-induced hypertension (therapeutic plasma magnesium concentration is 4 to 6 mEq·L^{-1}).

1. Patients with chronic renal dysfunction are at an increased risk for developing hypermagnesemia because excretion of magnesium is dependent on glomerular filtration rate.
2. **Manifestations** (Table 35–9)
3. **Treatment** of life-threatening hypermagnesemia (paralysis of respiratory muscles and heart block when plasma magnesium concentration is higher than 12 mEq·L^{-1}) is with calcium gluconate, 10 to 15 mg·kg^{-1} IV, followed by fluid loading and drug-induced diuresis.

IV. IRON

A. Approximately 80% of the iron in plasma (normal plasma iron concentration is 50 to 150 μg·dl^{-1}) enters the bone marrow to be incorporated into new erythrocytes.
B. **Iron deficiency** may be nutritional (most common cause) or the result of increased iron requirements (pregnancy, blood loss).
C. **Diagnosis** of iron deficiency is confirmed by decreased plasma concentrations of the iron-binding protein ferritin (lower than 12 μg·dl^{-1}).
D. **Treatment**
   1. Prophylactic use of oral iron preparations should be reserved for individuals at high risk for developing iron deficiency (parturients, lactating females, females with heavy menses, low-birth weight infants).
   2. An increase of 2 g·dl^{-1} or more in the plasma concentration of hemoglobin within 3 weeks of initiating oral iron therapy is evidence of a positive response to iron.
      a. There is no justification for continuing oral iron

Table 35–9
Manifestations of Hypermagnesemia

Sedation

Cardiac depression

Skeletal muscle weakness (inhibition of acetylcholine release and direct relaxant effect)

       therapy beyond 3 weeks if a favorable response in the hemoglobin concentration has not occurred.

    b. If a positive response to oral iron therapy does not occur within 3 weeks, continued bleeding, an infectious process, or impaired gastrointestinal absorption of iron should be considered.

3. Nausea and upper abdominal pain are the most frequent side effects of oral iron therapy.

    a. Hemochromatosis is unlikely to result from oral iron therapy that is administered to treat nutritional anemia.

    b. A plasma iron concentration of higher than 0.5 $mg \cdot dl^{-1}$ confirms the presence of life-threatening iron overdose.

4. For patients who cannot tolerate oral iron, the intravenous administration of iron (occasionally causes an allergic reaction) is preferred over painful intramuscular injection.

V. COPPER supplements should be given during prolonged hyperalimentation.

VI. ZINC is a cofactor of enzymes that may be deficient in diets that do not contain sufficient animal protein or in the presence of malabsorption syndromes.

    A. Zinc supplements should be given during prolonged hyperalimentation.

    B. Symptoms of zinc deficiency include suboptimal growth in children, hepatosplenomegaly, cutaneous rashes, and stomatitis.

VII. CHROMIUM deficiency may result in a diabetes-like syndrome, peripheral neuropathy, and encephalopathy.

VIII. SELENIUM deficiency, as may occur during prolonged hyperalimentation, has been associated with cardiomyopathy.

36

Blood Components and Substitutes

Blood components and certain drugs are most often administered systemically to overcome specific coagulation defects. (Updated and revised from Stoelting RK. Blood components and substitutes. In: Stoelting RK. Pharmacology and Physiology in Anesthetic Practice. 2nd ed. Philadelphia, JB Lippincott, 1991:570–9.) Blood substitutes lack coagulation activity, but are administered systemically to replace and maintain intravascular fluid volume.

I. BLOOD COMPONENTS

A. Administration of specific blood components is recommended in all circumstances other than acute hemorrhage (Table 36–1).
  1. In the presence of acute hemorrhage, whole blood is indicated to replace both oxygen-carrying capacity and intravascular fluid volume.
  2. A unit of whole blood can be divided into several components (Table 36–2).
  3. There are hazards associated with transfusion of blood components (Table 36–3).

B. **Packed Erythrocytes**
  1. Packed erythrocytes are the blood component of choice when the goal is to increase oxygen-carrying capacity in the absence of preexisting hypovolemia.
  2. One unit of packed erythrocytes typically increases the hemoglobin concentration 1 g·dl^{-1}.
  3. Administration of packed erythrocytes is facilitated by reconstituting them with crystalloid solutions (avoiding calcium-containing solutions) so as to decrease viscosity.

C. **Fresh Frozen Plasma**
  1. Fresh frozen plasma contains all procoagulants except platelets in a concentration of 1 unit·ml^{-1} and is specifically indicated for patients with **documented de-**

Table 36–1
Advantages of Blood Components

Replacement of only the deficient procoagulant cells or protein

Minimization of the likelihood of circulatory overload

Avoidance of transfusion of unnecessary donor plasma, which may contain undesirable antigens or antibodies

ficiencies of labile plasma coagulation factors (Table 36–4).

   a. The therapeutic response to fresh frozen plasma is determined by repeat measurement of the prothrombin time (PT) and/or partial thromboplastin time (PTT), as well as by continual assessment of the patient's clinical bleeding.

   b. In determining the need for additional fresh frozen plasma, the half-times of coagulation factors must be considered. (factor VII has a shorter half-time than the other factors such that the PT may become prolonged sooner than the PTT).

   2. A substantial sodium load is associated with the administration of fresh frozen plasma.

   a. Compatibility of ABO antigens is desirable, but cross-matching is not necessary.

   b. Life-threatening allergic reactions may occur, and transmission of diseases is possible.

D. Cryoprecipitated Antihemophiliac Factor

   1. Cryoprecipitate is useful for treating hypofibrinogenemia, von Willebrand's disease, and hemophilia A.

   2. Hemolytic anemia may occur when cryoprecipitated antihemophiliac factor is given to individuals with group A, B, or AB erythrocyte antigens.

   3. Multiple transfusions of cryoprecipitate may result in hyperfibrinogenemia.

   4. Desmopressin is a synthetic analogue of antidiuretic hormone that greatly increases factor VIII activity in patients with mild to moderate hemophilia and von Willebrand's disease.

   a. Decreases in blood pressure associated with evidence of peripheral vasodilation may occur with infusion of desmopressin.

   b. In contrast to blood components, desmopressin administration does not introduce the risk of transmission of viral diseases.

Table 36-2
Components Available from Whole Blood

Component	Content	Approximate Volume (ml)	Shelf Life
Packed erythrocytes	Erythrocytes Leukocytes Plasma Clotting factors	300	35 days in CPD-A 49 days in ADSOL
Fresh frozen plasma	Clotting factors	200-250 400-600 by plasma-pheresis from a single donor	Frozen—1 year Thawed—6 hours
Cryoprecipitate	Factor VIII	Lyophilized powder	Determined by manufacturer
Factor IX concentrate	Factor IX Some of factors II, VII, and X	Lyophilized powder	Determined by manufacturer

Fibrinogen	Fibrinogen		
Platelet concentrates	Platelets Leukocytes (few) Plasma Erythrocytes (few)	50	1-5 days
Granulocyte concentrates	Leukocytes Platelets Erythrocytes (few)	50-300	24 hours
Albumin	5% Albumin 25% Albumin	250 or 500 50 or 100	3 years
Plasma protein	Albumin Alpha- and beta-globulins	500	3 years
Immune globulin	Gamma-globulin	1-2	3 years

CPD-A, citrate-phosphate-dextrose-adenine; *ADSOL*, adenine-glucose-mannitol-sodium chloride

Table 36–3
Hazards of Transfusion of Blood Components

Transmission of viral diseases

Hemolysis due to ABO-incompatible plasma

Acute lung injury

Transmission of bacteria and/or endotoxins

Transmission of parasitic agents

Graft-versus-host disease

Allergic reactions

Immunosuppression

   c. Desmopressin has not been shown to decrease postoperative blood loss.
 E. Aminocaproic Acid
  1. Aminocaproic acid may be of benefit in the control of hemorrhage associated with primary fibrinolysis caused by increased plasminogen activation.
   a. A normal platelet count in the presence of hypofibrinogenemia supports the diagnosis of primary fibrinolysis.
   b. Aminocaproic acid, when administered to a patient with disseminated intravascular coagulation, may cause serious or even fatal thrombus formation.

Table 36–4
Clinical Indications for Fresh Frozen Plasma

Congenital or acquired deficiency of coagulation factors with active bleeding or prior to an operative or other invasive procedure (document need with prolonged prothrombin time, partial thromboplastin time, or coagulation factor assay)

Massive blood transfusion with evidence of coagulation deficiency and continued bleeding

Immediate reversal of warfarin effect

Deficiency of antithrombin III (when concentrate not available), protein C, or protein S

Plasma exchange for thrombotic thrombocytopenic purpura

(Adapted from Practice parameter for the use of fresh frozen plasma, cryoprecipitate, and platelets. JAMA 1994;271:777–81.)

  2. Aminocaproic acid has been used to treat hemorrhage in patients with hereditary angioedema.
- **F. Platelet Concentrates**
  1. One unit of platelet concentrate will increase the platelet count 5,000 to 10,000 cells mm^{-3} (Table 36–5).
  2. Administration of platelets (which contain large amounts of plasma) on the basis of ABO compatibility is desirable.
  3. For every 5 to 6 units of platelets, the patient is receiving a volume equivalent to 1 unit of fresh frozen plasma, including the coagulation factors.
- **G. Granulocyte concentrates,** administered to treat infection, may result in fever, pulmonary insufficiency (due to sequestration of granulocytes in the pulmonary capillaries), and cytomegalovirus infection (virus is concentrated in granulocytes).
- **H. Albumin**
  1. **Hypoalbuminemia** is the most frequent indication for the administration of albumin (25 g is equivalent osmotically to about 500 ml of plasma, but contains only about one seventh the amount of sodium present in the same volume of plasma).

Table 36–5
Clinical Implications of Platelet Counts

Platelet Count (cells·mm^{-3})	Response
<5000	Spontaneous hemorrhage (gastrointestinal, intracranial) likely
	Hemorrhage with trauma or invasive procedure likely
	Administer platelets
5000–10,000	Increased likelihood of spontaneous hemorrhage and hemorrhage with trauma or invasive procedure
10,000–50,000	Variably increased risk of bleeding with trauma or an invasive procedure
>50,000	Hemorrhge unlikely
5000–30,000	Platelets may be given prophylactically on the basis of significant bleeding risks

(Adapted from Practice parameter for the use of fresh frozen plasma, cryoprecipitate, and platelets. JAMA 1994;271:777–81.)

Table 36–6
Clinical Uses of Plasma Protein Fraction

Hypovolemic shock

Hypoproteinemia

Dehydration in infants due to diarrhea

       2. Coagulation factors and blood group antibodies are not present, and viral hepatitis is not a risk (when albumin is heated for 10 hours at 60°C).

  I. Plasma Protein Fraction

       1. Plasma protein fraction is a 5% pooled solution of stabilized human plasma proteins in saline containing at least 83% albumin (coagulation factors are absent, and heating to 60°C for 10 hours removes the risk of viral hepatitis).

          a. Each 100 ml of solution provides 5 g of proteins.

          b. The preparation is equivalent osmotically to an equal volume of plasma.

       2. Clinical Uses (Table 36–6)

  J. Immune globulin is prepared from large pools of human plasma and provides protection against the clinical manifestations of hepatitis A.

  II. TOPICAL HEMOSTATICS (Table 36–7)

III. BLOOD SUBSTITUTES are useful in restoring intravascular fluid volume until definitive treatment can be established

Table 36–7
Topical Hemostatics

Absorbable gelatin sponge (Gelfoam)

Absorbable gelatin film (Gelfilm)

Oxidized cellulose (Oxcel)

Oxidized regenerated cellulose (Surgical)

Microfibrillar collagen hemostat (Avitene)
    Attracts and entraps platelets to initiate formation of a platelet plug
    Effective in the presence of heparin and oral anticoagulants

Thrombin

(tend to be inexpensive, have long storage times, do not transmit viral diseases, and lack coagulation factors).

A. Dextran is a water-soluble glucose polymer (polysaccharide) that is synthesized by certain bacteria from sucrose.

    1. Clinical Uses

        a. High-molecular-weight dextrans (dextran-70) (20 $ml \cdot kg^{-1}$) remain in the intravascular space for 12 hours (and may serve as suitable alternatives to blood or plasma for expansion of intravascular fluid volume).

        b. Dextran-40 remains intravascular for only 2 to 4 hours, and is used most often to prevent thromboembolism by reducing blood viscosity.

    2. Hyskon (32% Dextran-70) is an electrolyte-free fluid that is used to distend the uterine cavity during hysteroscopic procedures (decreases the likelihood of tubal adhesions after reconstructive tubal surgery for infertility).

        a. Hyskon is absorbed from the endometrium in the same way fluid is absorbed from the prostate bed during transurethral prostatectomy.

        b. Pulmonary edema with and without coagulopathy has been ascribed to rapid intravascular absorption of Hyskon.

    3. Side Effects (Table 36–8)

B. Hetastarch (hydroxyethyl starch) is a synthetic colloid solution that is as effective as 5% albumin for expansion of intravascular fluid volume in the treatment of hypovolemia due to burns or hemorrhage (20 to 40 $ml \cdot kg^{-1}$).

    1. Large doses of hetastarch decrease the hematocrit, dilute plasma proteins, and interfere with the normal coagulation mechanism by diluting platelets and procoagulants.

    2. Hetastarch does not cause rouleaux formation, and cross-matching of blood is not impaired.

Table 36–8
Side Effects of Dextran

Allergic reactions

Increased bleeding time (decreased platelet adhesiveness, especially when dose is higher than 1500 ml)

Rouleaux formation (interferes with cross-matching of blood)

Noncardiogenic pulmonary edema

C. Stroma-free hemoglobin may be useful as a plasma volume expander (reflects the high molecular weight of hemoglobin), and has the potential capacity for delivering oxygen to tissues and carrying carbon dioxide away from these same tissues.

    1. Cross-matching is not necessary, and prolonged storage is possible.

    2. Renal dysfunction does not accompany administration of stroma-free hemoglobin solutions.

Chapter

37

Hyperalimentation Solutions

Hyperalimentation is designed to supply all the essential inorganic and organic nutritional elements necessary to prevent malnutrition in at-risk patients (Table 37-1). (Updated and revised from Stoelting RK. Hyperalimentation solutions. In: Pharmacology and Physiology in Anesthetic Practice. 2nd ed. Philadelphia, JB Lippincott, 1991:580-5.) Alimentation by the gastrointestinal tract (**enteral nutrition**) is preferred to intravenous alimentation (**parenteral nutrition**) as it avoids catheter-induced sepsis and maintains the absorptive activity of the small intestine.

I. ENTERAL NUTRITION

A. The ingredients and nutritional value of enteral alimentation solutions vary greatly (carbohydrates are the source of up to 90% of the calories, emphasizing the increased osmolarity of these solutions).

B. **Enteral tube feeding** may be necessary when patients are unable to consume nutritionally complete liquefied food orally.

1. The tip of the No. 4 to No. 8 French nasogastric tube used to deliver enteral nutrition (100 to 120 ml·h^{-1}) must be properly positioned in the stomach, duodenum, or jejunum.

a. Dislodgment of the tip can result in pulmonary aspiration.

b. Surgical placement of an esophagostomy or gastrostomy tube may be indicated for long-term feeding.

2. **Side Effects** (Table 37-2)

II. PARENTERAL NUTRITION is indicated for patients who are unable to ingest or digest nutrients or to absorb them from the gastrointestinal tract.

A. **Short-term parenteral therapy,** using isotonic solutions delivered through a peripheral vein, is acceptable when

Table 37–1
Indications for Hyperalimentation

Intestinal obstruction

Major burns

Trauma

Prolonged hypermetabolic states (infection, malabsorption states)

Gastrointestinal dysfunction (irradiation, chemotherapy)

Debilitated patients (those who have lost more than 20% of their
body weight) before operation

the daily caloric requirements are less than 2000 calories
and the anticipated need for nutritional support is brief (3
to 5 days postoperatively).

1. Glucose solutions with supplemental electrolytes are
commonly administered for short-term therapy (Table
37–3).
2. Peripheral infusion of fat emulsions may be selected
as a nonprotein source of calories to augment those
supplied by glucose (may result in thrombosis of the
peripheral vein).

B. **Long-term (total) parenteral nutrition (intravenous
hyperalimentation)** is indicated when daily caloric requirements are higher than 2000 calories or prolonged
nutritional support is required.
1. Total parenteral nutrition solutions contain a large proportion of calories from glucose and thus are hypertonic
(requires infusion through a central vein with high
blood flow to provide rapid dilution).
a. Daily volume of infusion is about 40 ml·kg^{-1}.

Table 37–2
Side Effects of Enteral Nutrition

Hyperglycemia and osmotic diuresis
  Hypovolemia
  Nonketotic coma

Hypophosphatemia

Cutaneous rashes

Pulmonary aspiration (maintain patients in a semisitting position
during feeding and for 1 hour after feeding)

Table 37–3
Contents of Various Crystalloid Solutions

	Glucose (mg·dl⁻¹)	Sodium (mEq·L⁻¹)	Chloride (mEq·L⁻¹)	Potassium (mEq·L⁻¹)	Magnesium (mEq·L⁻¹)	Calcium (mEq·L⁻¹)	Lactate (mEq·L⁻¹)	pH	Osmolarity (mOsm·L⁻¹)
5% Glucose in water	5000	0	0	0	0	0	0	5.0	253
5% Glucose in 0.45% sodium chloride	5000	77	77	0	0	0	0	4.2	407
5% Glucose in 0.9% sodium chloride	5000	154	154	0	0	0	0	4.2	561
0.9% Sodium chloride	0	154	154	0	0	0	0	5.7	308
Lactated Ringer's solution	0	130	109	4	0	3	28	6.7	273
5% Glucose in lactated Ringer's solution	5000	130	109	4	0	3	28	5.3	527
Normosol-R	0	140	98	5	3	0	*	7.4	295

*Contains 27 mEq·L⁻¹ of acetate and 23 mEq·L⁻¹ of gluconate.

       b. Daily weight gains greater than 0.5 kg may signify fluid retention.

       c. Serum electrolytes, blood glucose concentration, and blood urea nitrogen levels should be measured frequently during total parenteral nutrition.

    2. Side Effects (Table 37–4)

C. Preparation of Total Parenteral Nutrition Solutions

    1. Total parenteral nutrition solutions are prepared aseptically from commercially available solutions (hypertonic glucose, amino acids) with the addition of electrolytes, vitamins, and trace elements.

       a. Fat emulsions are not mixed with the total parenteral nutrition solutions.

       b. Isotonic fat solutions are administered intravenously through a separate peripheral vein or by a Y-connector into the same vein.

       c. Amino acids increase the blood urea nitrogen concentration and should be administered cautiously to patients with impaired renal function.

    2. Intralipid is an isotonic fat emulsion that is administered into a peripheral vein to prevent or correct essential fatty acid deficiency and to provide calories during total parenteral nutrition.

Table 37–4
Side Effects of Total Parenteral Nutrition

Sepsis (risk of contamination is a reason not to use central venous hyperalimentation catheter for administration of medications)

Fatty acid deficiency

Hyperglycemia (may result in osmotic diuresis and hypovolemia; nonketotic hyperosmolar hyperglycemic coma is a potential complication)

Hypoglycemia (a risk of abrupt discontinuation of parenteral nutrition solution infusion because pancreatic insulin release may continue)

Metabolic acidosis (liberation of hydrochloric acid during metabolism of amino acids in the parenteral nutrition solution)

Hypercarbia (metabolism of large quantities of glucose; may interfere with weaning from mechanical ventilation)

Fluid overload

Renal dysfunction

Hepatic dysfunction

Thrombosis of central veins

Chapter

38

Antiseptics and Disinfectants

Antiseptics (applied topically to living tissues to kill or prevent the growth of microorganisms) and disinfectants (applied topically to inanimate objects to destroy pathologic microorganisms and thus prevent transmission of infection) are of obvious importance in the perioperative preparation of the patient and surgeon (Table 38-1). (Updated and revised from Stoelting RK. Antiseptics and disinfectants. In: Pharmacology and Physiology in Anesthetic Practice. 2nd ed. Philadelphia, JB Lippincott, 1991:586-9.) Sterilization is the complete and total destruction of all microbial life, including vegetative bacteria, spores, fungi, and viruses (Table 38-1).

I. ALCOHOLS

   A. Applied to the skin (as before insertion of a needle), 70% ethyl alcohol kills nearly 90% of cutaneous bacteria within 2 minutes.

   1. A reduction in cutaneous bacterial count of greater than 75% is unlikely with a single wipe of an ethyl alcohol-wetted sponge followed by evaporation of the residual solution.

   2. Isopropyl alcohol has a slightly greater bactericidal activity than ethyl alcohol owing to its greater depression of surface tension.

   B. Alcohol is not fungicidal or virucidal.

II. CHLORHEXIDINE is used mainly for preoperative preparation of the surgeon (handwashing) and patient (skin prep).

III. IODINE kills bacteria, viruses and spores.

   A. A 1% tincture of iodine solution (alcohol vehicle facilitates spreading and penetration) kills 90% of cutaneous bacteria in 90 seconds.

Table 38–1
Classification of Antiseptics and Disinfectants

Antiseptics
  Alcohols (ethyl and isopropyl alcohol)
  Quaternary ammonium compounds (benzalkonium)
  Chlorhexidine
  Iodine
  Hexachlorophene

Disinfectants
  Aldehydes (formaldehyde, glutaraldehyde)
  Cresol
  Chlorine

Sterilization
  Ethylene oxide

1. The local toxicity of iodine is low, with cutaneous burns occurring only with concentrations higher than 7%.
2. In rare instances, an individual may be allergic to iodine and react to topical application (fever, generalized skin eruption).

B. Iodophors, such as povidone-iodine, provide increased solubility and a reservoir for sustained release of iodine.
  1. Iodophors are widely used as handwashes, for skin prep prior to surgical incision or needle insertion, and as treatment for minor cuts, abrasions, and burns.
  2. A standard surgical scrub with a 10% solution will decrease the usual cutaneous bacterial population by more than 90%, with a return to normal in about 6 to 8 hours.

IV. HEXACHOROPHENE provides delayed but sustained decreases in the cutaneous bacterial population following a hand scrub.

V. FORMALDEHYDE kills bacteria, fungi, and viruses; also used to disinfect inanimate objects, such as surgical instruments.

VI. GLUTARALDEHYDE is superior to formaldehyde as a disinfectant because it is rapidly effective against all microorganisms.

VII. ETHYLENE OXIDE is antimicrobial to all organisms and serves as an alternative to heat sterilization.
   A. Special sterilizing chambers are required because the gas must remain in contact with objects for several hours.
   B. Adequate **airing** of sterilized materials, such as plastic tracheal tubes, is necessary to ensure removal of residual ethylene chloride and thus minimize tissue irritation.

Section

2

PHYSIOLOGY

Chapter

39

Cell Structure and Function

The basic living unit of the body is the cell (estimated that the entire body consists of 75 trillion cells of which about 25 trillion are erythrocytes), and organs are masses of cells held together by intracellular supporting structures. (Updated and revised from Stoelting RK. Cell structure and function. In: Pharmacology and Physiology in Anesthetic Practice. 2nd ed. Philadelphia, JB Lippincott, 1991:593–605.) Almost every cell is within 25 to 50 μm of a capillary, assuring prompt diffusion of oxygen to cells.

I. ANATOMY OF A CELL

A. Principal components of cells include the cytoplasm, cell membrane, and nucleus.

1. **Cytoplasm** consists of water (70% to 85% of the cell substance); proteins, including enzymes (10% to 20% of the cell mass); and electrolytes.

2. **Cell membranes** (often a lipid bilayer) act as permeability barriers, allowing the cell to maintain a cytoplasmic composition different from extracellular fluid (Table 39-1).

   a. Proteins in the cell membrane function as microtubules, ion pumps, passive channels, receptors, and enzymes.

   b. Cell membranes are usually dynamic fluid structures.

3. **Nucleus** is made up, in large part, of chromosomes that carry the blueprint for heritable characteristics of the cell.

   a. The ultimate units of heredity are genes (a portion of a molecule of deoxyribonucleic acid [DNA] on the chromosomes).

   b. During normal cell division (mitosis), the chromosomes divide in such a way that each daughter cell receives a full complement (diploid number) of 46 chromosomes.

Table 39–1
Cell Membrane Composition

Phospholipids
   Lecithins (phosphatidylcholines)
   Sphingomyelins
   Amino phospholipids (phosphatidylethanolamine)

Proteins
   Structural proteins (microtubules)
   Transport proteins ($Na^+ - K^+$ ATPase)
   Channels
   Receptors
   Enzymes (adenylate cyclase)

      c. When a sperm and ovum unite, the resultant cell
      (zygote) has a full **(diploid)** complement of 46
      chromosomes.
  **B. Structure and Function of Deoxyribonucleic Acid
     and Ribonucleic Acid**
    1. The genetic message is determined by the sequence
      of four amino acids **(adenine, guanine, thymine,
      cytosine)** on the two nucleotide chains of DNA.
    2. Ribonucleic acid (RNA) (the type formed being deter-
      mined by DNA) is responsible for transferring the ge-
      netic message to the site of protein synthesis **(ribo-
      somes)** in cytoplasm.
    3. Highly differentiated cells, such as nerve and muscle
      cells, are not capable of reproduction to replace lost
      cells.
    4. Mutations occur when the amino acid sequence in the
      DNA molecule is altered by mutagenic chemicals or
      irradiation.
  C. Regulation of Gene Expression
    1. Genes may be activated by steroids and by proteins
      (transforming growth factor-B) manufactured by other
      genes in the cell.
    2. Oncogenes are genes that produce uncontrolled cell
      reproduction (tumors).
  D. Organelles are structures in the cytoplasm that have spe-
    cific roles in cellular function (Table 39–2).

Table 39–2
Organelles Present in Cytoplasm

Mitochondria (site of oxidative phosphorylation and synthesis of
adenosine triphosphate [ATP])

Endoplasmic reticulum (tubules in the cytoplasm to which
ribosomes attach and serve as sites for protein synthesis)

Lysosomes (serve as an intracellular digestive system)

Golgi apparatus (storage site for proteins)

Nucleolus (site of synthesis of ribosomes)

Centroles

II. TRANSFER OF MOLECULES ACROSS CELL MEMBRANES

A. **Endocytosis** and **exocytosis** are examples of processes
   that transfer molecules (such as nutrients) across, but not
   through, cell membranes.

B. **Phagocytosis** is uptake of particulate matter (bacteria,
   damaged cells), whereas **pinocytosis** is uptake of materials in solution in the extracellular fluid.

   1. The process of phagocytosis is initiated when antibod-
      ies attach to damaged tissue and foreign substances
      (opsonization), which results in acquirement of a
      positive charge.

   2. Typically, objects that have a negative charge are re-
      pelled by cell membranes, and thus are not vulnerable
      to phagocytosis.

III. TRANSFER OF MOLECULES THROUGH CELL MEMBRANES

A. Some molecules (oxygen, carbon dioxide, nitrogen) move
   through cell membranes by **diffusion,** whereas the passage of other molecules (glucose, amino acids) requires the
   presence of specific transport proteins in cell membranes.

   1. **Diffusion.** Because of the slowness of diffusion over
      macroscopic distances, organisms have developed cir-
      culatory systems to deliver nutrients (Table 39–3).

   2. **Lipid Bilayer**

      a. The lipid bilayer of cell membranes is the principal
         barrier to substances that permeate membranes by
         simple diffusion (highly lipid-soluble oxygen and
         carbon dioxide diffuse readily).

      b. Cell membranes are impermeable to charged water-

Table 39–3
Predicted Relationship Between Diffusion Distance and Time

Diffusion Distance (mm)	Time Required for Diffusion
0.001	0.5 ms
0.01	50 ms
0.1	5 s
1	498 s
10	14 h

soluble molecules, especially those with molecular weights higher than 200.

3. Protein Channels

    a. Charged ions are relatively insoluble in cell membranes such that their passage is thought to occur through protein channels (intermolecular spaces in proteins that extend through the entire cell membrane) (Table 39-4).

    b. Some channels are continuously open, whereas others are gated (opening or closing in response to alterations in membrane potential or binding of a ligand [acetylcholine]).

    c. Permeability of cell membranes to sodium (Na^+) and potassium (K^+) ions may change as much as 50- to 5000-fold during the course of nerve impulse transmission.

Table 39–4
Diameters of Ions, Molecules, and Channels

	Diameter (nm*)
Channel (average)	0.08
Water	0.03
Na^+ (hydrated)	0.51
K^+ (hydrated)	0.40
Cl^- (hydrated)	0.39
Glucose	0.86

*1 nm = 10A

4. **Protein-mediated transport** is responsible for movement of certain substances into or out of cells by way of specific carriers or channels.
   a. **Facilitated diffusion** is a mechanism that allows poorly lipid-soluble substances (glucose, amino acids) to pass through lipid bilayers.
   b. **Active transport,** as via the sodium pump, requires energy that is most often provided by hydrolysis of adenosine triphosphate (responsible for maintenance of the electrical potential difference across cell membranes that is essential for nerve conduction and skeletal muscle contraction).

IV. ELECTRICAL POTENTIALS ACROSS CELL MEMBRANES

A. Electrical potentials exist in nearly all cell membranes, reflecting principally the difference in transmembrane concentrations of Na^+ and K^+.
   1. This unequal distribution of ions is created and maintained by the energy-dependent sodium pump.
   2. The voltage difference across cell membranes (cytoplasm usually being electrically negative [about -70 mV] relative to the extracellular fluid) is known as the **resting membrane potential** (Fig. 39-1).

B. **Action Potential**
   1. An action potential is a rapid change in transmembrane potential followed by a return to the resting membrane potential.
   2. Propagation of the action potential along the entire length of a nerve axon or muscle cell is the basis of the signal-carrying ability of nerve cells and allows muscle cells to contract simultaneously (size and shape of the action potential varies among excitable tissues) (Fig. 39-1).
      a. An action potential is triggered when successive conductance increases to Na^+ and K^+ cause a **threshold potential** (about -50 mV) to be reached.
      b. Acetylcholine is an important chemical substance (neurotransmitter) that is capable of enlarging Na^+ channels.
      c. The initial inward rush of Na^+ leads to a positive charge inside the cell **(depolarization)** and the subsequent return of the electrical charge inside

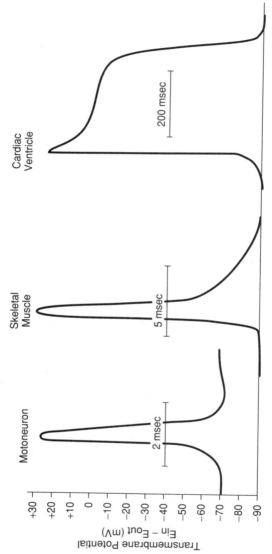

FIGURE 39-1. The transmembrane potential and duration of the action potential vary with the tissue site. (From Berne RM, Levy MN. Physiology, 2nd ed. St. Louis: CV Mosby, 1988; with permission.)

the cell toward the resting membrane potential is known as **repolarization.**

3. **Properties of Action Potentials**
   a. **Absolute refractory period** is the portion of the action potential during which the membrane is completely refractory to further stimulation.
   b. A **deficiency of calcium ions (Ca^{2+})** in the extracellular fluid prevents the sodium channels from closing between action potentials (sustained depolarization or tetany).
   c. A **deficiency of K^+** in the extracellular fluid increases the negativity of the resting membrane potential, resulting in **hyperpolarization** of skeletal muscle membranes, manifesting as skeletal muscle weakness.
   d. Local anesthetics decrease permeability of nerve cell membranes to Na^+, preventing achievement of a threshold potential that is necessary for generation of an action potential.

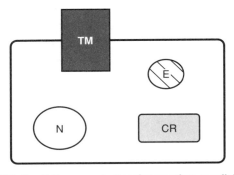

FIGURE 39–2.   Cell communication that manifests as cellular (physiologic), and ultimately as clinical responses, occurs via cytoplasmic receptors (CR), stimulation or inhibition of enzyme systems (E), and excitable transmembrane (TM) proteins. The location of each system is illustrated schematically in relation to the cell nucleus (N) and cell membrane. Examples of CRs may be steroid receptors, whereas E may be represented by phosphodiesterase inhibitors. Most clinically useful drugs and endogenously secreted hormones mediate their effects via excitable TM proteins. (From Schwinn DA. Adrenoceptors as models for G protein–coupled receptors: structure, function, and regulation. Br J Anaesth 1993;71:77–85; with permission.)

Table 39–5
Types of Excitable Transmembrane Proteins Involved in Cell Communication

	Examples
Voltage-sensitive ion channels	Sodium
	Potassium
	Calcium
	Chloride
Ligand-gated ion channels	Nicotinic cholinergic receptors
	Amino acid receptors
	Gamma-aminobutyric acid
	N-methyl-D-aspartate
Transmembrane receptors (signal transduction)	Adrenoceptors (alpha, beta)
	Muscarinic cholinergic
	Opioid
	Serotonin
	Dopamine

(Adapted from Schwinn DA. Adrenoceptors as models for G protein-coupled receptors: structure, function, and regulation. Br J Anaesth 1993;71:77–85.)

4. Conduction of Action Potentials

a. Action potentials are conducted along nerve or muscle fibers by local current flow that produces depolarization of adjacent areas of the membrane, resulting in a **nerve or muscle impulse** (entire action potential usually occurs in less than 1 ms).

b. Conduction velocity is greatly increased by **myelination** in which ion exchange occurs only at **nodes of Ranvier.**

c. Another property of conduction in myelinated fibers that enhances conduction velocity is called **saltatory conduction** because the impulse jumps from one node of Ranvier to the next.

V. INTRACELLULAR COMMUNICATION

A. Cells communicate with their environment in many different ways (Fig. 39–2).

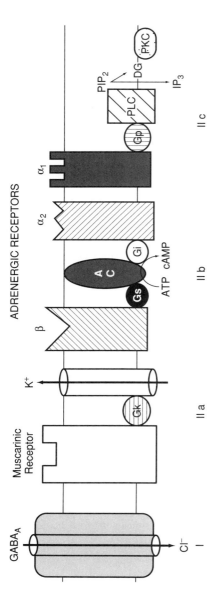

FIGURE 39–3. Schematic depiction of receptors on cell surfaces. Stimulation of the gamma-aminobutyric acid (GABA) receptor by an agonist (GABA$_A$) results in a flow of chloride ions (Cl⁻) into the cell along the associated ion channel (I). Stimulation of the muscarinic receptor by an agonist (acetylcholine) causes the coupling G protein (Gk) to facilitate conductance of potassium ions (K⁺) to the exterior of the cell (IIa). Adenylate cyclase (AC) activity can be enhanced via a stimulatory G protein (Gs) upon activation of a beta-adrenergic receptor by an agonist ligand, whereas this enzyme's activity can be attenuated via an inhibitory G protein (Gi) that is coupled to an alpha-2 adrenergic receptor, thus controlling the conversion of adenosine triphosphate (ATP) to cyclic adenosine monophosphate (cAMP) (IIb). On stimulation of the alpha-1 adrenergic receptor by an agonist ligand, the coupling protein (Gp) activates phospholipase C (PLP) to hydrolyze phosphatidylinositol biphosphate (PIP$_2$) to inositol triphosphate (IP$_3$) and diacylglycerol (DG), which then activates protein kinase C (PKC) (IIc). (From Maze M. Transmembrane signalling and the Holy Grail of anesthesia. Anesthesiology 1990;72:959–61; with permission.)

447

1. There are three basic types of transmembrane proteins (Table 39-5).
2. Transmembrane receptors located in lipid cell membranes interact with endogenous (hormones, neurotransmitters) or exogenous compounds (drugs), resulting in the initiation of a cascade of biochemical changes that lead to a cellular response (physiologic effect) (Figs. 39-3 and 39-4).
   a. Translation of information encoded in hormones, neurotransmitters, and drugs into a cellular response (most often via a change in transmembrane voltage and excitability) is known as **signal transduction.**
   b. Chemical messengers (first messengers, ligands) often exert their effects by increasing the concen-

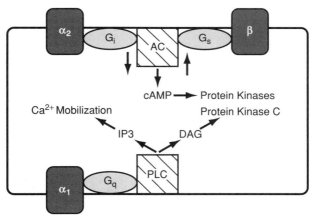

FIGURE 39-4. Transmembrane receptors (alpha-2, beta, alpha-1) are located in the cell membrane and bind drugs or hormones on the extracellular surface. Agonist-bound receptors interact with guanine nucleotide proteins (Gi [inhibitory], Gs [stimulatory], and Gq) and, ultimately, second messenger systems (adenyl cyclase [AC], phospholipase C [PLC], to activate a cascade of biochemical reactions and enzyme systems (protein kinases, inositol triphosphate [IP$_3$], diacylglycerol [DAG], and calcium ion [Ca^{2+}] mobilization) that manifest as physiologic and clinical effects. (From Schwinn DA. Adrenoceptors as models for G protein–coupled receptors: structure, function, and regulation. Br J Anaesth 1993;71:77–85; with permission.)

Table 39–6
Ligands that Act by Altering Intracellular Cyclic Adenosine Monophosphate (cyclic AMP) Concentrations

Increase in Cyclic AMP
Adrenocorticotrophic hormone
Catecholamines (beta-1 and beta-2 receptors)
Glucagon
Parathyroid hormone
Thyroid stimulating hormone
Follicle stimulating hormone
Vasopressin

Decrease in Cyclic AMP
Catecholamines (alpha-2 receptors)
Dopamine (dopamine-2 receptors)
Somatostatin

trations of second messengers (cyclic adenosine monophosphate, Ca^{2+}) in target cells (Tables 39–6 and 39–7; Fig. 39–4).
B. Receptors in cell membranes are not static components of the cell.
1. Excess circulating concentrations of ligand (norepinephrine owing to a pheochromocytoma) results in a decrease in the density of beta-adrenergic receptors in cell membranes **(downregulation).**
2. Drug-induced antagonism of beta receptors results in an increased density of receptors in cell membranes

Table 39–7
Ligands that Increase Intracellular Calcium Ion Concentration

Catecholamines (alpha-1 receptors)

Acetylcholine (muscarinic receptors)

Histamine (H-1 receptors)

Serotonin

Substance P

Vasopressin (V-1 receptors)

Oxytocin

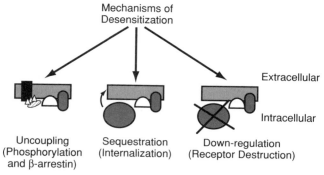

Mechanisms of
Desensitization

Extracellular

Intracellular

| Uncoupling
(Phosphorylation
and β-arrestin) | Sequestration
(Internalization) | Down-regulation
(Receptor Destruction) |

FIGURE 39–5. Three basic mechanisms for desensitization of receptors are uncoupling (preventing receptor interaction with G proteins), sequestration (mobilization of the receptor to intracellular vesicles over minutes to hours; can be recycled back to the cell membrane surface once agonist stimulation terminates), and down-regulation (destruction of sequestered receptors over a period of hours to days). (From Schwinn DA. Adrenoceptors as models for G protein–coupled receptors: structure, function, and regulation. Br J Anaesth 1993;71:77–85; with permission.)

(up-regulation) and the possibility of exaggerated sympathetic nervous system activity if the beta-antagonist drug is abruptly discontinued, as in the preoperative period.

3. **Desensitization** is waning of a physiologic response over time despite the presence of a constant stimulus (Fig. 39–5).

C. **Receptor Diseases** (Table 39–8)

Table 39–8
Receptor Diseases

Pseudohypoparathyroidism

Nephrogenic diabetes insipidus

Grave's disease

Myasthenia gravis

Chapter

40

Body Fluids

Total body fluid can be divided into intracellular and extracellular fluid depending on its location relative to the cell membrane (Fig. 40-1). (Updated and revised from Stoelting RK. Body fluids. In: Pharmacology and Physiology in Anesthetic Practice. 2nd ed. Philadelphia, JB Lippincott, 1991:606-11.) About 25 L of the 40 L of total body fluid present in an adult weighing 70 kg are contained inside the estimated 75 trillion cells of the body (**intracellular fluid**). The 15 L of fluid outside the cells is collectively referred to as **extracellular fluid** (divided into interstitial fluid and plasma by the capillary membrane). Loss of plasma (3 L) from the intravascular space is minimized by colloid osmotic pressure exerted by the plasma proteins.

I. TOTAL BODY WATER

A. Water is the most abundant single constituent in the body and is the medium in which all metabolic reactions occur (Table 40-1).

1. Total body water is less in females, obese patients, and elderly patients, reflecting the decreased water content of adipose tissue.

2. The normal daily water intake by an adult averages 2 L, of which about 1.2 L is excreted as urine.

   a. All gases that are inhaled become saturated with water vapor (47 mmHg at 37°C).

   b. This water vapor is subsequently exhaled, accounting for an average daily water loss through the lungs of 300 to 400 ml.

II. BLOOD VOLUME

A. The main priority of the body is to maintain intravascular fluid volume (average blood volume is 5 L [3 L plasma]), but this may vary greatly with age, weight, and gender.

1. In nonobese persons, the blood volume varies in direct proportion to body weight, averaging 70 ml·kg^{-1}.

2. The greater the ratio of fat to body weight, the less is

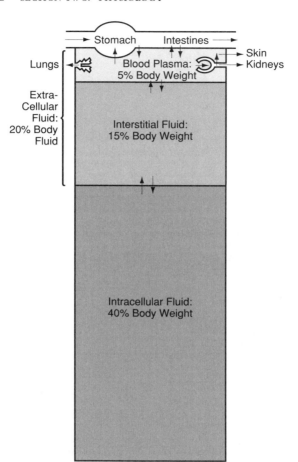

FIGURE 40–1. Body fluid compartments and the percentage of body weight represented by each compartment. The location relative to the capillary membrane divides extracellular fluid into plasma or interstitial fluid. Arrows represent fluid movement between compartments. (From Gamble JL. Chemical Anatomy, Physiology and Pathology of Extracellular Fluid, 6th ed. Boston: Harvard University Press, 1954; with permission.)

Table 40–1
Total Body Water, Age, and Gender

	Total Body Water	
Age (years)	*Male (percent)*	*Female (percent)*
18–40	61	51
40–60	55	47
Older than 60	52	46

the blood volume ($ml \cdot kg^{-1}$) because adipose tissue has a decreased vascular supply.

B. Hematocrit

1. The true hematocrit is about 96% of the measured value because 3% to 8% of plasma remains entrapped among the erythrocytes, even after centrifugation.
2. The hematocrit of blood in arterioles and capillaries is lower than that in larger arteries and veins (reflects axial streaming of erythrocytes in small vessels).

III. MEASUREMENT OF COMPARTMENTAL FLUID VOLUMES

A. The volume of a fluid compartment (blood volume, total body water) can be measured by the indicator dilution principle (interstitial fluid volume [15 L] minus plasma volume [3 L]).

B. **Blood volume** is most often calculated using the dilution principle and radioactive labeled chromium.

IV. CONSTITUENTS OF BODY FLUID COMPARTMENTS

A. The constituents of plasma, interstitial fluid, and intracellular fluid are identical but the quantity of each substance varies greatly among the compartments (Fig. 40–2).

1. The most striking differences are the low protein content in interstitial fluid compared with that of intracellular fluid and plasma, and the fact that sodium (Na^+) and chloride (Cl^-) ions are largely extracellular, whereas most of the potassium ions (K^+) are intracellular.
2. This unequal distribution of ions results in establish-

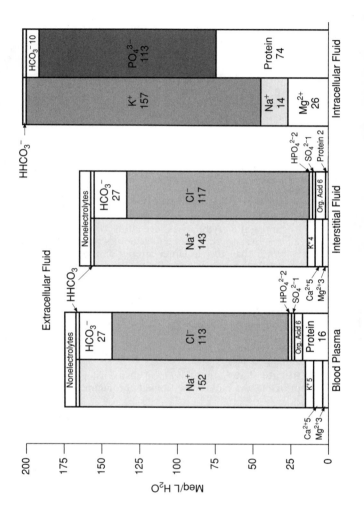

ment of a potential (voltage) difference across cell membranes.

B. The constituents of the extracellular fluid are carefully regulated by the kidneys so that the cells are bathed continually in a fluid containing the proper concentration of electrolytes.

1. Trauma is associated with progressive loss of K^+ through the kidneys (a patient undergoing surgery excretes about 100 mEq of K^+ in the first 48 hours postoperatively).

2. The plasma potassium concentration is not a good indicator of total body potassium because most K^+ are intracellular.

3. There is a correlation between the potassium and hydrogen ion content of plasma, the two increasing and decreasing together.

V. OSMOSIS

A. Osmosis is the movement of water across a semipermeable membrane (K^+, Na^+ cannot diffuse freely) from a compartment with lower nondiffusible solute (ion) concentration to one in which the solute concentration is higher (Fig. 40–3).

B. Osmotic pressure is the pressure on one side of the semipermeable membrane that is just sufficient to keep water from moving to a region of higher solute concentration (Fig. 40–3).

1. The osmotic pressure exerted by nondiffusible particles in solution is determined by the number of particles in solution (degree of ionization), not the type of particles (molecular weight).

   a. Thus, a 1-mol solution of glucose or albumin and a 0.5-mol solution of NaCl (which dissociates into two ions) should exert the same osmotic pressure.

   b. Osmole is the unit used to express osmotic activity in solutes (milliosmole is 1/1000 Osm).

2. The osmole concentration of a solution is called its **osmolality** when the concentration is expressed in osmoles per kilogram of water (**osmolarity** is the cor-

---

◄ **FIGURE 40–2.** Electrolyte composition of body fluid compartments. (From Leaf A, Newburgh LH. Significance of the Body Fluids in Clinical Medicine, 2nd ed. Springfield, IL: Thomas, 1955; with permission.)

Chapter

41

Central Nervous System

The brain is a complex collection of neural systems that regulate their own and each other's activity within relatively narrow limits (reflecting a balance between excitatory and inhibitory influences). (Updated and revised from Stoelting RK. Central nervous system. In: Pharmacology and Physiology in Anesthetic Practice. 2nd ed. Philadelphia, JB Lippincott, 1991:612–42.)

I. INTRODUCTION

   A. Anatomic divisions of the brain reflect the distribution of brain functions.
   B. The three principal components of the central nervous system are the cerebral hemispheres, brain stem, and spinal cord (Table 41-1).

II. CEREBRAL HEMISPHERES

   A. For each area of the cerebral cortex, there is a corresponding and connecting area to the thalamus such that stimulation of a small portion of the thalamus activates the corresponding and much larger portion of the cerebral cortex.
   B. The functional part of the cerebral cortex consists mainly of a 2- to 5-mm layer of neurons (50 to 100 billion neurons) covering the surface of the convolutions.
   C. **Anatomy of the Cerebral Cortex**
      1. The **sensorimotor cortex** is the area of the cerebral cortex that is responsible for receiving sensation from somatic sensory areas of the body and for controlling body movement (Fig. 41-1).
      2. **Topographic areas** of the cerebral cortex reflect the presence of specific sensory or motor neurons for receiving or transmitting information.

Table 41–1
Components of the Central Nervous System

Cerebral Hemispheres *(Cerebral Cortex)*
  Site where information is processed (sensory, motor, visual,
    auditory, olfactory)
  Anatomic regions (frontal, temporal, parietal, occipital)

Brain Stem *(connects cerebral cortex to spinal cord)*
  Controls subconscious activities (blood pressure, breathing)
  Anatomic regions (medulla, pons, thalamus, limbic system, basal
    ganglia, reticular activating system)

Spinal Cord *(extends from medulla oblongata to lower border of
  first or second lumbar vertebra)*
  Ascending and descending tracts
  Sensory information (dorsal portion)
  Motor outflow (ventral portion)

Motor Cortex

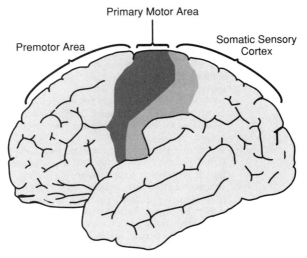

FIGURE 41–1. The sensorimotor cortex consists of the somesthetic cortex, the motor cortex, and pyramidal (Betz) cells. (From Guyton AC. Textbook of Medical Physiology, 7th ed. Philadelphia: WB Saunders, 1986; with permission.)

       a. In general, the size of the sensory or motor area is proportional to the preciseness of the function involved (lips, tongue, larynx, and digits are large areas in humans).

       b. Electrical stimulation during surgery can be used to identify specific areas of the motor cortex.

       c. The motor cortex is commonly damaged by loss of blood supply, as occurs during a **stroke.**

    3. Corpus callosum connects the two cerebral hemispheres for sharing of stored information.

    4. Dominant Versus Nondominant Hemisphere

       a. Based on genetic determination, the left hemisphere is dominant in 90% of right-handed and 70% of left-handed persons.

       b. Destruction of the dominant cerebral hemisphere results in loss of nearly all intellectual function.

       c. Prefrontal areas of the frontal lobes are important in **behavioral patterns.**

D. Memory is an important function of the cerebral cortex, especially the temporal lobes.

    1. Short-term memory may involve the presence of **reverberating circuits** or the phenomenon of **posttetanic potentiation.**

    2. Long-term memory does not depend on continued activity of the nervous system (anesthesia or hypothermia does not result in loss of long-term memory).

       a. It is assumed that long-term memory results from physical or chemical alterations in the synapses **(memory engram or memory trace).**

       b. If memory is to persist, the synapses must become permanently facilitated (consolidated), which requires at least 1 hour.

       c. Intraoperative awareness may depend on how long the painful stimulus is allowed to persist before the memory trace is disrupted by increasing the depth of anesthesia.

E. Pyramidal and Extrapyramidal Tracts

    1. Pathways for transmission of motor signals from the cerebral cortex to the anterior motor neurons of the spinal cord are through the pyramidal (corticospinal and extrapyramidal) tracts.

       a. All pyramidal tract fibers pass downward through the brain stem and then cross to the opposite side to terminate on motor neurons of the spinal cord.

       b. Impulses traveling via pyramidal tracts increase skeletal muscle tone, whereas the extrapyramidal tracts transmit inhibitory signals through the basal ganglia.

   2. Presence of the **Babinski sign** (upward extension of the first toe and outward fanning of the other toes) reflects selective damage to the pyramidal tracts.

F. Thalamocortical System

   1. The thalamocortical system serves as the pathway for passage of afferent impulses (with the exception of olfactory sensory signals) through the thalamus to the cerebral cortex.

   2. The thalamocortical system controls the activity level of the cerebral cortex.

III. BRAIN STEM

A. Limbic System and Hypothalamus

   1. Behavior associated with emotions is primarily a function of the limbic system (hippocampus and basal ganglia).

   2. Internal conditions of the body (core temperature, thirst, appetite) and activity of the reticular activity system are under the control of the hypothalamus.

B. Basal Ganglia (caudate nucleus, putamen, globus pallidus, substantia nigra)

   1. Impulses from the basal ganglia and the associated release of inhibitory neurotransmitters (dopamine, gamma-aminobutyric acid [GABA]) result in inhibition of skeletal muscles.

   2. Destruction of the basal ganglia results in skeletal muscle rigidity.

       a. Chorea reflects damage to the caudate and putamen nuclei that normally secrete GABA.

       b. Parkinson's disease reflects damage to the substantia nigra and loss of dopamine, which results in the predominance of the excitatory neurotransmitter acetylcholine (see Chapter 31).

Table 41–2
Dysfunction of the Cerebellum

Dysmetria (past-pointing)
Ataxia
Dysarthria
Intention tremor
Loss of equilibrium

      C. Reticular Activating System is a polysynaptic pathway that is intimately concerned with electrical activity of the cerebral cortex.

        1. It is likely that many of the injected and inhaled anesthetics used clinically exert depressant effects on the reticular activating system.

        2. Sleep and Wakefulness

          a. Sleep is a state of unconsciousness from which an individual can be aroused by sensory stimulation (anesthesia cannot be defined as sleep).

          b. Slow-wave sleep is characterized by high-voltage delta waves that occur at a frequency of less than 4 cycles·sec^{-1} (as determined by electroencephalography [EEG]) and a 10% to 30% decrease in blood pressure, heart rate, breathing frequency, and basal metabolic rate.

          c. Desynchronized sleep (rapid eye movement sleep) is characterized by active dreaming, irregular heart rate and breathing, and a desynchronized pattern of low-voltage beta waves on the EEG similar to those that occur during wakefulness.

      D. Cerebellum

        1. The cerebellum operates subconsciously to monitor and elicit corrective responses in motor activity (posture, equilibrium).

        2. Dysfunction of the Cerebellum (Table 41-2)

IV. SPINAL CORD

    A. Below the spinal cord, the vertebral canal is filled by the roots of the lumbar and sacral nerves **(cauda equina).**

    B. Gray matter of the spinal cord functions as the initial processor of incoming sensory signals from peripheral somatic receptors and as a relay station to send these signals to the brain. In addition, this area of the spinal cord is the site for final processing of motor signals that are being transmitted downward from the brain to skeletal muscles.

1. Anatomically, the gray matter of the spinal cord is divided into anterior, lateral, and dorsal horns consisting of nine separate laminae that have the shape of the letter "H" when viewed in cross-section (Fig. 41-2).

2. The anterior horn is the location of neurons that give rise to nerve fibers that leave the spinal cord via the anterior (ventral) nerve roots and innervate skeletal muscles.

3. Cells of the preganglionic neurons of the sympa-

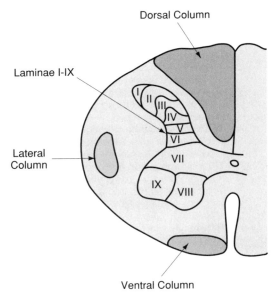

FIGURE 41-2. Schematic diagram of a cross-section of the spinal cord depicting anatomic laminae I to IX of the spinal cord gray matter and the ascending dorsal, lateral, and ventral sensory columns of the spinal cord white matter.

thetic nervous system are located in the lateral
horns of the thoracolumbar portions of the spinal
cord.

4. Cells located in the dorsal horns of the spinal cord
(**substantia gelatinosa, laminae II–III**) transmit
afferent tactile, temperature, and pain impulses to
the spinothalamic tract (dorsal column of the spinal
cord).

C. Spinal Nerve

1. Spinal nerves (31 pairs) are made up of **anterior
(ventral efferent motor fibers)** and **posterior
(dorsal sensory fibers) roots** which leave the
spinal cord through the **intervertebral foramen.**

2. Dermatomes and Myotomes
   a. Each spinal nerve innervates a segmental area of
   skin designated as a **dermatome** and a skeletal
   muscle known as a **myotome.**
   b. A **dermatome map** is useful in determining
   the level of spinal cord injury or level of sensory
   anesthesia produced by a regional anesthetic
   (Fig. 41–3) (extensive overlap between dermatomes is the reason three consecutive dorsal
   nerve roots need to be interrupted to produce
   complete denervation of a dermatome).
   c. Segmental innervation of myotomes is even less
   well defined than that of dermatomes.

D. Covering Membranes

1. The spinal cord is enveloped by membranes (dura,
arachnoid, pia) that are direct continuations of the
corresponding membranes surrounding the brain.

2. The epidural space does not extend beyond the
foramen magnum (drugs cannot travel cephalad
beyond this point), and a connective tissue band
(plica mediana dorsalis) may divide the epidural
space at the dorsal midline (consistent with the
occasional occurrence of unilateral analgesia following placement of local anesthetic solution into
the epidural space).

V. PATHWAYS FOR PERIPHERAL SENSORY
IMPULSES

A. Sensory information from somatic segments of the
body enters the gray matter of the spinal cord via the
dorsal nerve roots and is subsequently transmitted to
the brain by the dorsal-lemniscal system.

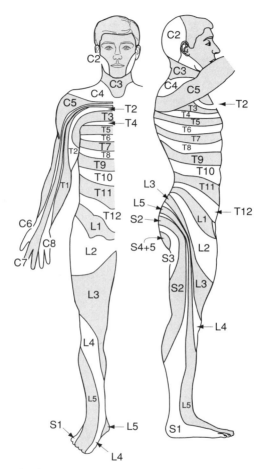

FIGURE 41–3. Dermatome map used to evaluate the level of sensory anesthesia produced by a regional anesthetic. (From Guyton AC. Textbook of Medical Physiology, 7th ed. Philadelphia: WB Saunders, 1986; with permission.)

B. Impulses in the dorsal column pathways cross in the spinal cord to the opposite side before passing upward to the thalamus.

C. All sensory information that enters the cerebral cortex, with the exception of that from the olfactory system, passes through the thalamus.

VI. PATHWAYS FOR PERIPHERAL MOTOR RESPONSES

A. Sensory information is integrated at all levels of the nervous system and causes appropriate motor responses (spinal cord elicits simple reflex responses, while responses from the cerebral cortex are more precise and complex).

   1. Transmission of large numbers of facilitatory impulses from the upper regions of the central nervous system (as occurs with a brain tumor or cerebrovascular accident) to the spinal cord results in exaggerated stretch reflex responses (knee jerk, ankle jerk).

   2. **Clonus** occurs when evoked muscle jerks oscillate as a reflection of facilitatory impulses from the brain (associated with recovery from general anesthesia).

   3. **Decerebrate rigidity** occurs with transection of the brain stem at the level of the pons (isolates the spinal cord from the rest of the brain, leading to diffuse facilitation of stretch reflexes).

   4. The motor system is often divided into **upper motor neurons** (destruction causes spastic paralysis) and **lower motor neurons** (neurons from the spinal cord that directly innervate skeletal muscles, destruction of these neurons results in flaccid paralysis, atrophy of skeletal muscles, and absence of stretch reflex responses).

   5. **Abdominal muscle spasm** occurs during general anesthesia in response to stimulation of the parietal peritoneum (skeletal muscle spasm is attenuated by volatile anesthetics and abolished by regional anesthesia or neuromuscular blocking drugs).

B. **Autonomic Reflexes**

   1. Segmental autonomic reflexes occur in the spinal cord and include changes in vascular tone, diaphoresis, and evacuation reflexes from the bladder and colon.

    2. Simultaneous excitation of all the segmental reflexes is the **mass reflex** (denervation hypersensitivity or autonomic hyperreflexia).

       a. The mass reflex (analogous to epileptic attacks that involve the central nervous system) occurs in response to painful stimulation to the skin below the level of spinal cord transection or distention of a hollow viscus (bladder).

       b. The principal manifestations of the mass reflex are **hypertension** (due to intense peripheral vasoconstriction below the level of spinal cord transection and reflecting an inability of vasodilating inhibitory impulses from the central nervous system to pass beyond the site of spinal cord transection) and **bradycardia** (due to carotid sinus activation by hypertension).

C. Spinal shock is a manifestation of the abrupt loss of spinal cord reflexes that immediately follows transection of the spinal cord.

    1. The immediate manifestations of spinal shock are **hypotension** owing to loss of vasoconstrictor tone and **absence of all skeletal muscle reflexes.**

    2. Within a few days to weeks, spinal cord neurons gradually regain their intrinsic excitability.

VII. ANATOMY OF NERVE FIBERS

A. Neurons function to relay information between the periphery and the central nervous system (Fig. 41-4).

    1. Transmission of impulses between responsive neurons at a synapse is mediated by the presynaptic release of a chemical mediator **(neurotransmitter)**, such as norepinephrine or acetylcholine.

    2. Nerve membranes of postsynaptic neurons are speculated to contain receptors that bind neurotransmitters that are released from presynaptic nerve terminals.

B. Classification of Afferent Nerve Fibers (Table 41-3)

    1. Myelin acts as an insulator that limits the flow of ions to areas where the myelin sheath is interrupted (nodes of Ranvier) (Fig. 41-5).

    2. Successive excitation of nodes of Ranvier by an

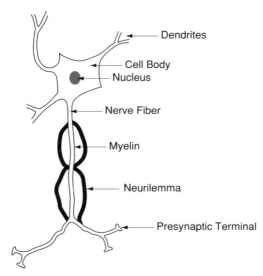

FIGURE 41–4.   Anatomy of a neuron.

impulse that jumps between successive nodes is termed **saltatory excitation** (greatly increases velocity of nerve conduction as compared with unmyelinated nerves) (Fig. 41-5).

VIII. NEUROTRANSMITTERS (Table 41-4)

A. Neurotransmitters are chemical mediators that are released into the synaptic cleft in response to the arrival of an action potential at the nerve ending.
1. **Excitatory neurotransmitters** (acetylcholine, glutamate, substance P) produce configurational changes of the postsynaptic protein receptor characterized by increased membrane permeability to most ions (decreased negativity of the resting transmembrane potential brings it nearer the threshold potential).
a. Glutamate is the major excitatory neurotransmitter in the central nervous system.
b. Block of the N-methyl-D-aspartate (NMDA) subtype of the glutamate receptor may contribute to the mechanism of action of ketamine.

Table 41–3
Classification of Peripheral Nerve Fibers

	Myelinated	Fiber Diameter (μm)	Conduction Velocity (m·sec⁻¹)	Function	Sensitivity to Local Anesthetic (Subarachnoid, Procaine)
A					
A-alpha	Yes	12–20	70–120	Innervation of skeletal muscles Proprioception	1%
A-beta	Yes	5–12	30–70	Touch Pressure	1%
A-gamma	Yes	3–6	15–30	Skeletal muscle tone	1%
A-delta	Yes	2–5	12–30	Fast pain Touch Temperature	0.5%
B	Yes	3	3–15	Preganglionic autonomic fibers	0.25%
C	No	0.4–1.2	0.5–2	Slow pain Touch Temperature Postganglionic sympathetic fibers	0.5%

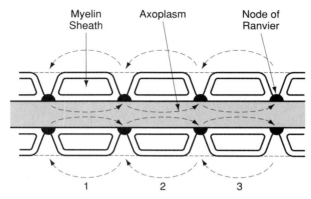

FIGURE 41–5. Saltatory conduction is transmission of nerve impulses that jump between successive nodes of Ranvier of myelinated nerves. (From Guyton AC. Textbook of Medical Physiology, 7th ed. Philadelphia: WB Saunders, 1986; with permission.)

   2. **Inhibitory neurotransmitters** (dopamine, norepinephrine, epinephrine, glycine, GABA, histamine) most likely produce **hyperpolarization** by increasing membrane permeability to chloride and potassium ions (increased negativity of the resting transmembrane potential).
      a. GABA is the major inhibitory neurotransmitter in the central nervous system (estimated that

Table 41–4
Chemicals that Act at Synapses as Neurotransmitters

Acetylcholine	Serotonin
Dopamine	Histamine
Norepinephrine	Vasopressin
Epinephrine	Oxytocin
Glycine	Prolactin
Gamma-aminobutyric acid	Cholecystokinin
Glutamate	Vasoactive intestinal peptide
Substance P	Gastrin
Endorphins	Glucagon

one third of all synapses are responsive to GABA).

b. GABA$_A$ receptors control chloride conductance through ion channels.

c. GABA$_B$ receptors result in inhibition of calcium channels or cause activation of potassium channels via G proteins.

d. There is increasing evidence that some anesthetic drugs (inhaled and injected) exert their hypnotic effects on neuronal membranes in the central nervous system by inhibitory effects exerted at GABA$_A$ receptors (see Chapter 1, Section VI B).

3. Some neurotransmitters function as **neuromodulators** in that they influence the sensitivity of receptors to other neurotransmitters.

B. General anesthetics depress excitable tissues at all levels of the nervous system by stabilizing neuronal membranes.

IX. **ELECTRICAL EVENTS DURING NEURONAL EXCITATION**

A. **Resting transmembrane potentials** of neurons in the central nervous system are about -70 mV, which is less than the -90 mV in large peripheral nerve fibers and skeletal muscles.

B. **Factors That Influence Neuron Responsiveness**

1. Neurons are highly sensitive to changes in the pH of surrounding interstitial fluids (alkalosis enhances neuron excitability).

2. Inhaled anesthetics may increase cell membrane threshold for excitation and thus decrease neuron activity throughout the body.

X. **CEREBRAL BLOOD FLOW**

A. Cerebral blood flow averages 50 ml·100 g^{-1}·min^{-1} of brain tissue (with gray matter blood flow exceeds that of white matter).

1. As in most other tissues of the body, cerebral blood flow parallels cerebral metabolic requirements for oxygen.

2. PaCO$_2$ (linear response) and PaO$_2$ (threshold response) influence cerebral blood flow, whereas

sympathetic and parasympathetic nerves play little or no role in the regulation of cerebral blood flow (Fig. 41-6).

B. Autoregulation

1. Cerebral blood flow is closely autoregulated between mean arterial pressures of about 60 and 140 mmHg (Fig. 41-6).

    a. Chronic hypertension shifts the autoregulation curve to the right (decreases in cerebral blood flow occur at mean arterial pressures higher than 60 mmHg).

    b. Autoregulation of cerebral blood flow is attenuated or abolished by hypercapnia, arterial hypoxemia, and volatile anesthetics.

2. Blood vessels surrounding cerebral infarcts and tumors are maximally vasodilated (**luxury perfusion**).

    a. If the $PaCO_2$ should increase, it is theoretically possible that the resulting vasodilation in normal blood vessels would shunt blood flow away from the diseased area (**intracerebral steal syndrome**).

    b. A decrease in $PaCO_2$ that constricts normal cerebral vessels could divert blood flow to diseased areas (**Robin Hood phenomenon**).

3. Increases in mean arterial pressure above the limits of autoregulation can cause leakage of intravascular

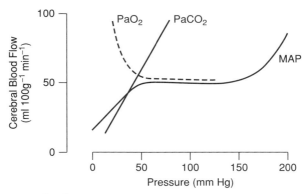

FIGURE 41–6. Cerebral blood flow is influenced by PaO_2, $PaCO_2$, and mean arterial pressure (MAP).

fluid through capillary membranes, resulting in cerebral edema and increased intracranial pressure.

C. Measurement of Cerebral Blood Flow

1. Cerebral blood flow changes within seconds in response to changes in local neuronal activity (reading increases blood flow in the occipital cortex).
2. Blood flow increases acutely at the site of origin of an epileptic attack.

XI. ELECTROENCEPHALOGRAM

A. The EEG is a recording of the brain waves that result from continuous electrical activity in the brain.

1. The character of the waves is greatly dependent on the level of activity of the cerebral cortex and the degree of wakefulness.
2. During periods of increased mental activity, brain waves usually become asynchronous.

B. Classification of Brain Waves (Table 41–5)

C. Clinical Uses

1. The EEG is useful in diagnosing different types of epilepsy and in determining the focus in the brain that is causing seizures.
2. Anesthetic drugs, depth of anesthesia, and $PaCO_2$ may influence EEG results.

D. Epilepsy is characterized by excessive activity of either a part or all of the central nervous system (Table 41–6).

XII. EVOKED POTENTIALS are the electrophysiologic response of the nervous system to sensory, motor, auditory, or visual stimulation.

Table 41–5
Classification of Brain Waves

	Frequency (cycles · sec⁻¹)	*Voltage (µv)*	*Event*
Alpha	8–12	50	Awake with eyes closed
Beta	13–30	<50	Increased mental activity
Theta	4–7		Sleep General anesthesia
Delta	<4		Deep sleep General anesthesia

Table 41–6
Classification and Manifestations of Epilepsy

Grand Mal Epilepsy
   Tonic-clonic seizure
   Postictal depression
   High-voltage, synchronous brain wave discharges over the entire
      cerebral cortex

Status Epilepticus
   Sustained grand mal seizure activity
   Treated with diazepam

Petit Mal Epilepsy
   Transient periods of unconsciousness
   Spike and dome pattern of brain waves

Focal Epilepsy
   Reflects presence of a localized lesion

Psychomotor Epilepsy
   Activated by methohexital or etomidate

A. **Somatosensory evoked potentials** are produced by
   application of a low-voltage electrical current that
   stimulates a peripheral nerve (median nerve at the
   wrist, posterior tibial nerve at the ankle). The resulting
   evoked potential reflects the intactness of sensory neural pathways from the peripheral nerve to the somatosensory cortex.
   1. Volatile anesthetics produce greater dose-depen-
      dent depression of somatosensory evoked poten-
      tials than do opioids (also true for motor, auditory,
      and visual evoked potentials).
   2. Acute hyperventilation of the lungs to produce a
      $PaCO_2$ near 20 mmHg does not alter the amplitude
      or latencies of evoked potentials.
B. **Motor evoked potentials** reflect the intactness of
   motor neural pathways from the peripheral nerve to
   the motor cortex (not possible to monitor in the presence of neuromuscular blockade).
C. **Auditory evoked potentials** arise from brain stem
   auditory pathways.
D. **Visual evoked potentials** are produced by flashes
   of light from light-emitting diodes that are mounted
   on goggles placed over a patient's closed eyes, as

during neurosurgical procedures involving visual pathways (transsphenoidal or anterior fossa surgery).

XIII. CEREBROSPINAL FLUID

- **A.** Cerebrospinal fluid (total volume of about 150 ml) functions to cushion the brain in the cranial cavity (Fig. 41-7).
- **B. Formation** of cerebrospinal fluid (30 ml·h^{-1}) occurs at the choroid plexuses.
  - **1.** The pH of cerebrospinal fluid is closely regulated and maintained at 7.32.
  - **2.** Changes in PaCO$_2$, but not in pH, promptly alter cerebrospinal fluid pH (reflecting the ease with which carbon dioxide crosses the blood–brain barrier).
    - **a.** Acute respiratory acidosis or alkalosis produces corresponding changes in cerebrospinal fluid pH.
    - **b. Active transport of bicarbonate ions** eventually returns cerebrospinal fluid pH to 7.32, despite persistence of alterations in the arterial pH.
- **C. Reabsorption** of cerebrospinal fluid into the venous circulation occurs through **arachnoid villi.**

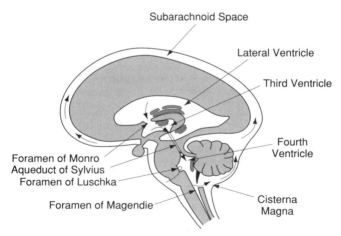

Subarachnoid Space

Lateral Ventricle

Third Ventricle

Fourth Ventricle

Foramen of Monro
Aqueduct of Sylvius
Foramen of Luschka

Foramen of Magendie

Cisterna Magna

FIGURE 41–7.   Circulation of cerebrospinal fluid.

D. Intracranial pressure (normally less than 15 mmHg) is regulated by the rate of formation and reabsorption of cerebrospinal fluid.

 1. **Volatile anesthetics,** by increasing cerebral blood flow, can increase intracranial pressure.
 2. Arterial blood pressure does not alter intracranial pressure, but phasic variations in blood pressure are transmitted as variations in intracranial pressure.

E. Papilledema occurs when swelling of the optic disc occurs in response to increased intracranial pressure.

F. Blood–brain barrier reflects the lack of permeability of capillaries in the central nervous system to circulating substances, such as electrolytes and exogenous drugs (maintains the internal consistency of the environment to which brain neurons are exposed).

 1. The exception to the existence of a blood–brain barrier is the area around the posterior pituitary and the chemoreceptor trigger zone.
 2. The blood–brain barrier is less developed in neonates and tends to break down in areas of the brain that are irradiated or infected or that are the site of tumors.

XIV. VISION

A. The eye is optically equivalent to a photographic camera in that it contains a lens system (focuses the image on the retina), a variable aperture system (pupil), and film (retina) (Fig. 41–8).

 1. **Anticholinergic drugs,** as administered for preoperative medication, may interfere with accommodation to nearby objects.
 2. The pupil may vary from 1.5 to 8 mm in diameter.
    a. Pupillary diameter and magnitude of the light reflex may be measured in the perianesthetic period in an attempt to quantify anesthetic effect and neurologic function.
    b. Inhaled anesthetics produce dose-dependent inhibition of the pupillary response to light.
 3. The lens loses its elastic nature with aging (denaturation of the lens' proteins) such that the ability to accommodate is almost totally absent (presbyopia) by 45 to 50 years of age.

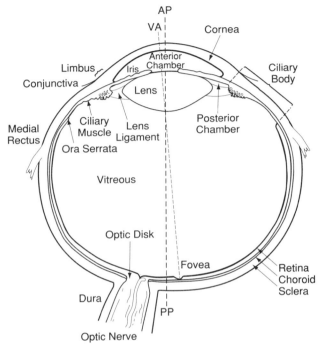

FIGURE 41–8. Schematic diagram of the eye. *AP*, anterior pole; *PP*, posterior pole; *VA*, visual axis. (From Ganong WF. Review of Medical Physiology, 13th ed. Norwalk, CT: Appleton and Lange, 1987; with permission.)

      4. Cataract formation reflects denaturation of proteins in the lens and deposition of calcium, which further increases the opacity of the lens and impairs vision (lens is then surgically removed and replaced by an artificial convex lens).

  B. Intraocular fluid consists of **aqueous humor** (front and sides of the lens) and **vitreous fluid** (between the lens and retina).

  C. Intraocular pressure (normally 15 to 25 mmHg) is determined principally by measuring resistance to outflow of aqueous humor from the anterior chamber into Schlemm's canal (glaucoma is associated with increased intraocular pressure sufficient to compress retinal artery inflow).

D. Retina is the light-sensitive portion of the eye containing the cones (color vision) and the rods (night vision).

1. When the cones and rods are stimulated, impulses are transmitted through successive neurons in the retina (viability can be documented by electroretinography) and optic nerve before reaching the cerebral cortex

2. The nutrient blood supply for the retina is largely derived from the central retinal artery, which accompanies the optic nerve (ophthalmic artery is the first branch of the internal carotid artery).

    a. This independent retinal blood supply prevents rapid degeneration of the retina should it become detached (allowing time for surgical correction).

    b. Ischemic optic neuropathy, manifesting as postoperative blindness or decreased visual acuity, has been associated with the intraoperative use of controlled hypotension combined with hemodilution.

E. Photochemicals (of which vitamin A is an important precursor) in rods and cones decompose upon exposure to light and stimulate fibers in the optic nerve.

F. Color Blindness

1. **Red-green** color blindness is present when red or green types of cones are absent.

2. Color blindness is a **sex-linked recessive trait** (X chromosome carries necessary genes) such that about 2% of males are color blind.

G. Visual Pathway

1. Impulses from the retina pass backward through the optic nerve (Fig. 41–9).

2. The **macula** is a small area in the center of the retina composed mainly of cones to permit detailed vision (**fovea** is the central portion of the macula).

3. At the **optic chiasm,** all the fibers from the nasal halves of the retina cross to the opposite side to join fibers from the opposite temporal retina to form the optic tracts.

H. Field of Vision

1. Anterior pituitary tumors may compress the optic

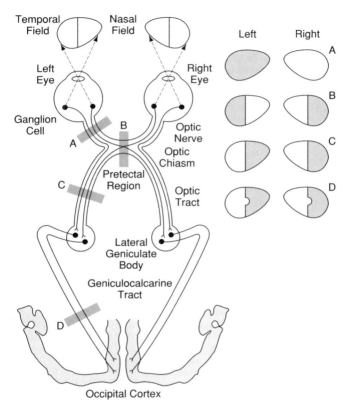

FIGURE 41–9.   Visual impulses from the retina pass to the optic chiasm where fibers from the nasal halves of the retina cross to the opposite side to join temporal fibers and form the optic tract. These fibers synapse in the lateral geniculate body before passing to the visual (occipital) area of the cerebral cortex. Visual field defects reflect lesions at various sites (A–D) in the nerve pathways. (From Ganong WF. Review of Medical Physiology, 13th ed. Norwalk CT: Appleton and Lange, 1987; with permission.)

chiasm, causing blindness in both temporal fields of vision **(bitemporal hemianopia).**

2. Infarction of the visual cortex may follow thrombosis of the posterior cerebral artery.

I. **Muscular control of eye movements** is controlled by three pairs of skeletal muscles (medial and lateral recti, superior and inferior recti, superior and inferior obliques), which are reciprocally innervated by cranial nerves III, IV, and VI.

1. Simultaneous movement of both eyes in the same direction is called **conjugate movement.**

2. **Nystagmus** is likely to occur when one of the vestibular apparatuses is damaged or when deep nuclei in the cerebellum are damaged.

J. **Innervation of the eye** is by the sympathetic (mydriasis) and parasympathetic (miosis) nervous system.

1. **Horner's syndrome** (miosis, ptosis, absence of sweating on the ipsilateral side) occurs with interruption of the sympathetic nervous system innervation **(stellate ganglion block)** of the eye.

2. Ptosis reflects the normal innervation of the superior palpebral muscle by the sympathetic nervous system.

XV. HEARING

A. The external ear, middle ear, and cochlea of the inner ear are concerned with hearing based on mechanical vibrations of sound waves in air (Fig. 41-10).

B. **Ossicle System**

1. The middle ear is an air-filled cavity that includes three bones (malleus, incus, and stapes).

2. Vibrations on any portion of the tympanic membrane are transmitted to the malleus.

a. The **eustachian tube** allows pressures on both sides of the tympanic membrane (external ear and nasopharynx) to be equalized during swallowing or chewing.

b. **Nitrous oxide** may increase middle ear pressure and has been associated with rupture of the tympanic membrane (could be more likely in the presence of scarring or inflammation of the eustachian tube).

C. **Cochlea** is a system of coiled tubes containing end organs to generate nerve impulses in response to sound vibrations.

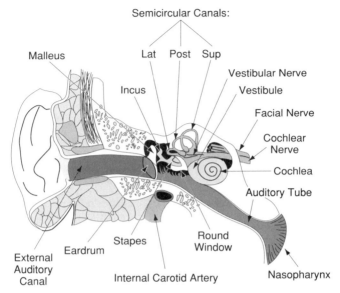

Semicircular Canals:

Lat Post Sup

Malleus

Incus

Vestibular Nerve

Vestibule

Facial Nerve

Cochlear Nerve

Cochlea

Auditory Tube

External Auditory Canal

Eardrum

Stapes

Round Window

Internal Carotid Artery

Nasopharynx

FIGURE 41–10. Schematic diagram of the outer and inner ear. (From Ganong WF. Review of Medical Physiology, 13th ed. Norwalk CT: Appleton and Lange, 1987; with permission.)

 D. **Deafness**
  1. **Nerve deafness** is due to an abnormality of the cochlear or auditory nerve.
  2. **Conduction deafness** is present when there is an abnormality in the middle ear (fibrosis of structures due to repeated infections, osteosclerosis).

XVI. EQUILIBRIUM

 A. Semicircular canals contain endolymph, which causes signals to be transmitted via the vestibular nerve nuclei and the cerebellum.
 B. The utricle and saccule contain cilia that transmit nerve impulses to the brain that are necessary for maintaining orientation of the head in space.
 C. Placement of ice water in the external ear causes cooling of the endolymph in the adjacent semicircular canals, manifesting as nystagmus.

XVII. CHEMICAL SENSES

A. **Taste** (sweet, sour, salty, bitter) is mainly a function of taste buds located principally in the papillae of the tongue (most of what is considered taste is actually smell).

B. **Smell** is a function of olfactory hairs that initiate impulses in olfactory nerve fibers.

XVIII. BODY TEMPERATURE

A. Heat is continually being produced in the body as a byproduct of metabolism.

   1. Body temperature is regulated within narrow limits (balance of heat production and loss), being lowest in the morning (36.1°C, reflecting a 10% to 15% decrease in basal metabolic rate during physiologic sleep) and highest in the evening (37.4°C). As a result, fever associated with disease states is superimposed on this circadian variation and tends to peak in the evening.

   2. An estimated 55% of the energy in nutrients becomes heat during the formation of adenosine triphosphate.

      a. The **calorie** is the unit used to express the quantity of energy released from different nutrients.

      b. The average daily caloric requirement for basal function is about 2000 calories (Table 41–7).

B. **Heat loss** (Table 41–8)

C. **Regulation of body temperature** is by nervous sys-

Table 41–7
Energy Expenditure for Various Forms of Physical Activity

Activity	Calories per Hour
Physiologic sleep	65
Awake at rest	77–100
Typing	140
Walking slowly (2.6 mph)	200
Swimming	500
Running (5.3 mph)	570
Walking up steps	1100

Table 41–8
Mechanism of Heat Loss

Radiation (contact of the body with a cooler environment)

Conduction

Convection

Evaporation (only mechanism that eliminates heat when environmental temperature is higher than that of the skin)

Diaphoresis (stimulation of the preoptic area of the hypothalamus)

tem feedback mechanisms that operate principally through the preoptic area in the hypothalamus.

1. Maintenance of body temperature at a value close to the optimum for enzyme activity assures a constant high rate of metabolism, rapid nervous system conduction, and skeletal muscle contraction.

   a. Protein denaturation begins at about 42°C, whereas ice crystals form in cells at about −1°C.

   b. **Chemical thermogenesis** (brown fat) is an important factor in maintaining normal body temperature in neonates.

2. **Fever** is produced to pyrogens (breakdown products of proteins and polysaccharide toxins secreted by bacteria) that cause the setpoint of the hypothalamic thermostat to increase (pyrexia is an abnormal increase in body temperature [hyperthermia] that reflects heat production that exceeds heat loss).

   a. Prostaglandins, released in response to pyrogens, are presumed to stimulate heat-sensitive neurons in the hypothalamus.

   b. Dehydration can cause fever, which in part reflects the lack of available fluid for sweating.

   c. An abnormal increase in core temperature may be due to pyrexia that results in hyperthermia (heat production exceeds heat loss) or fever (hypothalamic thermal setpoint rises).

   d. Fever occurs in about one third of hospitalized patients and is most often due to infection.

   e. Fever is best treated (especially when higher than 40°C) with drugs such as aspirin, which lower the hypothalamic setpoint (physical cooling methods are indicated when the hypothalamic setpoint is not increased).

        f. There is no evidence that fever is beneficial to host defense mechanisms (may cause seizures in children or precipitate congestive heat failure in elderly patients).

    3. Chills reflect the sudden resetting of the hypothalamic thermostat to a higher level.

  D. Cutaneous blood flow is highly variable (50 to 2800 ml·min^{-1}), reflecting its primary role in regulation of body temperature in response to alterations in the rate of metabolism and the temperature of the external surroundings.

    1. Nutritional requirements are so low for skin that this need does not significantly influence cutaneous blood flow.

    2. Cutaneous blood flow is largely regulated by the sympathetic nervous system.

    3. Inhaled anesthetics increase cutaneous blood flow, perhaps by inhibiting the temperature-regulating center of the hypothalamus.

    4. Skin color is principally due to the color of blood in the cutaneous capillaries and veins (Table 41–9).

  E. Perioperative Temperature Changes

    1. During anesthesia and surgery, exposure to the cold ambient temperature of the operating room and anesthetic-induced inhibition of thermoregulation combine to produce hypothermia (core temperature lower than 36°C).

    2. Volatile anesthetics produce dose-dependent and drug-specific changes in the **thermoregulatory threshold** (the zone between sweating and vasoconstriction thresholds which, under normal conditions, is about 0.2°C).

      a. Volatile anesthetics decrease (by about 2.5°C) the threshold temperature that triggers shivering and vasoconstriction and increase (by

Table 41–9
Factors that Influence Skin Color

Arterial blood flow through skin (pinkish hue)

Low blood flow due to cold (cyanosis)

Severe vasoconstriction (pallor)

Table 41–10
Changes in Core Temperature During Anesthesia

Initial Hypothermia (precipitous decrease in core temperature during first hour)

    Internal redistribution of heat from core to periphery (most important mechanism for initial hypothermia)

    Direct skin exposure to cool environment

    Cold skin prep solutions

    Induction of anesthesia (decreased metabolic heat production and vasodilation)

    Cold intravenous solutions

    Inhalation of dry gases

Linear Decrease (slow decrease in core temperature for 2 to 3 hours)

    Heat loss exceeds metabolic heat production

Plateau Phase (develops after the 2nd to 4th hour of anesthesia)

    Active thermoregulatory vasoconstriction (decreases cutaneous heat loss and conserves metabolic heat, preventing further hypothermia and sometimes leads to an increasing temperature)

(Data from Sessler DI. Temperature regulation and anesthesia. 44th Annual Refresher Course Lectures and Clinical Update Program. American Society of Anesthesiologists, October, 1993.)

---

        about 1°C) the threshold temperature that triggers sweating and vasodilation.

    b. Epidural and spinal anesthesia also widens the thermoregulatory threshold.

3. Widening the thermoregulatory threshold results in a broad temperature range over which active thermoregulatory responses are absent (within this range, patients are poikilothermic).

4. **Hypothermia** has a typical pattern **during general anesthesia** (Table 41-10).

5. **Consequences of Hypothermia** (Table 41-11)

6. **Prevention and Treatment of Hypothermia** (Table 41-12)

(text continues on page 489)

Table 41–11
Consequences of Intraoperative Temperature Decreases

Decreased anesthetic requirements (mean alveolar concentration [MAC])

Protection against cerebral ischemia (carotid endarterectomy, neurosurgery)

Delayed metabolism of drugs

Increased viscosity of blood

Prolongation of prothrombin time and plasma thromboplastin time

Inhibition of immune function (contributing to wound infection)

Decreased cutaneous blood flow (contributing to wound infection)

Postoperative shivering (preceded by core hypothermia and peripheral vasoconstriction indicating a thermoregulatory response; meperidine produces an anti-shivering effect)

Table 41–12
Prevention and Treatment of Hypothermia

Increase ambient temperature of operating room

Heat and humidify inhaled gases

Prevent cutaneous heat loss
  Forced air convective warming (most effective)
  Infrared irradiation (especially infants)
  Circulating water blankets (best when placed over patients, rather than under them, because little heat is lost to the operating table mattress; do not exceed 40°C)
  Surgical drapes

Table 41–13
Measurement of Body Temperature

Esophagus (lower 25% of the esophagus reflects blood and cerebral temperature)

Nasopharynx (may be influenced by temperature of inhaled gases)

Rectal

Bladder (dependent on urine flow)

Tympanic membrane

Pulmonary artery catheter

Skin (limited value as it does not reflect core temperature or reflect trends during malignant hyperthermia)

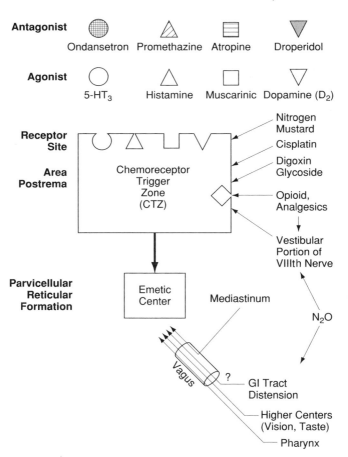

FIGURE 41–11. The chemoreceptor trigger zone and emetic center respond to a variety of stimuli resulting in nausea and vomiting. (From Watcha MF, White PF. Postoperative nausea and vomiting. Its etiology, treatment, and prevention. Anesthesiology 1992;77:162–84; with permission.)

Table 41–14
Characteristics and Events Associated with Postoperative Nausea and Vomiting

Patient-Related Factors
Age (peak incidence at 11 to 14 years of age)
Gender (premenopausal females, especially during 4th and 5th days of menstrual cycle)
Obesity (adipose tissue acts as a reservoir for inhaled anesthetics)
History of motion sickness or previous postoperative emesis
Preoperative anxiety

Operative Procedure
Laparoscopic gynecologic procedures
Strabismus surgery
Middle ear surgery
Tonsillectomy
Extracorporeal shock wave lithotripsy

Duration of Surgery *(long operations)*

Preanesthetic Medication *(opioids)*

Gastric Distention *(positive pressure ventilation of the lungs via a face mask)*

Anesthetic Technique
Volatile anesthetics (little difference between drugs)
Nitrous oxide (controversial)
Etomidate
Propofol (low incidence)
Opioids (not clearly linked to a specific opioid receptor; naloxone can cause nausea and vomiting)
Anticholinesterase drugs (increased gastric motility)
Regional anesthesia (incidence usually lower than after general anesthesia)

Postoperative Factors
Visceral or pelvic pain
Dizziness
Ambulation
Oral intake (controversial)
Opioids (alternative is ketorolac)
Neuraxial opioids (nalbuphine antagonizes emetic effects)

(Data from Watcha MF, White PF. Postoperative nausea and vomiting: Its etiology, treatment, and prevention. Anesthesiology 1992;77:162–84.)

   a. More than 50% of patients have a body temperature lower than 36°C (defined as hypothermia) when they are admitted to the postanesthesia care unit.

   b. Pediatric and elderly patients are particularly vulnerable to intraoperative decreases in body temperature.

F. Measurement of Body Temperature (Table 41-13)

   1. Measurement of core temperature during the first 30 minutes of general anesthesia is unlikely to be useful as body temperature is influenced by a variety of factors during this time.

   2. Core temperature is useful to measure during any period of general anesthesia lasting longer than 60 minutes.

XIX. NAUSEA AND VOMITING

A. The complex action of vomiting involves coordination of respiratory, gastrointestinal, and abdominal musculature in response to several stimuli received at the chemoreceptor trigger zone (no effective blood–brain barrier and thus can be activated by stimuli received through the blood as well as the cerebrospinal fluid) and emetic center (medullary vomiting center) (Fig. 41-11).

B. Nausea and vomiting are among the most common postoperative complaints (affecting an estimated 20% to 30% of patients) and can occur after general, regional, or local anesthesia (Table 41-14).

   1. Persistent nausea and vomiting (severe in 0.1% of patients) may result in postoperative complications (Table 41-15).

Table 41–15
Complications of Persistent Postoperative Nausea and Vomiting

Dehydration

Electrolyte imbalance

Delayed discharge after outpatient surgery

Tension on suture lines

Increased bleeding under skin flaps

Risk of aspiration

2. Routine antiemetic prophylaxis of all patients undergoing elective operations is not recommended as fewer than 30% of patients experience symptoms, and of those who do, many have only transient nausea or only one to two episodes of vomiting (see Chapter 26).

Chapter

42

Autonomic Nervous System

The sympathetic and parasympathetic nervous systems usually function as physiologic antagonists such that activity of organs innervated by both divisions of the autonomic nervous system represent a balance of the influence of each component (Table 42-1). (Updated and revised from Stoelting RK. Autonomic nervous system. In: Pharmacology and Physiology in Anesthetic Practice. 2nd ed. Philadelphia, JB Lippincott, 1991:643-53.) An understanding of the anatomy and physiology of the autonomic nervous system is essential for predicting the pharmacologic effects of drugs that act on either the sympathetic or the parasympathetic nervous system (Table 42-2).

I. ANATOMY OF THE SYMPATHETIC NERVOUS SYSTEM

- **A.** Nerves of the sympathetic nervous system arise from the thoracolumbar (T1 to L2) segments of the spinal cord (Fig. 42-1).
- **B.** These nerve fibers pass to the **paravertebral sympathetic chains** (22 pairs of ganglia) located lateral to the spinal cord.
- **C.** **Postganglionic neurons** exit from paravertebral ganglia to travel to various peripheral organs.

II. ANATOMY OF THE PARASYMPATHETIC NERVOUS SYSTEM

- **A.** Nerves of the parasympathetic nervous system leave the central nervous system through cranial nerves III, V, VII, IX, and X (vagus) and from the sacral portions of the spinal cord (Fig. 42-2).
- **B.** About 75% of all parasympathetic nervous system fibers are in the vagus nerves passing to the thoracic and abdomi-

(text continues on page 497)

Table 42-1
Responses Evoked by Autonomic Nervous System Stimulation

	Sympathetic Nervous System Stimulation	*Parasympathetic Nervous System Stimulation*
Heart		
Sinoatrial node	Increased heart rate	Decreased heart rate
Atrioventricular node	Increased conduction velocity	Decreased conduction velocity
His-Purkinje system	Increased automaticity, conduction velocity	Minimal effect
Ventricles	Increased contractility, conduction velocity, automaticity	Minimal effect; slight decrease in contractility(?)
Bronchial Smooth Muscle	Relaxation	Contraction
Gastrointestinal Tract		
Motility	Decrease	Increase
Secretion	Decrease	Increase
Sphincters	Contraction	Relaxation
Gallbladder	Relaxation	Contraction
Urinary Bladder		
Smooth muscle	Relaxation	Contraction
Sphincter	Contraction	Relaxation

Eye		
Radial muscle	Mydriasis	
Sphincter muscle		Miosis
Ciliary muscle	Relaxation for far vision	Contraction for near vision
Liver	Glycogenolysis Gluconeogenesis	Glycogen synthesis
Pancreatic Beta Cell Secretion	Decrease	
Salivary Gland Secretion	Increase	Marked increase
Sweat Glands	Increase*	
Apocrine Glands	Increase	
Arterioles		
Coronary	Constriction (alpha) Relaxation (beta)	Relaxation(?)
Skin and mucosa	Constriction	
Skeletal muscle	Constriction (alpha) Relaxation (beta)	Relaxation
Pulmonary	Constriction	Relaxation

*The postganglionic sympathetic fibers to sweat glands are cholinergic.

Table 42–2
Mechanisms of Action of Drugs that Act on the Autonomic Nervous System

Mechanism	Site	Drug
Inhibition of neurotransmitter synthesis	SNS	Alpha-methyltyrosine
False neurotransmitter	SNS	Alpha-methyldopa
Inhibition of uptake of neurotransmitter	SNS	Tricyclic antidepressants, cocaine, ketamine(?)
Displacement of neurotransmitter from storage sites	SNS PNS	Amphetamine, guanethidine Carbachol
Prevention of neurotransmitter release	SNS PNS	Bretylium Botulinum toxin
Mimicking of action of neurotransmitter at receptor	SNS alpha-1 alpha-2 beta-1 beta-2	 Phenylephrine, methoxamine Clonidine, dexmedetomidine Dobutamine Terbutaline, albuterol
Inhibition of action of neurotransmitter on postsynaptic receptor	SNS alpha-1 alpha-2 alpha-1, alpha-2 beta-1 beta-1, beta-2 PNS M-1 M-1, M-2 N-1 N-2	 Prazosin Yohimbine Phentolamine Metoprolol, esmolol Propranolol Pirenzipine Atropine Hexamethonium d-Tubocurarine
Inhibition of metabolism of neurotransmitter	SNS PNS	Monoamine oxidase inhibitors Neostigmine, pyridostigmine, edrophonium

SNS, sympathetic nervous system; *PNS,* parasympathetic nervous system.

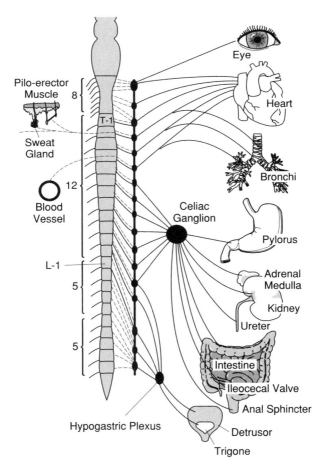

FIGURE 42–1. Anatomy of the sympathetic nervous system. Dashed lines represent postganglionic fibers in gray rami leading into spinal nerves for subsequent distribution to blood vessels and sweat glands. (From Guyton AC. Textbook of Medical Physiology, 7th ed. Philadelphia, WB Saunders, 1986; with permission.)

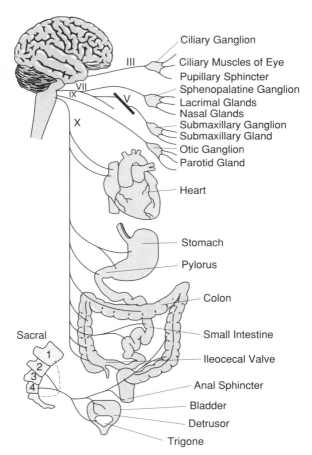

FIGURE 42–2. Anatomy of the parasympathetic nervous system. (From Guyton AC. Textbook of Medical Physiology, 7th ed. Philadelphia, WB Saunders, 1986; with permission.)

nal regions of the body (heart, lungs, esophagus, stomach, small intestine, liver, gallbladder, pancreas, upper portions of the ureters).

C. In contrast to the sympathetic nervous system, preganglionic fibers of the parasympathetic nervous system pass uninterrupted to ganglia near or in the innervated organ.

III. PHYSIOLOGY OF THE AUTONOMIC NERVOUS SYSTEM

A. Postganglionic fibers of the sympathetic nervous system release **norepinephrine** as the neurotransmitter and are classified as **adrenergic fibers.**

   1. Postganglionic fibers of the sympathetic nervous system that innervate sweat glands release acetylcholine as the neurotransmitter.

   2. All preganglionic neurons of the sympathetic and parasympathetic nervous systems release acetylcholine as the neurotransmitter and are classified as cholinergic fibers.

B. Postganglionic fibers of the parasympathetic nervous system secrete **acetylcholine** as the neurotransmitter and are classified as **cholinergic fibers.**

C. Norepinephrine as a Neurotransmitter

   1. **Synthesis** of norepinephrine involves a series of enzyme-controlled steps that begin in the cytoplasm of postganglionic sympathetic nerve endings (varicosities) and are completed in the synaptic vesicles.

   2. **Storage and Release**

     a. Norepinephrine is stored in synaptic vesicles for subsequent release **(exocytosis)** in response to an action potential.

     b. Adrenergic fibers can sustain output of norepinephrine during prolonged periods of stimulation.

   3. **Termination of Action** (Table 42-3)

D. Acetylcholine as a Neurotransmitter

   1. **Synthesis** of acetylcholine occurs in the cytoplasm of varicosities of the preganglionic and postganglionic parasympathetic nerve endings (choline acetyltransferase catalyzes the combination of choline with acetyl coenzyme A to form acetylcholine).

   2. **Storage and release** of acetylcholine is from synaptic vesicles in response to an action potential.

   3. **Metabolism**

     a. Rapid hydrolysis of acetylcholine by **acetylcholin-**

Table 42–3
Termination of Action of Norepinephrine

Uptake (accounts for 80% of released norepinephrine and is blocked by drugs such as cocaine and tricyclic antidepressants)

Metabolism (vanillylmandelic acid is the principal urinary metabolite)
   Cytoplasm (monoamine oxidase enzyme)
   Liver (catechol-O-methyltransferase enzyme)

Dilution on Diffusion from Receptors

___

   esterase (true cholinesterase) accounts for the brief effect at receptors (1 msec or less).
   b. Plasma cholinesterase (pseudocholinesterase) is not important in the hydrolysis of acetylcholine (absence of this enzyme produces no effects until drugs, such as succinylcholine or mivacurium, are administered).

IV. INTERACTIONS OF NEUROTRANSMITTERS WITH RECEPTORS

   A. Norepinephrine Receptors (Table 42–4) (see Chapter 12)
   B. Acetylcholine receptors are classified as **nicotinic** (autonomic ganglia, neuromuscular junction) and **muscarinic** (heart, salivary glands) (see Chapter 12).

V. RESIDUAL AUTONOMIC NERVOUS SYSTEM TONE

   A. Sympathetic nervous system tone normally keeps blood vessels about 50% constricted (permits alterations in systemic vascular resistance).
   B. Acute denervation of the sympathetic nervous system, as produced by a regional anesthetic, results in immediate maximal vasodilation.

VI. ADRENAL MEDULLA

   A. The adrenal medulla is innervated by preganglionic fibers that pass directly from the spinal cord to cells that are analogous to postganglionic neurons.
      1. Stimulation of the sympathetic nervous system causes release of epinephrine (80%) and norepinephrine.

Table 42–4
Responses Evoked by Selective Stimulation of Adrenoceptors

Alpha-1 (Postsynaptic) Receptors
Vasoconstriction
Mydriasis
Relaxation of gastrointestinal tract
Contraction of gastrointestinal sphincters
Contraction of bladder sphincter

Alpha-2 (Presynaptic) Receptors
Inhibition of norepinephrine release

Alpha-2 (Postsynaptic) Receptors
Platelet aggregation
Hyperpolarization of cells in the central nervous system

Beta-1 (Postsynaptic) Receptors
Increased conduction velocity
Increased automaticity
Increased contractility

Beta-2 (Postsynaptic) Receptors
Vasodilation
Bronchodilation
Gastrointestinal relaxation
Uterine relaxation
Bladder relaxation
Glycogenolysis
Lipolysis

Dopamine-1 (Postsynaptic) Receptors
Vasodilation

Dopamine-2 (Presynaptic) Receptors
Inhibition of norepinephrine release

    2. Catecholamines released by the adrenal medulla act as hormones and not as neurotransmitters.
B. Synthesis
    1. Most of the formed norepinephrine is converted to epinephrine by the action of phenylethanolamine-N-methyltransferase.
    2. Activity of this enzyme is enhanced by cortisol.
C. Release of epinephrine and norepinephrine from the adrenal medulla is triggered by liberation of acetylcholine from preganglionic cholinergic fibers.

1. Responses evoked by release of epinephrine and norepinephrine into the circulation are similar to direct sympathetic nervous system stimulation with the difference being a prolonged duration of action (10 to 30 seconds) compared with the brief duration of action on receptors that is produced by norepinephrine acting as a neurotransmitter (Table 42–1) (see Chapter 12).

2. This prolonged effect of circulating epinephrine and norepinephrine released by the adrenal medulla reflects the time necessary for metabolism in the liver (Table 42–3).

3. Circulating norepinephrine and epinephrine released by the adrenal medulla and acting as hormones can substitute for sympathetic nervous system innervation of an organ.

Chapter

43
Pain

Pain (nociception) is a protective mechanism that occurs when tissues are being damaged causing the individual to react to remove the painful stimulus. (Updated and revised from Stoelting RK. Pain. In: Pharmacology and Physiology in Anesthetic Practice. 2nd ed. Philadelphia, JB Lippincott, 1991:654–60.)

I. CLASSIFICATION OF PAIN (Table 43–1)

A. Organic pain may be subdivided into nociceptive (somatic and visceral pain due to peripheral stimulation of nociceptors at these sites) and neuropathic (non-nociceptive pain, such as that associated with peripheral nerve involvement by a tumor).

B. Nociceptive pain is usually responsive to opioids or non-steroidal antiinflammatory drugs, whereas patients experiencing neuropathic pain frequently respond poorly to opioids but may benefit from tricyclic antidepressants.

II. TYPES OF PAIN

A. Two qualitatively different types of pain can be readily appreciated.

1. **Fast pain** starts abruptly with the stimulus (surgical skin incision) and ends promptly when the stimulus is removed (small, myelinated type A-delta fibers with conduction velocities of 12 to 30 m·sec^{-1} are responsible for transmission).

2. **Slow pain** is characterized as a throbbing, burning, or aching sensation that is poorly localized and may continue long after removal of the stimulus (unmyelinated type C fibers with conduction velocities of 0.5 to 2 m·sec^{-1} are responsible for transmission).

3. A subjective perception of the different conduction velocities and functions of A-delta and C fibers is the phenomenon of **first pain** (A-delta fibers) and **second pain** (C fibers).

4. When a finger touches a hot stove, there is an initial

Table 43–1
Pathophysiologic Classification of Pain

Organic Pain
   Nociceptive (somatic and visceral)
   Neuropathic (deafferentation)

Psychologic Pain

(Adapted from Ashburn MA, Lipman AG. Management of pain in the cancer patient. Anesth Analg 1993;76:402–16.)

rapid, sharp, and brief sensation (first pain) leading to instant withdrawal. This is followed by a more prolonged, burning, and usually more unpleasant sensation (second pain).

B. Nerve fibers for temperature follow the same pathways as fibers for pain (heat stimulus causes pain in almost all subjects when skin temperature is higher than 43°C **[pain threshold]**).

III. PAIN RECEPTORS

A. Pain receptors **(nociceptors)** are naked afferent nerve endings of myelinated A-delta and unmyelinated C fibers that encode the occurrence, intensity, duration, and location of noxious stimuli and signal pain sensation.

   1. Pain receptors are widespread in superficial layers of the skin (mechanosensitive pain receptors, mechanothermal receptors, polynodal pain receptors), periosteum, joint surfaces, skeletal muscles, and tooth pulp.

   2. Most other deep tissues are not richly supplied with pain receptors, although widespread tissue damage can summate to cause aching pain in these areas.

   3. In contrast to sensory receptors, pain receptors do not adapt (protective).

B. Skeletal muscle spasm is a common cause of pain and may become the basis for a myofascial pain syndrome (stimulation of mechanosensitive pain receptors, as well as ischemia, that stimulates polynodal pain receptors).

C. Autonomic Nervous System Responses

   1. Painful stimulation may evoke reflex increases in sympathetic nervous system efferent activity.

2. **Reflex sympathetic dystrophy** is an extreme example of pain associated with increases in sympathetic nervous system activity.

IV. TRANSMISSION OF PAIN SIGNALS

A. Pain signals are transmitted from peripheral pain receptors via A-delta and C fibers to the dorsal horn of the spinal cord where they synapse with cells in the **substantia gelatinosa.**
   1. Spinothalamic tracts are the principal ascending pathways responsible for cephalad transmission of pain impulses.
   2. Impulses travel from the thalamus to the somatosensory areas of the cerebral cortex.
   3. Stimulation of the reticular activating system by burning and aching pain awakens the patient from sleep and produces generalized activation of the nervous system.
   4. Perception of nociceptive input is modulated at every level of the afferent sensory pathway from the peripheral nerve to cerebral cortex.
B. **Conceptual Model of Pain Transmission**
   1. A conceptual model of pain transmission includes ascending excitatory afferent pain pathways, descending inhibitory pain pathways, and a variety of neuromodulators and neurotransmitters (Fig. 43–1).
   2. Transmission of pain impulses may be modulated by activation of descending inhibitory pain pathways that pass from the brain to the spinal cord.
      a. Endorphins may be responsible for activating these descending inhibitory pathways (opioid receptors in the substantial gelatinosa).
      b. The net effect of activating these descending inhibitory pathways and releasing inhibitory neurotransmitters is to inhibit transmission of pain impulses from pain receptors via ascending afferent fibers.
C. **Sites Amenable to Surgical Section of Pain Pathways** (Fig. 43–2)
D. **Gate Control Theory**
   1. Conceptually, the dorsal horn of the spinal cord may function as the gate controlling the subsequent synaptic transmission of pain impulses via the spinothalamic tract.
   2. Activation of large afferent fibers (transcutaneous

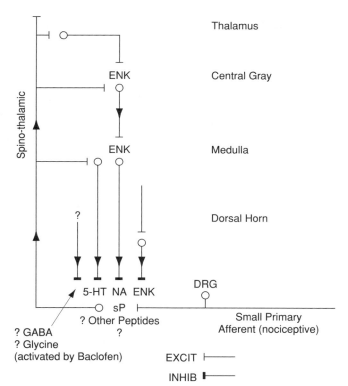

FIGURE 43–1. A conceptual model of pain transmission includes ascending excitatory and descending inhibitory pain pathways and a variety of neurotransmitters. Primary afferent pain (nociceptive) signals travel by the dorsal root ganglion (*DRG*) to cells in the dorsal horn of the spinal cord where substance P acts as the excitatory neurotransmitter. The endogenous endorphin (*ENK*) system is activated by pain signals that reach the thalamus. Activation of descending inhibitory pain pathways by ENK results in inhibition of dorsal horn neurons in the spinal cord through the release of inhibitory neurotransmitters that may include serotonin (*5-HT*), norepinephrine (*NA*), endorphins (ENK), gamma-aminobutyric acid (*GABA*), and glycine. (From Cousins MJ, Mather LE. Intrathecal and epidural administration of opioids. Anesthesiology 1984;61:276–310; with permission.)

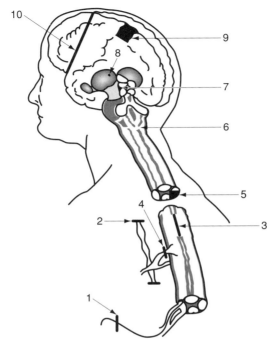

FIGURE 43–2. Diagram of various surgical procedures designed to interrupt pain pathways. 1—nerve section; 2—sympathectomy for visceral pain; 3—myelotomy to section spinothalamic fibers in the anterior white commissure; 4—posterior rhizotomy; 5—anterior cordotomy; 6—medullary tractotomy; 7—mesencephalic tractotomy; 8—thalamotomy; 9—gyrectomy; 10—prefrontal lobotomy. (From Ganong WF. Review of Medical Physiology, 13th ed. Norwalk, CT: Appleton and Lange, 1987; with permission.)

electrical nerve stimulation) may produce a counterirritant effect by inhibition of smaller pain fibers.

V. PERIPHERAL EVENTS IN TISSUE TRAUMA AND POSTOPERATIVE PAIN

A. Tissue injury leads to nociception by **direct damage to nerve endings, inflammation, and hyperalgesia** (Fig. 43–3).

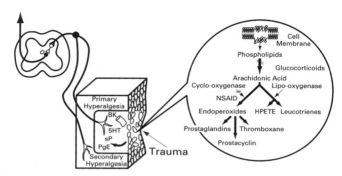

FIGURE 43–3.   Trauma to tissue leads to the local release of multiple chemical substances (substance P[*sP*], bradykinin [*BK*], serotonin [*5HT*], prostaglandins [*PgE*] from a cascade of arachidonic acid metabolites) from afferent nerve endings, resulting in vasodilation, increased vascular permeability (inflammation), and sensitization of nociceptors (primary hyperalgesia). (From Dahl JB, Kehlet H. Nonsteroidal anti-inflammatory drugs: Rationale for use in severe postoperative pain. Br J Anaesth 1991;66:703–12; with permission.)

    B. The primary afferent nerve ending serves a dual function (transmission of neural stimuli and release of mediators of inflammation [prostaglandins, histamine, bradykinin, serotonin, substance P]) at the site of trauma.

        1. Activation of nociceptive afferents may also elicit spinal cord reflexes that markedly increase the activity of postganglionic sympathetic nervous system efferents.

        2. Hyperalgesia is an altered functional state of the nervous system characterized by extreme sensitivity to painful stimuli (decrease in pain threshold) and, often, spontaneous pain.

        3. Primary hyperalgesia refers to changes that occur within the site of injury (sensitization of nociceptors), whereas secondary hyperalgesia refers to changes in the peripheral and central nervous system.

VI. REACTION TO PAIN

    A. Pain threshold is similar, but people's reaction to pain varies greatly (psychic reactions and reflex motor responses).

   1. Anxiety makes pain less tolerable.
   2. The preoperative level of anxiety may be a useful predictor of the likely intensity of postoperative pain.
B. Administration of an opioid prior to the painful surgical stimulus (preoperative medication or intravenous medication at the time of induction of anesthesia) **(preemptive analgesia)** may decrease the intensity of postoperative pain.
   1. It is hypothesized that painful afferent signals alter central processing so that, postoperatively, input from the damaged cells travels to sensitized spinal cord cells which amplify the peripheral signal and contribute to enhanced postoperative pain.
   2. Support for the concept of preemptive analgesia is derived from animal data demonstrating that the dose of systemic morphine required to abolish established noxious stimulus–induced central hyperactivity is greater than the dose required to prevent it.

VII. VISCERAL PAIN

A. Pain receptors in viscera are sparsely distributed such that surgical incision is not associated with intense pain.
B. Visceral pain typically radiates, and may be referred to surface areas of the body far removed from the painful viscus but with the same dermatome origin as the diseased viscus.
   1. Often, visceral pain occurs in cycles corresponding to rhythmic contractions of smooth muscle.
   2. Distention of a hollow viscus results in aching, diffuse or cramping pain due to stretch of the tissues, and possibly, ischemia due to compression of blood vessels.
   3. Pain impulses from most of the abdominal and thoracic viscera are conducted through afferent fibers that travel with the sympathetic nervous system.
   4. Parenchyma of the brain, liver, and alveoli of the lungs are devoid of pain receptors.

VIII. SOMATIC PAIN

A. Somatic pain is sharp, stabbing, well-localized pain that typically arises from skin, skeletal muscles, and the peritoneum.

B. Pain from a surgical skin incision, the second stage of labor, or peritoneal irritation is somatic pain.

IX. EMBRYOLOGIC ORIGIN AND LOCALIZED PAIN

A. The position of the spinal cord to which visceral afferent fibers pass for each organ depends on the segment (dermatome) of the body from which the organ developed embryologically.

B. This explains the phenomenon of referred pain to a site distal from tissues causing the pain (heart originates in the neck, and the referred pain of myocardial ischemia is to the neck and arm).

Chapter

44

Systemic Circulation

The systemic circulation supplies blood to all the tissues of the body except the lungs. (Updated and revised from Stoelting RK. Systemic circulation. In: Pharmacology and Physiology in Anesthetic Practice. 2nd ed. Philadelphia, JB Lippincott, 1991:661–78.)

I. COMPONENTS OF THE SYSTEMIC CIRCULATION
(Table 44-1)

II. PHYSICAL CHARACTERISTICS OF THE SYSTEMIC CIRCULATION

A. The systemic circulation contains 80% of the blood volume, of which about 64% is in the veins (Fig. 44-1).

B. **Progressive Declines in Blood Pressure** (Fig. 44-2)
   1. Resistance to blood flow in the aorta and other large arteries is minimal, and mean arterial pressure decreases only 3 to 5 mmHg as blood travels into arteries as small as 3 mm in diameter.
      a. Arterioles account for about 50% of the resistance in the entire systemic circulation.
      b. As a result, blood pressure decreases to about 30 mmHg at the point where blood enters the capillaries.
      c. At the venous end of the capillaries, the intravascular pressure has decreased to about 10 mmHg.
   2. The decrease in blood pressure from 10 mmHg to nearly 0 mmHg as blood traverses veins indicates that these vessels impart far more resistance to blood flow than would be expected for vessels of their large sizes (reflecting compression of veins by external forces).

C. **Pulse pressure in arteries** reflects the intermittent injection of blood into the aorta by the heart (Table 44-2; Fig. 44-3).
   1. **Factors that alter pulse pressure** include left ventricular stroke volume, velocity of blood flow,

Table 44–1
Components of the Systemic Circulation

Arteries (transport blood to tissue under high pressure)

Arterioles (dilate or constrict to control blood flow into the capillaries)

Capillaries (serve as sites for transfer of oxygen to tissues)

Venules and veins (serve as conduits for transmitting blood to the right atrium)

and compliance of the arterial tree (aging often decreases distensibility of the arterial walls and pulse pressure increases).

2. **Transmission of the Pulse Pressure**
   a. There is often enhancement of the pulse pressure as the pressure wave is transmitted peripherally (Fig. 44-4).
   b. Systolic blood pressure in the radical artery is sometimes as much as 20% to 30% above that in the central aorta **(mean arterial pressure is similar regardless of the site of blood pressure measurement).**

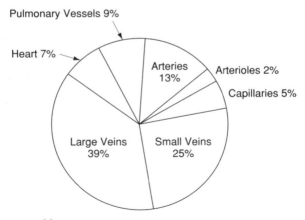

FIGURE 44–1. Distribution of blood volume in the systemic and pulmonary circulation. (From Guyton AC. Textbook of Medical Physiology, 7th ed. Philadelphia: WB Saunders, 1986; with permission.)

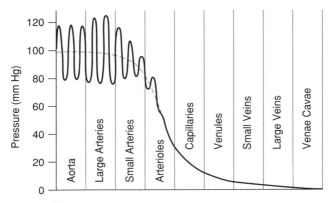

FIGURE 44–2. Blood pressure decreases as blood travels from the aorta to large veins. (From Guyton AC. Textbook of Medical Physiology, 7th ed. Philadelphia: WB Saunders, 1986; with permission.)

Table 44–2
Normal Pressures in the Systemic Circulation

	Mean Value (mmHg)	Range (mmHg)
Systolic blood pressure*	120	90–140
Diastolic blood pressure*	80	70–90
Mean arterial pressure	92	77–97
Left ventricular end-diastolic pressure	6	0–12
Left atrium	8	2–12
a wave	10	4–16
v wave	13	6–20
Right atrium	5	3–8
a wave	6	2–10
c wave	5	2–10
v wave	3	0–8

*Measured in the radial artery

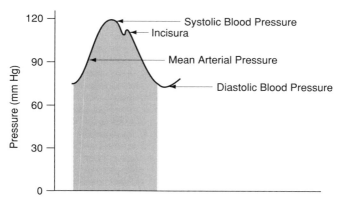

FIGURE 44–3. Schematic depiction of blood pressure recorded from a large systemic artery. Mean arterial pressure is equal to the area under the blood pressure curve divided by the duration of systole.

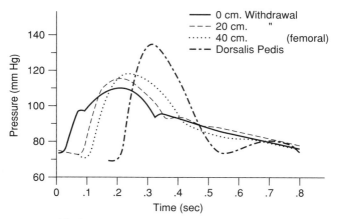

FIGURE 44–4. There is enhancement of the pulse pressure as the blood pressure is transmitted peripherally. (From Guyton AC. Textbook of Medical Physiology, 7th ed. Philadelphia: WB Saunders, 1986; with permission.)

c. Reversal of the usual relationship between aortic and radial artery blood pressures can occur during hypothermic cardiopulmonary bypass (failure to appreciate this change may lead to inappropriate treatment in the early period following termination of cardiopulmonary bypass). The discrepancy between blood pressure measurements obtained from the central aorta and radial artery has been shown to develop shortly after the institution of cardiopulmonary bypass and is not influenced by rewarming or by drug-induced (nitroprusside, phenylephrine) changes in systemic vascular resistance (Fig. 44–5).

3. **Pulsus paradoxus** is an exaggerated decrease in systolic blood pressure (greater than 10 mmHg) during inspiration in the presence of increased intrapericardial pressures.

4. **Pulsus alternans** is alternating weak and strong cardiac contractions causing a similar alteration in the strength of the peripheral pulse (heart block).

5. **Pulse deficit** is the presence of a cardiac contraction that pumps insufficient blood to create a peripheral pulse.

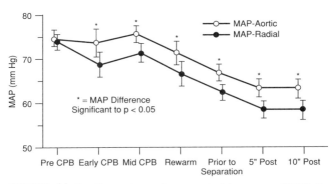

FIGURE 44–5. Comparison of mean arterial pressure (*MAP*) recorded from the central aorta (*aortic*) or radial artery at various times before (*Pre*), during, and following (*Post*) cardiopulmonary bypass (*CPB*). (From Rich GF, Lubanski RE, McLoughlin TM. Differences between aortic and radial artery pressure associated with cardiopulmonary bypass. Anesthesiology 1992;63–6; with permission.)

6. Measurement of blood pressure by auscultation usually gives values that are within 10% of those determined by direct measurements from the arteries.

7. **Right atrial pressure** (commonly designated the central venous pressure) is regulated by a balance between venous return and the ability of the right ventricle to eject blood.

8. **Peripheral Venous Pressure**

   a. Most large veins are compressed at multiple extrathoracic sites.

   b. It is important to recognize that veins inside the thorax are not collapsed because of the distending effect of negative intrathoracic pressure.

9. **Effect of Hydrostatic Pressure**

   a. Pressure in veins below the heart is increased and that in veins above the heart is decreased by the effect of gravity (Fig. 44–6).

   b. As a guideline, pressure changes about **0.77 mmHg for every centimeter** the vessel is above or below the heart (negative pressure may exist in veins above the heart, leading to extrainment of air).

10. **Venous Valves and the Pump Mechanism**

    a. Valves in veins are arranged so that the direction of blood flow can only be toward the heart.

    b. **Varicose veins** result when valves are destroyed and veins are chronically distended by increased venous pressure.

11. **Reference Level for Measuring Venous Pressures**

    a. Hydrostatic pressure does not alter venous or arterial pressures that are measured at the level of the **tricuspid valve** (external reference points are one third the distance from the anterior chest and about one fourth the distance above the lower end of the sternum).

    b. The potential error introduced by measuring pressure above or below the tricuspid valve is greatest with venous pressures that are normally low.

    c. A venous pressure measurement expressed in mmHg can be converted to cm H_2O by multiplying the pressure by 1.36.

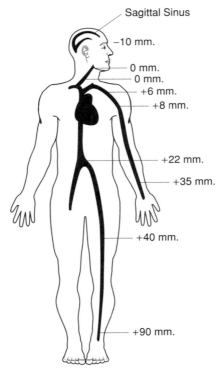

FIGURE 44–6. Effect of hydrostatic pressure on venous pressure throughout the body. (From Guyton AC. Textbook of Medical Physiology, 7th ed. Philadelphia: WB Saunders, 1986; with permission.)

III. PHYSICAL CHARACTERISTICS OF BLOOD

    A. The percentage of blood comprising erythrocytes is the hematocrit, which to a large extent determines the viscosity of blood.

    B. When the hematocrit increases to 60% to 70%, viscosity of blood is increased about 10-fold compared with water.

IV. DETERMINANTS OF TISSUE BLOOD FLOW

    A. Tissue blood flow is directly proportional to the pressure difference between two points and inversely propor-

$$\frac{\text{Blood Flow}}{(Q)} = \frac{\text{Pressure Difference Between Two Points (P)}}{\text{Resistance to Flow (R)}}$$

$$\Delta P = Q \times R$$

$$R = \Delta P / Q$$

FIGURE 44–7. The relationship between blood flow, pressure, and resistance to flow can be expressed as a variant of Ohm's law.

tional to resistance to flow through the vessel (Fig. 44-7).

1. Rearrangement of this formula emphasizes that pressure is directly proportional to flow multiplied by resistance.
2. Resistance (cannot be measured but rather is calculated) is directly proportional to pressure (also viscosity) and inversely proportional to flow (and also to the fourth power of the radius of the vessel).
   a. Systemic vascular resistance is calculated as the difference between mean arterial pressure and right atrial pressure divided by cardiac output.
   b. Pulmonary vascular resistance is calculated as the difference between mean pulmonary artery pressure and left atrial pressure divided by cardiac output.
   c. Resistance is expressed in units or dynes·sec·cm^{-5} if the calculated value is multiplied by 80.
B. **Vascular Distensibility**
   1. Increases in systemic blood pressure can cause the vascular diameter to increase which, in turn, decreases resistance to blood flow.
   2. When the heart is abruptly stopped, the pressure in the entire circulatory system (**mean circulatory pressure**) equilibrates at about 7 mmHg.
C. **Vascular Compliance**
   1. Compliance of veins is much greater than that of arteries (when mean arterial pressure is 100 mmHg, the volume of blood in veins is about 2500 ml and that in the arteries is about 750 ml).
   2. Sympathetic nervous system activity can greatly alter the distribution of blood volume.

V. CONTROL OF TISSUE BLOOD FLOW

A. Total tissue blood flow or cardiac output is about 5 $L \cdot min^{-1}$, with large amounts being delivered to the heart, brain, liver, and kidneys (Table 44–3).

B. **Local control of blood flow** is most often based on the need for delivery of oxygen to the tissues.

C. **Autoregulation of blood flow** is a local mechanism for control of blood flow in which a specific tissue is able to maintain a relatively constant blood flow over a wide range of mean arterial pressure.

D. **Long-term local control of blood flow** involves a change in vascularity of tissues.

E. **Autonomic nervous system control of blood flow** is characterized by a rapid response time and ability to regulate blood flow to certain tissues at the expense of other tissues.

F. **Vasomotor center,** which is located in the pons and medulla, transmits sympathetic nervous system impulses through the spinal cord to all blood vessels.

Table 44–3
Tissue Blood Flow

	Approximate Blood Flow		*Cardiac Output*
	($ml \cdot min^{-1}$)	*($ml \cdot 100\ g^{-1} \cdot min^{-1}$)*	*(% of total)*
Brain	750	50	15
Liver	1450	100	29
Portal vein	1100		
Hepatic artery	350		
Kidneys	1000	320	20
Heart	225	75	5
Skeletal muscles (at rest)	750	4	15
Skin	400	3	8
Other tissues	425	2	8
TOTAL	5000		100

(Adapted from Guyton AC. Textbook of Medical Physiology, 7th ed. Philadelphia: WB Saunders, 1986; with permission.)

1. **Mass reflex** is characterized by stimulation of all portions of the vasomotor center, resulting in generalized vasoconstriction and an increase in cardiac output in an attempt to maintain tissue blood flow.
2. **Syncope** may reflect profound skeletal muscle vasodilation and resulting hypotension.

G. **Hormone control of blood flow** is via vasoconstricting (norepinephrine) and vasodilating (histamine, carbon dioxide) factors.

VI. REGULATION OF BLOOD PRESSURE

A. Blood pressure is maintained over a narrow range by reciprocal changes in cardiac output and systemic vascular resistance.

B. **Rapid-Acting Mechanisms for the Regulation of Blood Pressure** (Table 44-4)
1. **Baroreceptors** adapt in 1 to 3 days to whatever blood pressure level they are exposed to, emphasizing that these reflexes are probably of no importance in the long-term regulation of blood pressure.
2. **Vasomotor or Traube-Hering waves** are cyclic increases and decreases in blood pressure that presumably reflect oscillation in the reflex activity of baroreceptors.

C. **Moderately Rapid-Acting Mechanisms for the Regulation of Blood Pressure**
1. There are at least three hormonal mechanisms that provide either rapid or moderately rapid control of

Table 44-4
Rapid-Acting Mechanisms for Regulation of Blood Pressure

Baroreceptor reflexes (important for maintaining blood pressure when an individual changes from the supine to standing position; blunted by volatile anesthetics)

Chemoreceptor reflexes (important for stimulating breathing when the PaO_2 is lower than 60 mmHg; inhibited by subanesthetic concentrations of volatile anesthetics)

Atrial reflexes (stretching of atria evokes vasodilation and tachycardia)

Central nervous system ischemic reflex (intense outpouring of sympathetic nervous system activity when ischemia of medullary vasomotor center occurs [Cushing reflex])

blood pressure (catecholamines, renin-angiotensin, antidiuretic hormone).
   2. In addition to hormonal mechanisms, there are two intrinsic mechanisms (capillary fluid shift and stress relaxation of blood vessels) which begin to react within minutes of changes in blood pressure.
D. **Long-term mechanisms for the regulation of blood pressure,** unlike the short-term regulatory mechanisms, have a delayed onset but do not adapt, providing a sustained regulatory effect.
   1. **Renal–body fluid system** can return blood pressure to normal by changes in sodium ion (Na^+) and water excretion by the kidneys.
   2. **Renin-angiotensin system** stimulates the kidneys to retain Na^+ and water.

VII. REGULATION OF CARDIAC OUTPUT AND VENOUS RETURN

A. Because the circulation is a closed circuit, the cardiac output (5 L·min^{-1} in a 1.7 m^2 adult) must equal venous return.
B. **Determinants of Cardiac Output**
   1. Venous return is more important than myocardial contractility in determining cardiac output.
      a. **Metabolic requirements** of tissues control cardiac output through alterations in resistance to tissue blood flow.
      b. Any factor that interferes with venous return (hemorrhage, venodilation due to regional anesthesia, positive pressure ventilation of the lungs) can lead to decreased cardiac output.
      c. The optimal therapy for hypotension resulting from spinal anesthesia is appropriate positioning of the patient and intravenous infusion of fluids to improve venous return.
   2. Decreases in systemic vascular resistance (anemia, exercise, hyperthyroidism, arteriovenous shunts) can increase cardiac output.
   3. **Increased blood volume** increases cardiac output by increasing the gradient for flow to the right atrium and by distending blood vessels, which decreases resistance to flow.
   4. **Sympathetic nervous system stimulation** increases myocardial contractility and heart rate beyond that possible from venous return alone (al-

though the effect is transient owing to autoregulation and fluid shift out of the capillaries).

C. **Ventricular Function Curves** (Frank-Starling curves) depict the cardiac output at different atrial (ventricular end-diastolic) filling pressures (Fig. 44-8).

    1. A point is reached where further stretching of the cardiac muscle results in a decrease in cardiac output.

    2. Clinically, ventricular function curves are used to **estimate myocardial contractility.**

D. **Circulatory shock** is characterized by inadequate tissue blood flow and oxygen delivery to cells, resulting in generalized deterioration of organ function.

    1. **Hemorrhage** is the most common cause of shock owing to decreased venous return.

    2. **Loss of plasma** in the absence of blood loss (gastrointestinal obstruction, burns) may result in shock (in contrast to hemorrhage, selective loss of plasma greatly increases viscosity of blood).

    3. **Neurogenic shock** occurs in the absence of blood loss when vascular capacity increases greatly, as may occur with acute blockade of the peripheral sympathetic nervous system by spinal or epidural anesthesia.

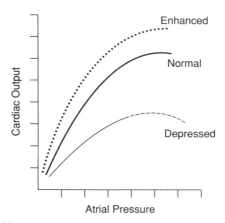

FIGURE 44–8. Ventricular function curves (Frank-Starling curves) depict the volume of forward ventricular ejection (cardiac output) at different atrial filling pressures and varying degrees of myocardial contractility.

4. **Septic shock** is characterized by profound peripheral vasodilation, increased cardiac output, and disseminated intravascular coagulation.
   a. Causes of septic shock are most often a release
      of endotoxins from ischemic portions of the gas-
      trointestinal tract or from bacteremia owing to
      extension of urinary tract infections.
   b. The end-stages of septic shock are not greatly
      different from the end-stages of hemorrhagic
      shock.
5. Decreased cardiac output associated with shock
   decreases tissue oxygen delivery (Table 44–5).
E. **Measurement of Cardiac Output**
   1. **Fick method** calculates the cardiac output as oxy-
      gen consumption (respirometer) divided by the ar-
      teriovenous difference for oxygen (venous blood
      from the right ventricle or pulmonary artery).
   2. **Indicator dilution method** measures cardiac out-
      put as a function of the arterial concentration of a
      known dose of dye previously injected into the
      central venous circulation.
      a. It is necessary to extrapolate the dye curve to
         zero because recirculation of the dye occurs be-
         fore the downslope of the curve reaches base-
         line.
      b. **Early recirculation** of the dye may indicate
         the presence of a right-to-left intracardiac shunt
         (foramen ovale).
   3. **Thermodilution method** of determining cardiac
      output involves measuring the change in blood tem-
      perature between two points (right atrium and pul-
      monary artery) following injection of a known vol-

Table 44–5
*Manifestations of Decreased Tissue Oxygen Delivery During
Shock*

Skeletal muscle weakness
Decreased body temperature
Impaired mental clarity
Decreased urine output
Acute tubular necrosis
Myocardial depression

ume of saline (room temperature or colder) at the proximal right atrial port.

  a. The change in blood temperature, as measured at the distal pulmonary artery port, is inversely proportional to pulmonary blood flow, which is equivalent to cardiac output.

  b. A computer converts the area under the temperature-time curve to its equivalent in cardiac output.

  c. The advantages of this method compared with the other methods are its relative simplicity, safety of repeated measurements, and absence of any influence of recirculation.

VIII. FETAL CIRCULATION (Fig. 44-9)

  A. In utero, the placenta acts as the fetal lung, and oxygenated blood (saturation about 80%) from the placenta passes through a single umbilical vein to the fetus.

   1. Most of the oxygenated blood entering the fetal right atrium from the inferior vena cava preferentially passes through the foramen ovale into the left atrium, thus bypassing the lungs (allowing perfusion of the fetal brain with maximum available concentrations of oxygen).

   2. Fetal hemoglobin differs from adult hemoglobin in binding oxygen less avidly, thus maximizing oxygen transfer to tissues despite low hemoglobin saturations with oxygen.

   3. Blood is returned to the placenta for oxygenation by two umbilical arteries.

  B. The principal changes in fetal circulation at birth are increased systemic vascular resistance and blood pressure owing to cessation of blood flow through the placenta.

   1. Expansion of the lungs decreases pulmonary vascular resistance, leading to a marked increase in pulmonary blood flow.

   2. These alterations in systemic and pulmonary vascular resistance change the pressure gradient across the foramen ovale, causing the flaplike valve to occlude this opening.

    a. In the absence of permanent closure of the foramen ovale, events that increase right atrial pressure above left atrial pressure (positive pressure

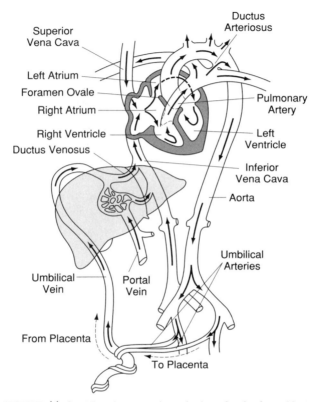

FIGURE 44–9. The placenta acts as the lung for the fetus. Most of the oxygenated blood reaching the fetal heart via the umbilical vein and inferior vena cava is diverted through the foramen ovale and pumped out the aorta to the head. Most of the deoxygenated blood returned via the superior vena cava is pumped through the pulmonary artery and ductus arteriosus to the feet and the umbilical arteries. (From Ganong WF. Review of Medical Physiology, 13th ed. Norwalk, CT: Appleton and Lange, 1987; with permission.)

ventilation of the lungs, especially with positive end-expiratory pressure) may introduce an unexpected right-to-left intracardiac shunt at this site.

   b. Arterial hypoxemia may be the initial manifestation of this intracardiac shunt when right atrial pressure is acutely increased.

C. Flow through the **ductus arteriosus** decreases after birth owing to constriction of the muscular wall of this vessel in response to exposure to higher concentrations of oxygen (failure to close is associated with excessive pulmonary blood flow).

Chapter

45

Capillaries and Lymph Vessels

Capillaries serve as the site for transfer of oxygen and nutrients to tissues and receipt of metabolic products, whereas lymph vessels represent an alternate route by which excess fluids can flow from interstitial fluid spaces into the blood. (Updated and revised from Stoelting RK. Capillaries and lymph vessels. In: Pharmacology and Physiology in Anesthetic Practice. 2nd ed. Philadelphia, JB Lippincott, 1991:679–84.)

I. CAPILLARIES

A. Anatomy of the Microcirculation

1. Arterioles give rise to metarterioles, which give rise to capillaries (unlikely that any functional cell is more than 50 μm away from a capillary) (Fig. 45–1).
2. Capillary walls are about 0.5 mm thick and consist of a single layer of endothelial cells that include interdigitated junctions and pores for transfer of molecules (Table 45–1).
   a. Oxygen and carbon dioxide are both lipid-soluble and readily pass through endothelial cells.
   b. Plasma proteins have diameters that exceed the width of capillary pores.

B. Blood flow in capillaries is intermittent (vasomotion), rather than continuous.

1. Oxygen is the most important determinant of the degree of opening and closing of metarterioles and precapillary sphincters (nutritive blood flow).
2. Nonnutritive blood flow is characterized by direct vascular connections between arterioles and venules.

C. Fluid movement across capillary membranes occurs by filtration, diffusion, and pinocytosis via endothelial vesicles.

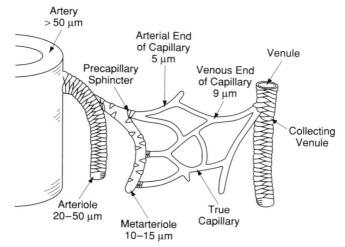

FIGURE 45–1. Anatomy of the microcirculation. (From Ganong WF. Review of Medical Physiology, 13th ed. Norwalk, CT: Appleton and Lange, 1987; with permission.)

1. **Filtration**
    a. Four different pressures determine whether fluid will move outward across capillary membranes **(filtration)** or inward across capillary membranes **(reabsorption)** (Table 45-2).
    b. The net effect of these four pressures is a positive filtration pressure at the arterial end of capillaries,

Table 45–1
Permeability of Capillary Membranes

	Molecular Weight	Relative Permeability
Water	18	1.0
Sodium chloride	58.5	0.96
Glucose	180	0.6
Hemoglobin	66,700	0.01
Albumin	69,000	0.0001

Table 45–2
Filtration of Fluid at the Arterial Ends of Capillaries

Pressures Favoring Outward Movement

Capillary pressure	25 mm Hg
Interstitial fluid pressure	−6.3 mm Hg
Interstitial fluid colloid osmotic pressure	5 mm Hg
Total	36.3 mm Hg

Pressure Favoring Inward Movement

Plasma colloid osmotic pressure	28 mm Hg
Net Filtration Pressure	8.3 mm Hg

causing fluid to move outward across cell membranes into interstitial fluid spaces.

c. At the venous end of capillaries, the net effect of these four pressures is a positive reabsorption pressure that causes fluid to move inward across capillary membranes into capillaries (Table 45–3).

d. Overall, the mean values of the four pressures acting across capillary membranes are nearly identical such that the amount of fluid filtered nearly equals the amount reabsorbed (Table 45–4).

e. Any fluid that is not reabsorbed enters the lymph vessels.

2. **Diffusion** is the most important mechanism for trans-

Table 45–3
Reabsorption of Fluid at the Venous Ends of Capillaries

Pressures Favoring Outward Movement

Capillary pressure	10 mm Hg
Interstitial fluid pressure	−6.3 mm Hg
Interstitial fluid colloid osmotic pressure	5 mm Hg
Total	21.3 mm Hg

Pressure Favoring Inward Movement

Plasma colloid osmotic pressure	28 mm Hg
Net Reabsorption Pressure	6.7 mm Hg

Table 45–4
Mean Values of Pressures Acting Across Capillary Membranes

Pressures Favoring Outward Movement	
Capillary pressure	17 mm Hg
Interstitial fluid pressure	−6.3 mm Hg
Interstitial fluid colloid osmotic pressure	5 mm Hg
Total	28.3 mm Hg
Pressure Favoring Inward Movement	
Plasma colloid osmotic pressure	28 mm Hg
Net Overall Filtration Pressure	0.3 mm Hg

fer of nutrients between the plasma and the interstitial fluid.

    a. Oxygen, carbon dioxide, and anesthetic gases are examples of lipid-soluble molecules that can diffuse directly through capillary membranes independently of pores.

    b. Typically, only slight partial pressure differences suffice to maintain adequate transport of oxygen between the plasma and interstitial fluid.

  3. Pinocytosis is the process by which capillary endothelial cells ingest small amounts of plasma or interstitial fluid followed by migration to the opposite surface where the fluid is released.

II. LYMPH VESSELS

  A. The most important function of the lymphatic system is return of protein into the circulation and maintenance of a low-protein concentration in the interstitial fluid.

  B. Anatomy

    1. The terminal lymph vessels are the thoracic duct and the right lymphatic duct (Fig. 45-2).

    2. Avoidance of possible damage to the thoracic duct is often a reason to select the right side of the neck as the preferred site for placement of a venous catheter into the internal jugular vein.

    3. The central nervous system is devoid of lymphatics.

  C. Formation

    1. Lymph is interstitial fluid that flows into lymphatic vessels.

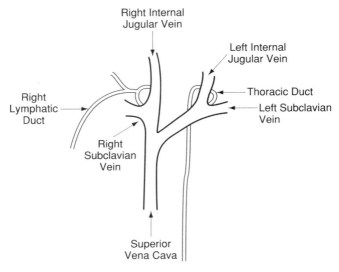

FIGURE 45–2. Depiction of the thoracic duct and right lymphatic duct as they enter the venous system.

Table 45–5
Causes of Increased Interstitial Fluid Volume

Increased Capillary Pressure
Cardiac failure
Local histamine release
Angioneuritic edema

Decreased Plasma Protein Concentrations
Renal failure
Nutritional factors

Obstruction of Lymph Vessels
Radical mastectomy (usually transient, as new lymph vessels
develop)

>   **2.** Bacteria that enter lymphatics are removed by lymph
>   nodes.
>   **D.** **Flow** of lymph through the thoracic duct occurs at a rate
>   of about 100 ml·h^{-1} (increased when there is a decrease
>   in the negative value of interstitial fluid pressure).

III. EDEMA is the presence of excess interstitial fluid in peripheral tissues that exceeds the ability of lymph vessels to transport the excess fluid (Table 45–5).

>   **A.** Fluid that collects in potential spaces (pericardium, pleu-
>   ral space, peritoneal space [ascites]) is called a **transudate**
>   (**exudate** if it contains bacteria).

Chapter

46

Pulmonary Circulation

The pulmonary circulation is a low-pressure, low-resistance system in series with the systemic circulation. (Updated and revised from Stoelting RK. Pulmonary circulation. In: Pharmacology and Physiology in Anesthetic Practice. 2nd ed. Philadelphia, JB Lippincott, 1991:685–91.)

I. ANATOMY

A. The thickness of the right ventricle is one third that of the left ventricle, reflecting the difference in pressures between the two ventricles.

   1. Pulmonary capillaries supply the estimated 300 million alveoli, providing a gas-exchange surface of about 70 m^2.

   2. Blood passes through pulmonary capillaries in about 1 second (increasing cardiac output may shorten transit time to less than 0.5 sec), during which time it is oxygenated and excess carbon dioxide is removed.

   3. Despite the presence of autonomic nervous system innervation, the resting pulmonary vasomotor tone is minimal, and pulmonary vessels are almost maximally dilated in the normal resting state.

B. **Bronchial Circulation**

   1. Bronchial arteries from the thoracic aorta provide oxygenated nutrient blood to supporting tissues of the lungs and then empty deoxygenated blood into the left atrium (cardiac output of the left ventricle exceeds that of the right ventricle by an amount equal to the bronchial blood flow).

   2. The entrance of deoxygenated blood into the left atrium dilutes oxygenated blood and accounts for an **anatomic shunt** that is equivalent to 1% to 2% of the cardiac output.

C. **Pulmonary lymph vessels** remove particulate matter entering the alveoli.

II. INTRAVASCULAR PRESSURES

A. Pressures in the pulmonary circulation are about one fifth those present in the systemic circulation (Fig. 46–1) (see Table 44–2).
   1. Overall, the resistance to blood flow in the pulmonary circulation is about one tenth the resistance in the systemic circulation.
   2. When the left ventricle fails, the mean pulmonary artery pressure also increases as a reflection of increased left atrial pressure.
B. **Measurement of left atrial pressure** can be estimated via a balloon-tipped catheter (Swan-Ganz catheter) that has been floated into a small pulmonary artery.

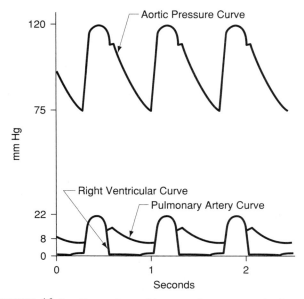

FIGURE 46–1. Comparison of intravascular pressures in the systemic and pulmonary circulations. (From Guyton AC. Textbook of Medical Physiology, 7th ed. Philadelphia: WB Saunders, 1986; with permission.)

1. Inflation of the balloon on the catheter prevents flow around the catheter; the resulting pulmonary artery occlusion pressure (wedge pressure) is only 2 to 3 mmHg higher than the left atrial pressure.
2. In the absence of pulmonary hypertension, the pulmonary artery end-diastolic pressure correlates with the pulmonary artery occlusion pressure.

III. INTERSTITIAL FLUID SPACE

A. The interstitial fluid space in the lung is minimal, and a continued negative pulmonary interstitial pressure dehydrates interstitial fluid spaces of the lungs and pulls alveolar epithelial membranes toward capillary membranes (minimizing diffusion distance).
B. Another consequence of negative pressure in pulmonary interstitial spaces is that it pulls fluid from alveoli through alveolar membranes and into interstitial fluid spaces, thus keeping the alveoli dry.

IV. PULMONARY BLOOD VOLUME

A. Blood volume in the lungs is about 450 ml, of which about 70 ml is in the capillaries.
B. Pulmonary blood volume may be increased in certain situations (Table 46–1).

V. PULMONARY BLOOD FLOW AND DISTRIBUTION

A. Optimal oxygenation is dependent on matching ventilation to pulmonary blood flow so as to minimize **shunt** or **dead space effect** (Fig. 46–2).

Table 46–1
Situations Associated with Increased Pulmonary Blood Volume

Cardiac failure

Mitral stenosis

Exercise (distensibility of pulmonary arteries and opening of previously collapsed alveoli protect against the development of pulmonary edema)

Change from standing to supine position (manifests as decreased vital capacity and orthopnea in the presence of left ventricular failure)

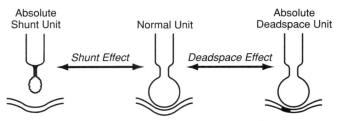

Absolute Shunt Unit   Normal Unit   Absolute Deadspace Unit

Shunt Effect   *Deadspace Effect*

FIGURE 46–2. Gas exchange is maximally effective in normal lung units with optimal ventilation: perfusion (V/Q) relationships. The continuum of V/Q relationships is depicted by the ratios between normal and absolute shunt or dead space units.

B. Hypoxic Pulmonary Vasoconstriction

    1. Alveolar hypoxia evokes vasoconstriction in the corresponding arterioles, diverting blood flow away from poorly ventilated alveoli (locally mediated mechanism).

        a. As a result, the shunt effect is minimized and the resulting PaO_2 is maximized.

        b. Drug-induced inhibition of hypoxic pulmonary vasoconstriction (nitroprusside, nitroglycerin) could result in unexpected decreases in PaO_2.

    2. The present consensus is that potent volatile anesthetics are acceptable choices for thoracic surgery requiring one-lung ventilation (implies that hypoxic pulmonary vasoconstriction is maintained).

C. Effect of Breathing. Spontaneous inspiration increases venous return to the heart, whereas a mechanically delivered inspiration impedes venous return.

D. Hydrostatic Pressure Gradients

    1. Blood flow to the lungs in the upright position is mainly gravity-dependent.

    2. The amount of blood flow to the various areas of the lungs along the vertical axis of the lungs depends on the relationship between pulmonary artery pressure (decreases 1.25 $mmHg \cdot cm^{-1}$ of vertical distance up the lung), alveolar pressure, and pulmonary venous pressure.

    3. Traditionally, the lung is divided into three blood flow zones, reflecting the impact of alveolar pressure, pulmonary artery pressure, and pulmonary venous pressure on the caliber of pulmonary blood vessels (Fig. 46–3).

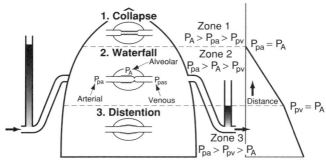

FIGURE 46–3. The lung is divided into three pulmonary blood flow zones, reflecting the impact of alveolar pressure (P_A), pulmonary artery pressure (P_{pa}), and pulmonary venous pressure (P_{pv}) on the caliber of pulmonary blood vessels. (From West JB, Dollery CT, Naimark A. Distribution of blood flow in isolated lung: Relation to vascular and alveolar pressures. J Appl Physiol 1964; 19:713–8; with permission.)

Table 46–2
Events that Obstruct Pulmonary Blood Flow

Pulmonary embolism
   Tachypnea
   Dyspnea
   Pulmonary artery hypertension and right ventricular failure
   Anticoagulation to prevent extension of the clot
Pulmonary emphysema
   Destruction of alveoli accompanied by concomitant loss of
    pulmonary vasculature
   Supplemental oxygen may lower pulmonary artery pressure
Anthracosis
   Fibrosis of supportive lung tissues
Atelectasis

   VI. PULMONARY EDEMA is present when there are excessive quantities of fluid, either in pulmonary interstitial spaces or in alveoli.

      A. The most common cause of acute pulmonary edema is a greatly increased pulmonary capillary pressure resulting from left ventricular failure.

      B. Local capillary damage following inhalation of acidic gastric fluid or irritant gases may result in acute pulmonary edema.

C. Enlargement of lymph vessels sufficient to allow lymph flow to increase up to 20 times is the most likely reason that pulmonary edema does not occur in the presence of chronically increased left atrial pressures.

VII. EVENTS THAT OBSTRUCT PULMONARY BLOOD FLOW (Table 46–2).

Chapter

47

Heart

The heart can be characterized as a pulsatile four-chamber pump composed of two atria (conduits or primer pumps) and two ventricles (power pumps). (Updated and revised from Stoelting RK. Heart. In: Pharmacology and Physiology in Anesthetic Practice. 2nd ed. Philadelphia, JB Lippincott, 1991:692–706.)

I. CARDIAC PHYSIOLOGY

A. Systole means contraction and is the time interval between closure of the tricuspid and mitral valves and closure of the pulmonary and aortic valves (**diastole** is the period of relaxation corresponding to the interval between closure of the pulmonary and aortic valves and closure of the tricuspid and mitral valves).

B. Cardiac muscle is a syncytium in which cells are so tightly bound together that when one of these cells become excited, the action potential spreads to all of them.

   1. As a result, stimulation of a single atrial cell causes the atria or ventricles to contract as a single unit.

   2. A specialized conduction pathway (**atrioventricular node**) is responsible for conducting the action potential from the atrial syncytium into the ventricular syncytium.

C. Cardiac Action Potential

   1. The normal cardiac action potential results from time-dependent changes in the permeability of cardiac muscle cell membranes to multiple ions during phases 0 to 4 of the cardiac action potential (Fig. 47-1) (Table 47-1).

   2. In **nonpacemaker** contractile atrial and ventricular cardiac cells, phase 4 is constant during diastole.

   3. In **pacemaker** cardiac cells, spontaneous phase 4 depolarization occurs until threshold potential is reached, resulting in self-excitation.

   a. Heart rate is determined by the slope of phase 4

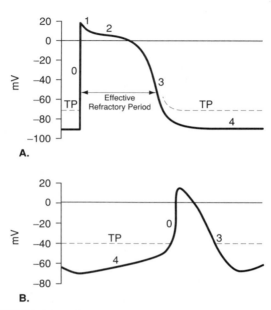

FIGURE 47–1.   Cardiac action potential recorded from a ventricular contractile cell (A) or atrial pacemaker cell (B). *TP*, threshold potential.

Table 47–1
Ion Movement During Phases of the Cardiac Action Potential

Phase	Ion	Movement Across Cell Membrane
0	Sodium	In
1	Potassium	Out
	Chloride	In
2	Calcium	In
	Potassium	Out
3	Potassium	Out
4	Sodium	In

depolarization, threshold potential, and the resting transmembrane potential.

   b. Norepinephrine increases and vagal stimulation decreases the rate of spontaneous phase 4 depolarization.

  4. Cardiac muscle is absolutely refractory to stimulation during phases 1, 2, and part of phase 3 of the cardiac action potential.

D. Cardiac cycle consists of a period of relaxation (diastole) followed by a period of contraction (systole) (Fig. 47-2).

  1. Atrial pressure curves consist of a waves (reflect atrial contraction and so are absent in the presence of atrial fibrillation), c waves, and v waves (retrograde flow into the atria via an incompetent tricuspid or mitral valve results in a large v wave).

  2. Atria as Pumps

    a. Atrial contraction accounts for about 30% of the blood that enters the ventricle during each cardiac cycle.

    b. This component of ventricular filling is lost during atrial fibrillation and contributes to the reduction of stroke volume that accompanies this cardiac dysrhythmia.

  3. Ventricles as Pumps

    a. During diastole, filling of the ventricles with blood from the atria normally increases the volume of blood in each ventricle to about 130 ml **(end-diastolic volume).**

    b. Subsequent ventricular ejection creates a stroke volume of about 70 ml.

    c. The ratio of stroke volume to end-diastolic volume is the ejection fraction (measure by echocardiography).

    d. An ejection fraction less than 0.4 is a reflection of left ventricular dysfunction, as may accompany myocardial ischemia or myocardial infarction.

  4. Function of the Heart Valves

    a. Heart valves open passively along a pressure gradient and close when a backward pressure gradient develops owing to high pressure in the pulmonary artery and aorta.

    b. Papillary muscles are attached to the tricuspid and mitral valves by chordae tendineae (rupture of a chorda tendinea or dysfunction of a papillary

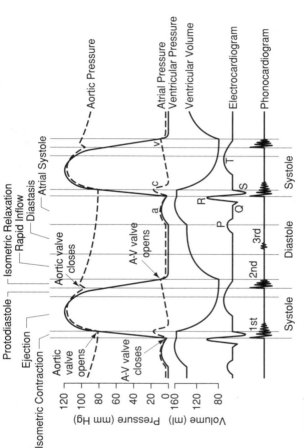

FIGURE 47–2. Events of the cardiac cycle, including changes in intravascular pressures, ventricular volume, electrocardiogram results, and phonocardiogram results. (From Guyton AC. Textbook of Medical Physiology, 7th ed. Philadelphia: WB Saunders, 1986; with permission.)

muscle, as may accompany myocardial ischemia, results in an incompetent valve and appearance of large v waves during ventricular contraction).

E. Work of the heart is dependent on energy derived mainly from metabolism of fatty acids.

F. Intrinsic Autoregulation of Cardiac Function

   1. The intrinsic ability of the heart to adapt to changing venous return (preload) reflects the increased stretch of cardiac muscle produced by increased filling of the ventricles from the atria **(Frank-Starling law of the heart)** (see Fig. 44-8).

   2. The most important factor determining cardiac output is the atrial pressure created by venous return.

G. Neural Control of the Heart

   1. The atria are abundantly innervated by the sympathetic and parasympathetic nervous system, but the ventricles are supplied principally by the sympathetic nervous system (Fig. 47-3).

   2. Maximal sympathetic nervous system stimulation can increase cardiac output by about 100% above normal.

II. CORONARY BLOOD FLOW

A. Unique features of coronary blood flow include interruption of blood flow during systole (mechanical compression of vessels by myocardial contraction) and maximum oxygen extraction that results in a coronary venous oxygen saturation of about 30% (PO_2 of 18 to 20 mmHg).

B. Anatomy of the Coronary Circulation

   1. The two coronary arteries that supply the myocardium arise from the sinuses of Valsalva (resting coronary blood flow is 225 to 250 ml·min^{-1}) (Fig. 47-4).

   2. Coronary artery disease manifesting as atherosclerosis involves large epicardial (conductance) arteries and not the coronary arterioles.

   3. Coronary blood flow, especially to the left ventricle, occurs predominantly during diastole when cardiac muscle relaxes and no longer obstructs blood flow through ventricular capillaries (Fig. 47-5).

      a. During systole, blood flow through the subendocardial arteries of the left ventricle falls almost to zero (subendocardial region of the left ventricle is the most common site for myocardial infarction).

      b. Tachycardia, with an associated decrease in the

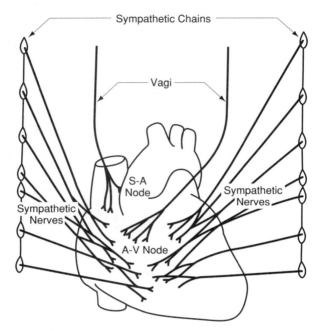

FIGURE 47–3. Innervation of the atria is from the sympathetic and parasympathetic (*vagi*) nervous systems, whereas the ventricles are supplied principally by the sympathetic nervous system. (From Guyton AC. Textbook of Medical Physiology, 7th ed. Philadelphia: WB Saunders, 1986; with permission.)

    time for coronary blood flow to occur during diastole, further jeopardizes the adequacy of myocardial oxygen delivery, particularly if coronary arteries are narrowed by atherosclerosis.

c. The impact of systole on coronary blood flow through the right ventricle is minimal.

d. Most of the venous blood that has perfused the left ventricle enters the right atrium via the coronary sinus.

e. A small amount of coronary blood flows back into the heart through Thebesian veins that can empty into any cardiac chamber (may contribute to the inherent anatomic shunt).

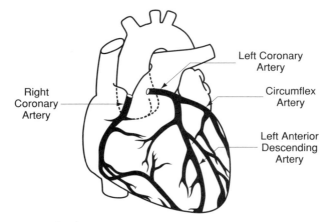

FIGURE 47–4. Anatomy of the coronary circulation.

C. Determinants of Coronary Blood Flow

1. A striking feature of coronary blood flow is the parallelism between the local metabolic needs of cardiac muscle for nutrients (especially oxygen) and the magnitude of coronary blood flow.

   a. **Adenosine** is the most potent local endogenous vasodilator substance.

   b. **Acadesine** is a purine nucleoside analogue that, when administered as a continuous intravenous infusion, may decrease the incidence and/or severity of myocardial ischemia (as may follow cardiopulmonary bypass) by increasing the availability of adenosine in ischemic tissues.

   c. Increased oxygen needs must be met by increased coronary blood flow, since oxygen extraction is already nearly maximal.

2. **Myocardial Oxygen Consumption**

   a. Myocardial oxygen consumption of the normothermic contracting myocardium is 10 ml·100 g^{-1}·min^{-1} (decreases to 5 ml·100 g^{-1}·min^{-1} in the arrested distended or beating empty heart and to 1 ml·100 g^{-1}·min^{-1} in the arrested nondistended heart).

   b. The fact that electromechanical arrest of the normothermic heart decreases myocardial oxygen consumption by 90% (from 10 ml·100 g^{-1}·min^{-1} to

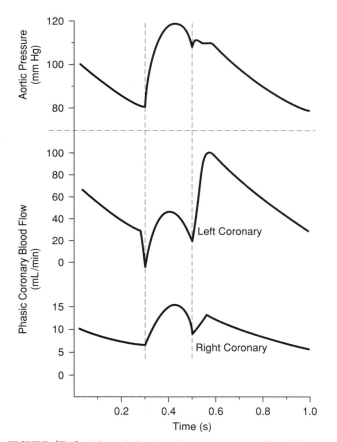

FIGURE 47–5. Phasic left and right coronary artery blood flow in relation to aortic pressure. (From Berne RM, Levy MD. Review of Medical Physiology, 13th ed. Norwalk, CT: Appleton and Lange, 1987; with permission.)

1 ml·100 g^{-1}·min^{-1}) is the reason that purposeful lowering of myocardial temperature to less than 15°C during cardiopulmonary bypass (presumed to offer added protection to ischemic myocardium), is able to lower myocardial oxygen consumption only an additional 5% (hypothermia introduces risk of damage to cell membranes).

    c. Sympathetic nervous system stimulation with associated increases in heart rate, blood pressure, and myocardial contractility results in increased myocardial oxygen consumption.

    d. Increases in heart rate that shorten diastolic time for coronary blood flow are likely to increase myocardial oxygen consumption more than elevations in blood pressure, which are likely to offset increased oxygen demands by enhanced pressure-dependent coronary blood flow.

    e. Increasing venous return (volume work) by optimizing intravascular fluid volume is the least costly means of increasing cardiac output in terms of myocardial oxygen consumption.

    f. When myocardial oxygenation is jeopardized, the heart produces lactate, with increases in coronary sinus lactate concentration being considered a conclusive indicator of global myocardial ischemia.

  3. Nervous System Innervation

    a. Coronary arteries contain alpha (predominant in epicardial coronary arteries), beta, and histamine (H-1, H-2) receptors.

    b. H-1 receptors mediate coronary artery vasoconstriction, whereas H-2 (beta receptors also) mediate coronary artery vasodilation.

D. Coronary artery steal is an absolute decrease in collateral-dependent myocardial perfusion at the expense of an increase in blood flow to a normally perfused area of myocardium as may follow drug-induced vasodilation of coronary arterioles (Fig. 47–6).

  1. Drugs that produce arteriolar vasodilation (nitroprusside, isoflurane) can redistribute coronary blood flow under certain conditions, possibly leading to myocardial ischemia in patients with coronary artery disease.

  2. Coronary artery steal is most likely to occur in those patients with steal-prone anatomy (occlusion of a coronary artery with significant stenosis of the collat-

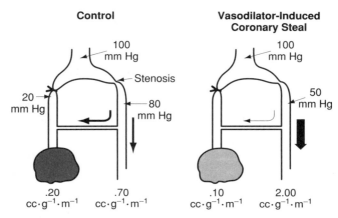

Control

**Vasodilator-Induced
Coronary Steal**

FIGURE 47–6. Schematic depiction of vasodilator-induced coronary artery steal. Following distal coronary artery vasodilation, flow increases to the normally perfused area, and there is a significant pressure drop across the stenosis that reduces the pressure gradient across the collateral bed. (From Cason BV, Verrier ED, London MJ, Mangano DT, Hickey RF. Effects of isoflurane and halothane on coronary vascular resistance and collateral myocardial blood flow: Their capacity to induce coronary steal. Anesthesiology 1987;67:665–75; with permission.)

eral supplying vessel), which is estimated to be present in about 23% of patients with coronary artery disease (Fig. 47–7).

III. DYNAMICS OF HEART SOUNDS

A. First and Second Heart Sounds

1. Closure of the mitral and tricuspid valves (first heart sound) and aortic and pulmonary valves (second heart sound) creates sudden pressure differentials such that blood vibrates, creating a transmitted sound that can be heard through a stethoscope (Fig. 47–8).

2. The loudness of the first heart sound is directly proportional to the force of ventricular contraction (rate of development of pressure differences across the mitral and tricuspid valves).

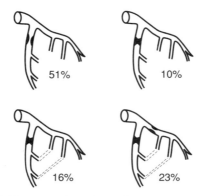

FIGURE 47–7. Anatomic variants of coronary artery disease and their incidence based on coronary angiograms. Steal-prone anatomy was present in 23% (*lower right*) of patients studied because arteriolar dilation decreases pressure distal to the stenosis and reduces flow through the high-resistance collaterals. (Buffington CW, Davis KB, Gillespie S, Pettinger M. The prevalence of steal-prone coronary anatomy in patients with coronary artery disease: An analysis of the coronary artery surgery registry. Anesthesiology 1988;69:721–7; with permission.)

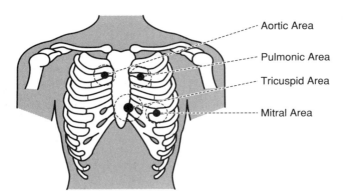

FIGURE 47–8. Optimal sites for auscultation of heart sounds due to opening or closure of specific cardiac valves. (From Guyton AC. Textbook of Medical Physiology, 7th ed. Philadelphia: WB Saunders, 1986; with permission.)

Table 47–2
Heart Murmurs

	*Timing of Murmur**
Aortic stenosis	Systole
Aortic regurgitation	Diastole
Mitral stenosis	Diastole
Mitral regurgitation	Systole
Patent ductus arteriosus	Continuous
Atrial septal defect	Systole
Ventricular septal defect	Systole

*Pulmonary or tricuspid stenosis or regurgitation produce murmurs during the cardiac cycle that correspond to the similar aortic or mitral valve abnormality.

    B. Third heart sound may be heard at the beginning of the middle third of diastole.

    C. Fourth heart sound is caused by rapid inflow of blood into the ventricles due to atrial contraction.

    D. Abnormal heart sounds (murmurs) occur in the presence of abnormalities of the cardiac valves or congenital anomalies (Table 47-2).

IV. CONDUCTION OF CARDIAC IMPULSES

    A. Cardiac impulses are transmitted over a specialized conduction system in the heart, with normal impulses being spontaneously generated at the **sinoatrial node** so as to maintain resting heart rate at about 70 beats·min^{-1} (Fig. 47-9).

        1. The self-excitatory impulse travels from the sinoatrial node to the **atrioventricular node,** where it is delayed before passing into the ventricles.

        2. In the ventricles, the cardiac impulse travels via the **atrioventricular bundle** (bundle of His), which divides initially into the **left and right bundle branches.**

        3. Bundle branches divide into a complex network of conducting fibers known as **Purkinje fibers,** which ramify over the subendocardial surfaces of both ventricles.

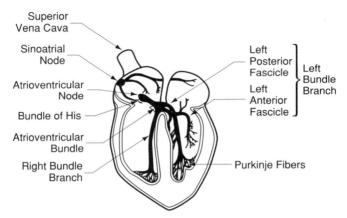

FIGURE 47–9. Anatomy of the conduction system for transmission of cardiac impulses.

B. Cardiac Pacemakers

1. A cardiac pacemaker cell is one that undergoes spontaneous phase 4 depolarization to reach threshold potential and thus undergoes self-excitation.

   a. The role of the sinoatrial node as the normal cardiac pacemaker reflects the higher intrinsic discharge rate of this node (70 to 80 beats·min^{-1}) relative to that of atrioventricular nodal fibers (40 to 60 beats·min^{-1}) and of Purkinje fibers (15 to 40 beats·min^{-1}).

   b. A cardiac pacemaker other than the sinoatrial node is called an **ectopic pacemaker.**

2. Stimulation of the parasympathetic nervous system results in the release of **acetylcholine,** which hyperpolarizes cardiac muscle cell membranes and depresses the intrinsic discharge rate of the sinoatrial node.

3. Stimulation of the sympathetic nervous system results in the release of **norepinephrine** (increases permeability of cardiac muscle cell membranes to sodium and calcium), which speeds the rate of spontaneous phase 4 depolarization and thus increases the intrinsic rate of discharge of the sinoatrial node.

Table 47–3
Circulatory Effects of Heart Disease

Valvular Heart Disease *(volume overload due to regurgitant lesions or pressure overload due to stenotic lesions)*

Aortic stenosis or regurgitation
  Left ventricular hypertrophy
  Myocardial ischemia
  Often asymptomatic (listen for murmur in preoperative evaluation)
Mitral stenosis or regurgitation
  Pulmonary edema
  Atrial fibrillation
  Pulmonary hypertension

Congenital Heart Disease *(circulatory effects due to increased or decreased pulmonary blood flow because of left-to-right or right-to-left intracardiac shunts)*

Patent ductus arteriosus
  Decreased exercise tolerance
  Increased pulmonary blood flow that may lead to pulmonary hypertension
Atrial septal defect
  Increased pulmonary blood flow that may lead to pulmonary hypertension
Tetralogy of Fallot
  Decreased pulmonary blood flow
  Arterial hypoxemia

V. CIRCULATORY EFFECTS OF HEART DISEASE
(Table 47–3)

VI. MYOCARDIAL INFARCTION

  A. The four major causes of death following a myocardial infarction are decreased cardiac output, pulmonary edema, ventricular fibrillation, and rupture of the heart.
      1. **Decreased cardiac output** occurs immediately after a myocardial infarction (cardiogenic shock is likely when more than 40% of the left ventricular muscle is infarcted).
      2. **Ventricular fibrillation** is a common cause of sudden death related to acute myocardial infarction, especially in the first few minutes following the infarction.

B. The ability of the heart to increase its cardiac output following recovery from a myocardial infarction is commonly less (decreased ejection fraction) than in a normal, undamaged heart.

VII. ANGINA PECTORIS occurs when myocardial oxygen requirements exceed delivery (distribution of pain into the neck and arms reflects the embryonic origin of the heart), such that both these structures receive pain fibers from the same spinal cord segments (T2 to T5).

VIII. CARDIAC FAILURE manifests as decreased cardiac or pulmonary edema, with selective left ventricular failure occurring 30 times more often than selective right ventricular failure.

A. Any increased stress, such as exercise, sepsis, or trauma, may unmask decreased cardiac reserve in patients vulnerable to cardiac failure.

B. Inhaled anesthetics produce exaggerated decreases in myocardial contractility when administered in the presence of cardiac failure.

Chapter

48

The Electrocardiogram and Analysis of Cardiac Dysrhythmias

The electrocardiogram (ECG) is vital for the detection and analysis of cardiac dysrhythmias. (Updated and revised from Stoelting RK. The electrocardiogram and analysis of cardiac dysrhythmias. In: Pharmacology and Physiology in Anesthetic Practice. 2nd ed. Philadelphia, JB Lippincott, 1991:707–18.)

I. ELECTROCARDIOGRAM

A. Body fluids are good conductors, making it possible to record the sum of the action potentials of myocardial fibers on the surface of the body as the ECG (Fig. 48-1).

  1. The normal ECG consists of a P-wave (atrial depolarization), a QRS complex (ventricular depolarization), and a T-wave (ventricular repolarization).

  2. The atrial T-wave (atrial repolarization) is obscured on the ECG by the larger QRS complex.

B. Recording the Electrocardiogram

  1. Paper used for recording the ECG is designed such that each horizontal line corresponds to 0.1 mV and each vertical line corresponds to 0.04 second (Fig. 48-1).

  2. The duration of events during conduction of the cardiac impulse can be calculated from a recording of the ECG (Table 48-1).

C. Electrocardiogram Leads

  1. The ECG is recorded using a unipolar lead (exploring electrode) or bipolar leads (two active electrodes).

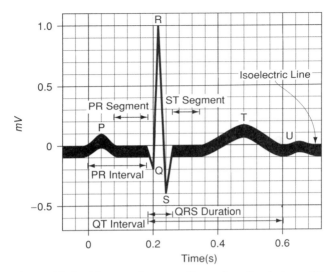

FIGURE 48–1. The normal waves and intervals on the electrocardiogram.

Table 48–1
Intervals and Corresponding Events on the Electrocardiogram

	Average	*Range*	*Event in Heart*
P-R interval*	0.18 sec	0.12–0.20 sec	Atrial depolarization and conduction through the atrioventricular node
QRS duration	0.08 sec	0.05–0.1 sec	Ventricular depolarization
Q-T interval*	0.40 sec	0.26–0.45 sec	Ventricular depolarization plus repolarization
S-T segment	0.32 sec		Ventricular repolarization

*Dependent on heart rate.

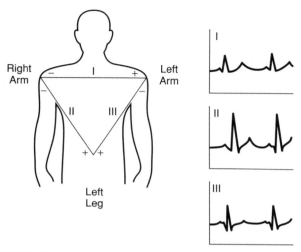

FIGURE 48–2. Standard limb leads for the electrocardiogram and typical recordings.

2. **Standard limb leads** are placed on the left and right arms and the left leg (Fig. 48-2).
   a. Polarity is positive for the ECG recorded from the standard limb leads.
   b. P-waves are prominent in lead II since the direction of atrial depolarization parallels this lead.
3. **Chest leads** are precordial unipolar leads (V_1 through V_6) that are recorded by placing an electrode on the anterior surface of the chest over one of six separate sites (Table 48-2).

Table 48–2
Placement of Precordial Leads

V_1	Fourth intercostal space at the right sternal border
V_2	Fourth intercostal space at the left sternal border
V_3	Equidistant between V_2 and V_4
V_4	Fifth intercostal space in the left midclavicular line
V_5	Fifth intercostal space in the left anterior axillary line
V_6	Fifth intercostal space in the left midaxillary line

4. **Augmented limb leads** are unipolar leads similar to the standard limb lead recordings except that the recording from the right arm lead (aVR) is inverted.

D. Interpretation of the Electrocardiogram

1. Abnormalities of the heart can be detected by analyzing the contours of the different waves in the various ECG leads.

2. When one ventricle of the heart hypertrophies, the axis of the heart shifts toward the enlarged ventricle.

3. **Abnormalities of the QRS complex,** characterized by prolongation to greater than 0.1 second, may reflect ventricular hypertrophy or blockade of the Purkinje fibers.

4. **Decreased voltage in the standard limb leads** may reflect abnormal conditions around the heart (pericardial effusion, pulmonary emphysema) that interfere with the conduction of electric currents from the heart to the surface of the body.

5. **Current of injury** is due to the inability of damaged areas of the heart (as from myocardial ischemia or infarction) to undergo repolarization during diastole.

   a. Specific leads of the ECG are more likely than other leads to reflect myocardial ischemia that develops in areas of the myocardium supplied by an individual coronary artery (Table 48-3).

   b. An estimated 80% to 90% of S-T segment information contained in a conventional 12-lead ECG is present in lead V_5.

   c. A Q-wave occurs because there is no electrical activity in the infarcted area.

   d. The most sensitive indicator of myocardial ischemia is the appearance of new motion wall abnormalities (normal wall motion becoming hypokinetic, or hypokinetic wall motion becoming akinetic or dyskinetic and lasting at least 1 minute) on transesophageal echocardiography (more sensitive than exercise electrocardiography).

6. **Abnormalities of the T-wave,** as reflected by inversion or biphasic T-wave or elevation of the S-T segment, is most often due to myocardial ischemia.

7. **His bundle electrocardiogram** is recorded from an electrode inserted through a vein and positioned near the tricuspid valve (used to measure conduction times accurately).

Table 48–3
Relationship of Electrocardiogram Lead Reflecting Myocardial Ischemia to Area of Myocardium Involved

Electrocardiogram Lead	Coronary Artery Responsible for Ischemia	Area of Myocardium Supplied by Coronary Artery
II, III, aVF	Right coronary artery	Right atrium Interatrial septum Right ventricle Sinoatrial node Atrioventricular node Inferior wall of left ventricle
$V_3 - V_5$	Left anterior descending coronary artery	Anterior and lateral wall of left ventricle
I, aVL	Circumflex coronary artery	Lateral wall of left ventricle Sinoatrial node Atrioventricular node

II. CARDIAC DYSRHYTHMIAS

   A. Cardiac dysrhythmias are observed to occur in 60% or more of patients undergoing anesthesia and surgery when continuous methods of monitoring are utilized.
   1. **Anesthesia** produced by halogenated anesthetics may evoke a nodal rhythm and/or increased ventricular automaticity.
   2. Halothane, but not isoflurane, slows the rate of sinoatrial node discharge and prolongs His-Purkinje and ventricular conduction times.
   3. Light anesthesia may be responsible for the initiation of cardiac dysrhythmias during anesthesia and surgery.
   B. **Mechanisms**
   1. **Automaticity** is enhanced by sympathetic nervous system activation (arterial hypoxemia, acidosis, release of catecholamines) and decreased by parasympathetic nervous system activity (acetylcholine hyperpolarizes cardiac cell membranes).
      a. Vagal stimulation may decrease the vulnerability of the heart to develop ventricular fibrillation.
      b. **Ectopic pacemaker** manifests as a premature con-

Table 48–4
Causes of Heart Block

Excessive parasympathetic nervous system stimulation

Drug-induced (digitalis, propranolol) depression of impulse
  conduction

Myocardial infarction

Atherosclerotic plaques

Age-related degenerative process

---

traction of the heart (possibly reflecting an irritable
area of cardiac muscle, such as that due to a local
area of myocardial ischemia).

2. **Excitability** is the ability of a cardiac cell to respond
   to a stimulus by depolarizing its cell membrane.

   a. A measure of excitability is the difference be-
      tween the resting transmembrane potential and
      threshold potential of the cardiac cell membrane
      (the smaller the difference, the greater the excit-
      ability).

   b. Once a cell depolarizes, it is initially refractory to
      all stimuli (absolute refractory period); that is fol-
      lowed by a period during which a greater-than-
      normal stimulus can cause cardiac cell membranes
      to depolarize (relative refractory period).

3. **Conduction abnormalities** manifest as development
   of heart block, reentry circuits, or preexcitation syndromes.

   a. **Heart block** is most likely to occur at the atrioven-
      tricular bundle, or one of the bundle branches (Table
      48–4).

   b. **Reentry** implies reexcitation of cardiac tissue by

Table 48–5
Accessory Pathways and Preexcitation Syndromes

	Connections
Kent's bundle	Atrium to ventricle
Mahaim bundle	Atrioventricular node to ventricle
Atrio-Hissian fiber	Atrium to His bundle
James fiber	Atrium to atrioventricular node

Table 48–6
Types of Cardiac Dysrhythmias

Sinus Tachycardia *(heart rate higher than 100 beats·min⁻¹)*

Sympathetic nervous system stimulation
Fever
Carotid sinus activation

Sinus Bradycardia *(heart rate lower than 60 beats·min⁻¹)*

Atrioventricular Heart Block

First-degree (P-R interval longer than 0.2 sec)
Second-degree
    Wenckebach (progressive prolongation of P-R interval until a
    beat is dropped)
    Mobitz (nonconducted atrial impulse without prior change in
    P-R interval)
Third-degree (P-waves are dissociated from the QRS complex and
    heart rate depends on the site of the ectopic pacemaker;
    treatment is insertion of an artificial cardiac pacemaker)

Premature Atrial Contractions *(abnormal P-wave and
shortened P-R interval)*

Premature Nodal Contractions *(absence of a P-wave preceding
the QRS complex)*

Premature Ventricular Contractions

Ectopic pacemaker in the ventricles (consider myocardial
    ischemia)
QRS complex wide, followed by a compensatory pause

Atrial Paroxysmal Tachycardia

Regular rhythm and abnormal P-waves
Ectopic pacemaker in the atria
Typically abrupt in onset (single beat)

Nodal Paroxysmal Tachycardia *(resembles atrial paroxysmal
tachycardia except P-waves are not identifiable)*

Ventricular Tachycardia

Resembles a series of ventricular premature contractions that
    occur at a rapid and regular rate
Treatment is electrical cardioversion if hemodynamically
    significant
Predisposes to ventricular fibrillation

(continued)

Table 48–6 *(continued)*

Atrial Flutter

P-waves have a saw-toothed appearance

Conduction of atrial impulses to the ventricle is 2:1, 3:1, or 4:1

Atrial Fibrillation

Normal QRS complexes at a rapid and irregular rate in the absence of identifiable P-waves

Pulse deficit

Treated with digitalis, which prolongs the refractory period of the ventricles

Ventricular Fibrillation

Total incoordination of contraction with cessation of any effective pumping activity

Electrical defibrillation is the only effective treatment.

return of the same cardiac impulse using a circuitous pathway (probably responsible for most cardiac dysrhythmias). These circuits can be eliminated by speeding conduction through normal tissue so the cardiac fiber is still refractory, or by prolonging the refractory period of normal cells so the returning impulse cannot reenter).

c. **Preexcitation syndromes** are present when the atrial impulse bypasses the atrioventricular node to produce early excitation of the ventricle (P-R interval shorter than 0.12 second) (Table 48-5).

C. **Types of Cardiac Dysrhythmias** (Table 48-6)

D. Percutaneous catheter ablation (localized destructive energy delivered via an intracardiac catheter to the endocardium adjacent to the area of aberrant conduction) is a technique for selectively interrupting cardiac conduction pathways (ablation of supraventricular bypass tracts, atrioventricular node ablation, ablation of ventricular reentry pathways) in patients with symptomatic tachycardia that is refractory to drug therapy.

Chapter

49
Lungs

The human lungs perform oxygenation, ventilation, and metabolic functions. (Updated and revised from Stoelting RK. Lungs. In: Pharmacology and Physiology in Anesthetic Practice. 2nd ed. Philadelphia, JB Lippincott, 1991:719-31.)

I. ANATOMY

A. The human thorax is composed of 12 thoracic vertebral bodies, 12 pairs of ribs, and the sternum, which are sufficiently rigid to protect the organ systems contained within but pliable enough to allow the lungs to act as a bellows.

1. The **suprasternal notch** is in the same plane as the midportion of the second thoracic vertebra, which corresponds to the **midportion of the trachea** (desirable location for the distal tip of a tracheal tube).

2. The adult trachea is 10 to 12 cm in length, beginning at the level of the sixth cervical vertebra (cricoid cartilage) and extends downward to its bifurcation at the carina opposite the fifth thoracic vertebra.

a. The bifurcation of the trachea gives rise to the right main stem bronchus (extends 2.5 cm prior to its initial division) and the left mainstem bronchus (extends 5 cm prior to its initial division).

b. In adults, the angle of the takeoff of the right main stem bronchus is such that accidental endobronchial intubation or aspiration of foreign material is more likely to involve this bronchus than the left main stem bronchus.

c. The short length of the right main stem bronchus is the reason for the common recommendation to use a left endobronchial tube when a double-lumen tube is selected.

3. The opposing lung and chest wall recoil forces produce a subatmospheric pressure of approximately

Table 49–1
Innervation of the Larynx

Sensory Innervation

Glossopharyngeal nerve (tongue, pharynx, tonsils)

Superior laryngeal nerve branch of the vagus nerve (epiglottis and mucous membranes to level of the false vocal cords)

Recurrent laryngeal nerve branch of the vagus nerve (vocal cords and upper trachea)

Motor Innervation

Recurrent laryngeal nerve (all muscles except cricothyroid muscle)

Superior laryngeal nerve (cricothyroid muscle)

−4 mmHg in the potential space between visceral and parietal pleura during quiet breathing.

B. Respiratory Passageways

1. Airway smooth muscles are principally under the bronchoconstricting neural influence of the vagus nerve (explains the bronchodilating effects of inhaled anticholinergics).

2. Inhaled gases are warmed, filtered, and humidified by the extensive vascular surfaces of the nasal turbinates and septum (bypassed with a translaryngeal tracheal tube or tracheostomy).

3. **Innervation of the Larynx** (Table 49-1)

4. **Cough Reflex**
   a. The medulla initiates a series of responses characterized by inhalation followed by closure of the glottis and contraction of abdominal muscles.
   b. Depressant drugs (opioids, volatile anesthetics) and increasing age are associated with depression of the cough reflex.

II. MECHANICS OF BREATHING

A. The diaphragm is the principal muscle of breathing, accounting for approximately 75% of the air that enters the lungs during spontaneous inspiration.

1. It is estimated that the diaphragm moves 10 to 12 cm vertically during each inspiration.

2. The diaphragm is innervated by the phrenic nerve, which arises from the third, fourth, and fifth cervical nerves.

3. During quiet breathing, the contribution of intercostal muscle contraction to inspiration is small.

4. Overall, the oxygen cost of breathing is usually less than 5% of minute oxygen consumption.

5. During exhalation, the elastic recoil of the lungs, chest wall, and abdominal structures compresses the lungs.

   a. Abdominal muscles of exhalation are active only during forced exhalation maneuvers (coughing to clear secretions) or obstruction to the flow of gas.

   b. Paralysis of abdominal muscles, such as that produced by regional anesthesia, does not influence alveolar ventilation but may compromise the patient's ability to cough and clear secretions.

B. Alveolar Volume and Distribution of Ventilation

1. Alveolar volume is not uniform throughout the lungs because of differences in the distending pressures to which alveoli are subjected (distending negative pleural pressure is greatest at the apex of the lung).

2. Distribution of ventilation in the lungs and the volume at which airways in lung bases begin to close can be assessed by the single breath nitrogen washout test (Fig. 49-1).

   a. The first gases exhaled from large airways are considered to represent dead space gases (phase I).

   b. The beginning of alveolar gas exhalation is re-

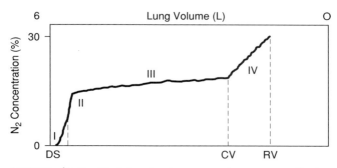

FIGURE 49–1. Single-breath nitrogen washout curve reflecting dead space volume (phase I), exhalation of alveolar gas (phases II and III), and airway closure in the lung bases (phase IV).

flected by an increase in the exhaled nitrogen concentration (phase II) followed by a plateau (phase III).

   c. If the nitrogen concentration continues to increase during phase III, it can be assumed that alveoli are filling and emptying at different rates.

3. **Pneumothorax** occurs when air enters the pleural space via a rupture in the lung or a hole in the chest wall.

   a. There is a shift of the mediastinum toward the intact lung, with kinking of the great vessels and development of arterial hypoxemia and severe dyspnea.

   b. **Tension pneumothorax** is present when pressure in the pleural space increases above atmospheric pressure (life-saving treatment is decompression of the pneumothorax).

   c. Air from a closed pneumothorax diffuses along a partial pressure gradient into venous blood, being completely absorbed in 1 to 2 weeks.

III. SURFACE TENSION AND PULMONARY SURFACTANT

A. Surface tension results from attraction of molecules in the fluid lining the alveoli.

B. **Pulmonary surfactant** is a lipoprotein secreted by type II alveolar cells (pneumocytes) lining the alveoli.

   1. Pulmonary surfactant decreases surface tension of fluids lining the alveoli, thus preventing collapse of alveoli as they become smaller.

      a. As alveoli become larger and surfactant is spread more thinly on the fluid surface, the surface tension becomes greater.

      b. Thus, surfactant helps to stabilize the size of alveoli, causing larger alveoli to contract more and small ones to contract less (net effect is maintenance of alveoli in any area of the lung at about the same size).

   2. Absence or an inadequate amount of pulmonary surfactant results in alveolar collapse (characteristic of respiratory distress syndrome of the neonate).

   3. Surfactant therapy (delivered by inhalation) decreases morbidity and mortality from respiratory distress syndrome in the neonate.

IV. COMPLIANCE

   A. Compliance is expressed as the increase in the gas volume of the lungs for each unit increase in alveolar pressure (about 130 ml for every 1 cm H_2O).
   B. Any condition that destroys lung tissue or blocks bronchioles causes decreased pulmonary compliance.

V. LUNG VOLUMES AND CAPACITIES (Table 49-2 and Fig. 49-2)

   A. A lung capacity is the sum of two or more lung volumes.
      1. Lung volumes and capacities are decreased in adult females, in the supine position (abdominal contents press upward against the diaphragm plus an increase in blood volume), and in small and asthenic individuals.
      2. Gas volumes tend to increase in diseases associated with airway obstruction and air trapping (asthma, emphysema).
   B. **Functional residual capacity** (FRC) provides a buffer in the alveoli such that abrupt alterations in PaO_2 and $PaCO_2$ are less likely to occur.
      1. In the presence of a decreased FRC (parturient, obesity), transient interruptions in breathing (as may

Table 49-2
Lung Volumes and Capacities

	Abbreviation	*Normal Adult Value*
Tidal volume	V_T	500 ml (6-8 ml·kg^{-1})
Inspiratory reserve volume	IRV	3000 ml
Expiratory reserve volume	ERV	1200 ml
Residual volume	RV	1200 ml
Inspiratory capacity	IC	3500 ml
Functional residual capacity	FRC	2400 ml
Vital capacity	VC	4500 ml (60-70 ml·kg^{-1})
Forced exhaled volume in 1 sec	FEV_1	80%
Total lung capacity	TLC	5900 ml

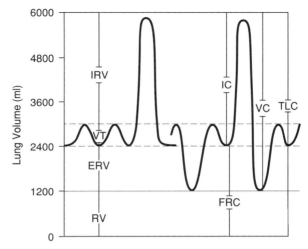

FIGURE 49–2. Schematic diagram of breathing excursions at rest and during maximal inhalation and/or exhalation. (See Table 49-2 for an explanation of abbreviations.) Lung capacities are the sum of two or more lung volumes.

occur during direct laryngoscopy) may result in rapid decreases in PaO_2.

2. **Effects of Anesthesia**
   a. Following induction of anesthesia and placement of a tracheal tube, there is a decrease in the FRC of approximately 450 ml that is similar whether or not skeletal muscle paralysis is present (consistent with the increase in right-to-left shunt that accompanies general anesthesia).
   b. Positive end-expiratory pressure may restore FRC (and decrease shunt), but the beneficial effect on PaO_2 may be offset by associated decreases in cardiac output.
C. **Vital capacity** is decreased in patients with bronchial asthma, chronic bronchitis, and heart failure associated with excess fluid in the lungs.
D. **Forced exhaled vital capacity** is the volume of gas that can be exhaled rapidly and maximally after 1 (FEV_1) and 3 seconds (FEV_3), starting from total lung capacity (Fig. 49-3).

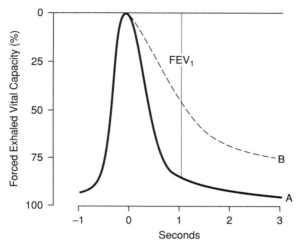

FIGURE 49–3. Schematic diagram of forced exhaled volume in normal patients (*A*) and in individuals with obstructive airway disease (*B*). Normal individuals can exhale approximately 80% of the vital capacity in 1 second (FEV_1) compared with a rate of approximately 50% in 1 second in individuals with obstructive airway disease.

      1. A normal patient can exhale approximately 80% of the vital capacity in 1 second.
      2. In the presence of obstructive airway disease, the FEV_1 is less than 50%.

VI. MINUTE VENTILATION is the total amount of gas moved into the lungs each minute (tidal volume multiplied by breathing frequency).

    A. Alveolar ventilation is the volume of gas that enters areas of the lung capable of participating in gas exchange with pulmonary capillary blood (dead space volume is subtracted).
      1. The $PaCO_2$ and, to a lesser extent, the PaO_2 are determined by alveolar ventilation.
      2. The frequency of breathing and tidal volume are important only insofar as they influence alveolar ventilation.
    B. Dead space (comprising both anatomic dead space

[nasal passageways, pharynx, trachea] and physiologic dead space [due to absent or poor blood flow through corresponding capillaries resulting in wasted ventilation]) is the fraction of inhaled gases (about 150 ml) that does not normally participate in gas exchange with pulmonary capillary blood.

1. Chronic lung disease tends to selectively increase physiologic dead space.
2. Conceptually, rebreathing dead space gas (oxygen and anesthetic not removed and devoid of carbon dioxide) is similar to delivering fresh gases from the anesthesia machine. This is the reason anesthetic breathing systems are designed to preferentially conserve dead space gas and to eliminate alveolar gas.

VII. CONTROL OF VENTILATION

A. Control of ventilation is designed to make adjustments in alveolar ventilation so as to maintain an optimal and unchanging PaO_2, $PaCO_2$, and concentration of hydrogen ions (H^+).
   1. The major factor in regulation of ventilation is the $PaCO_2$ (a 50% increase in $PaCO_2$ evokes a 10-fold increase in alveolar ventilation).
   2. Fine control of ventilation is provided by the respiratory center (depressed by anesthetic drugs) and peripheral chemoreceptors.
B. **Respiratory center** is located bilaterally in the medulla and pons and consists of inspiratory, pneumotoxic, and expiratory areas (Fig. 49-4).
C. **Chemical control** of breathing is influenced by the effects of changes in $PaCO_2$, PaO_2, and H^+ concentration as sensed by a chemosensitive area in the medulla or peripheral chemoreceptors.
   1. **Chemosensitive area** (medullary chemoreceptors) is located in the medulla and responds to changes in H^+ concentration (Fig. 49-5).
      a. H^+ ions do not easily cross the blood–brain barrier to enter the cerebrospinal fluid such that changes in blood pH have less effect on stimulating the chemosensitive areas than does carbon dioxide, which readily crosses the blood–brain barrier.
      b. It is estimated that 75% to 80% of the ventilatory response to carbon dioxide ($2.5 \ L \cdot min^{-1}$ for every 1 mmHg increase in $PaCO_2$) reflects activation of the medullary chemosensitive area.

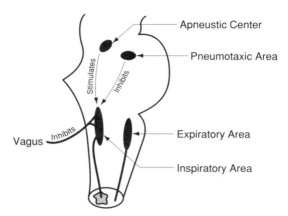

FIGURE 49–4. The respiratory center is located bilaterally in the reticular substance of the medulla oblongata and pons. (Redrawn from Guyton AC. Textbook of Medical Physiology, 7th ed. Philadelphia: WB Saunders, 1986; with permission.)

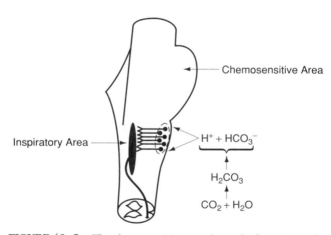

FIGURE 49–5. The chemosensitive area, located a few microns below the ventral surface of the medulla, transmits stimulatory impulses to the inspiratory area. This chemosensitive area is highly responsive to hydrogen ions (H^+) in the cerebrospinal fluid. (From Guyton AC. Textbook of Medical Physiology, 7th ed. Philadelphia: WB Saunders, 1986; with permission.)

      c. After several hours, the stimulant effect of carbon dioxide on ventilation mediated by the medullary chemoreceptors wanes, reflecting active transport (ion pump) of bicarbonate ions into the cerebrospinal fluid from the blood to return the cerebrospinal fluid pH to a normal value of 7.32.

  2. Chemoreceptors are **carotid and aortic bodies,** located outside the central nervous system, which are responsive to changes in PO_2, PCO_2, and H^+ concentration.

      a. It is the PaO_2 and not the arterial hemoglobin saturation with oxygen (SaO_2) that determines stimulation of peripheral chemoreceptors (reason anemia does not stimulate ventilation).

      b. Normally, peripheral chemoreceptors become stimulated when the PaO_2 decreases below approximately 60 mmHg (response to arterial hypoxemia is greatly attenuated by injected and inhaled anesthetics, even at subanesthetic concentrations [0.1 MAC]).

  3. Together, the respiratory center, peripheral and central chemoreceptors, and cerebral input constitute the physiologic control system that regulates breathing (the functional integrity of this control can be tested by determining the ventilatory response to hypercapnia and/or hypoxia).

VIII. EFFECTS OF SLEEP ON BREATHING

  A. Reductions in the level of environmental stimulation, as occur during sleep, are associated with modest increases in $PaCO_2$, and the ventilatory response to carbon dioxide is decreased, as reflected by rightward displacement of the carbon dioxide response curve.

  B. Phasic and tonic activity of skeletal muscles (especially upper airway muscles) decreases during sleep, resulting in brief periods of upper airway obstruction even in normal individuals.

IX. APNEIC PERIODS DURING SLEEP

  1. Sleep apneas are classified as central (cessation of respiratory efforts) or obstructive (despite respiratory efforts, air flow ceases because of total upper airway obstruction).

2. Recurrent episodes of hypoxemia and hypercarbia may lead to polycythemia and pulmonary hypertension.
3. Apnea lasting more than 10 seconds and associated with decreases in SaO_2 to less than 75% is common in elderly males and premature infants.

Table 49–3
Metabolic Functions of the Lung

Synthesized and Used in the Lung
Surfactant

Synthesized and Released into the Blood
Prostaglandins
Histamine
Kallikrein
Von Willebrand factor
Tissue plasminogen activator

Partially Removed from the Blood
Prostaglandins
Bradykinin
Serotonin
Norepinephrine
Acetylcholine
Fentanyl
Propranolol
Lidocaine
Atrial natriuretic factor
Adenosine
Imipramine

Not Removed from the Blood
Epinephrine
Dopamine
Prostacyclin
Morphine
Histamine
Angiotensin II
Vasopressin

Activated in the Lung
Angiotensin I
Arachidonic acid

X. PERIODIC BREATHING possibly a manifestation of central nervous system disease.

- **A. Cheyne-Stokes** breathing (cyclic waxing and waning pattern of ventilation interrupted by periods of apnea) is the most common form of periodic breathing.
  1. Cyclic increases and decreases in $PaCO_2$ are the presumed mechanisms for this form of periodic breathing.
  2. Congestive heart failure (delay in blood flow from the lungs to the brain) and brain stem damage may be associated with Cheyne-Stokes respiration.
- **B. Ataxic (Biot's) breathing** is characterized by an unpredictable sequence of breaths varying in rate and depth, most likely reflecting damage to the reticular formation in the medulla.
- **C. Apneustic breathing** involves repetitive gasps with sustained pauses at full inspiration, most likely reflecting damage to the pons.

XI. NONVENTILATORY FUNCTION OF THE LUNGS (Table 49-3)

- **A.** Most exogenous substances removed by passage through the pulmonary circulation are not metabolized, but instead are bound to components by lung tissue.
- **B.** Drugs most effectively bound to lung tissue are lipid-soluble and have pK values higher than 8. First-pass pulmonary uptake of some injected drugs is sufficiently great to influence the peak arterial concentration of these drugs.

Chapter

50

Pulmonary Gas Exchange and Blood Transport of Gases

The pulmonary function of the lungs is to provide for the optimal exchange of oxygen and carbon dioxide between the ambient environment and pulmonary capillaries. (Updated and revised from Stoelting RK. Pulmonary gas exchange and blood transport of gases. In: Pharmacology and Physiology in Anesthetic Practice. 2nd ed. Philadelphia, JB Lippincott, 1991:732–44.)

I. PULMONARY GAS EXCHANGE

- **A.** Gas exchange is greatly dependent on the matching of regional alveolar ventilation with pulmonary capillary perfusion ($\dot{V}/\dot{Q}$).
- **B. Partial Pressure**
  - **1.** The partial pressure (P) that a gas exerts is due to the constant impact of molecules in motion against a surface.
    - **a.** The higher the concentration of gas molecules or the higher the temperature, the greater is the sum of the forces of all the molecules striking the surface at any instant.
    - **b.** In a mixture of gases, the partial pressure that each gas contributes to the total partial pressure is directly proportional to its relative concentration (Table 50-1).
  - **2.** When a gas-liquid or gas-tissue interface exists, gas molecules dissolve in the liquid or tissue until equilibrium (partial pressures equal in both phases) is achieved.
  - **3.** The concentration of a gas in a liquid is determined by multiplying the partial pressure the gas exerts by its **solubility coefficient** (Henry's law).
- **C. Vapor pressure of water** is the pressure that water

Table 50–1
Partial Pressures of Respiratory Gases at Sea Level (760 mmHg)

Respiratory Gas	Inhaled Air (mm Hg)	Alveolar Gas (mm Hg)	Exhaled Gases (mm Hg)
Oxygen	159	104	120
Carbon dioxide	0.3	40	27
Nitrogen	597	569	566
Water	3.7	47	47

molecules exert to escape into the gas phase (47 mm Hg at 37°C).

D. **Composition of alveolar gases** is different than that of inhaled gases because oxygen is being absorbed, carbon dioxide is being added, and dry inhaled gases are humidified by the addition of water vapor.

   1. **Alveolar partial pressure of oxygen** (PAO_2) is determined by alveolar ventilation and rate of oxygen absorption ($250 \ ml \cdot min^{-1}$).

      a. The inspired partial pressure of oxygen is diluted by the alveolar carbon dioxide ($PACO_2$, 40 mm Hg) and P_{H_2O} (47 mm Hg), which are both independent of P_B.

      b. Breathing supplemental oxygen offsets the dilutional effect of carbon dioxide and water vapor.

   2. **Alveolar partial pressure of carbon dioxide** is determined by delivery of carbon dioxide to the alveoli by pulmonary capillary blood ($200 \ ml \cdot min^{-1}$) and alveolar ventilation (when delivery is constant, the $PACO_2$ is directly proportional to alveolar ventilation).

E. **Composition of exhaled gases** is determined by the proportion that is alveolar gas and the proportion that is dead space gas.

   1. Because gas exchange does not occur in conducting airways, the composition of dead space gas resembles the composition of inhaled gas.

   2. Collection of the last portion of exhaled alveolar gas (end-tidal sample) is a method for analyzing the composition of alveolar gas, including anesthetic concentrations (minimum alveolar concentration [MAC]).

   3. Contamination of the end-tidal gas sample with inhaled gases invalidates the interpretation of the obtained values.

Table 50–2
Calculation of the Physiologic Dead Space to Tidal Volume Ratio

$V_D/V_T = PaCO_2 - P_{ET}CO_2/PaCO_2$
V_D/V_T = ratio of physiologic dead space to tidal volume
$PaCO_2$ = arterial partial pressure of CO_2 (mm Hg)
$P_{ET}CO_2$ = mixed exhaled partial pressure of CO_2 (mm Hg)

F. Gas Diffusion from Alveoli to Blood

1. The average diameter of the pulmonary capillaries is only 8 μm, which means that erythrocytes must squeeze through the vessels in single file such that the distance for diffusion of oxygen and carbon dioxide is minimized (60 to 140 ml of blood spread over 70 m²).

2. Based on solubility, carbon dioxide diffuses across the membrane approximately 20 times as rapidly as oxygen.

G. Ventilation-to-perfusion ratio ($\dot{V}/\dot{Q}$ ratio) determines the composition of the alveolar gas and the effectiveness of gas exchange, especially for oxygen across the alveolar capillary membrane.

1. Physiologic shunt ($\dot{V}/\dot{Q}$ is 0) refers to the 2% to 5% of the cardiac output that normally bypasses the lungs.

2. **Physiologic dead space** ($\dot{V}/\dot{Q}$ = infinity) is the same as **wasted ventilation** (Table 50-2).

II. BLOOD TRANSPORT OF OXYGEN AND CARBON DIOXIDE

A. Oxygen Uptake into the Blood

1. After diffusion from alveoli into pulmonary capillary blood, oxygen is transported principally in combination with hemoglobin to tissue capillaries, where it is released along a partial pressure gradient for use by cells (Fig. 50-1).

2. Rapid equilibration of pulmonary capillary blood with the PAO_2 provides an important safety factor for transfer of oxygen when blood flow through the lungs is accelerated, as during exercise (pulmonary diffusing capacity does not limit exercise).

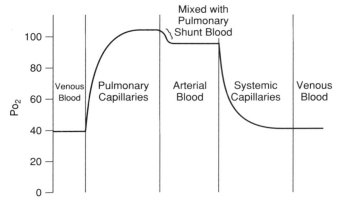

FIGURE 50–1. Changes in the PO_2 as blood traverses the systemic and pulmonary circulations. (From Guyton AC. Textbook of Medical Physiology, 7th ed. Philadelphia: WB Saunders, 1986; with permission.)

  B. Diffusion of oxygen from the capillaries is dependent on the partial pressure gradient for oxygen between tissues, capillaries, and the interstitial fluid PO_2.

  C. Diffusion of carbon dioxide from the cells reflects continuous formation of carbon dioxide in cells, which maintains a partial pressure gradient for its diffusion into capillary blood.

  D. Blood Transport of Oxygen

    1. Approximately 97% of oxygen transported from alveoli to tissues is carried to tissues in chemical combination with hemoglobin (1.34 ml of oxygen for each gram of hemoglobin) while approximately 3% of oxygen is transported in the dissolved state (0.003 ml·mm Hg^{-1}).

    2. Under resting conditions, approximately 5 ml of oxygen is released to the tissues for every 100 ml of blood (250 ml·min^{-1} of oxygen when cardiac output is 5 L·min^{-1}).

    3. Hemoglobin

      a. Types of hemoglobin are designated A through S, depending on the genetically determined sequence of amino acids in the globin portion of the molecule (substitution of valene for glutamic acid results in hemoglobin S and **sickle cells**).

      b. Myoglobin is capable of binding only one mole-

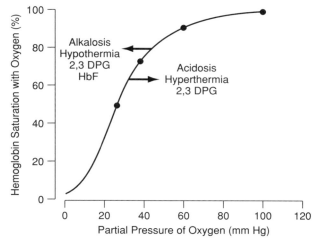

FIGURE 50–2. Oxyhemoglobin dissociation curve for hemoglobin A at a pH of 7.4 and 37°C. Changes in pH, body temperature, concentration of 2,3-diphosphoglycerate (2,3 DPG), and the presence of different types of hemoglobin shift the oxyhemoglobin dissociation curve to the left or right of its normal position.

    cule of oxygen, which cannot be released until the PO_2 has decreased to very low values.

  4. **Oxyhemoglobin dissociation curve** depicts the percentage of hemoglobin saturation with oxygen at different partial pressures of oxygen (Fig. 50-2).
    a. The S-shape of the oxyhemoglobin dissociation curve means that increasing the PaO_2 above 100 mm Hg increases the concentration of oxygen in the blood only slightly.
    b. The steep portion of the oxyhemoglobin dissociation curve means that small changes in the PaO_2 result in the transfer of large amounts of oxygen from hemoglobin to tissues.
  5. **Shift of the Oxyhemoglobin Dissociation Curve** (Fig. 50-2)
    a. A convenient indicator of the position of the oxyhemoglobin dissociation curve is the PO_2 which produces 50% saturation of hemoglobin with oxygen (P_{50}) (P_{50} is approximately 26 mmHg, and this is

increased when the oxyhemoglobin dissociation curve is shifted to the right).

   b. When the oxyhemoglobin dissociation curve is shifted to the left, the PO_2 must decrease to a lower level before oxygen is released from hemoglobin to tissues.

   c. **Bohr effect** is the pH-dependent shift in the position of the oxyhemoglobin dissociation curve caused by carbon dioxide entering or leaving the blood.

   d. **2,3-Diphosphoglycerate** decreases the affinity of hemoglobin for oxygen by shifting the oxyhemoglobin dissociation curve to the right.

6. **Carbon monoxide** combines with hemoglobin more avidly (230 times more) than does oxygen (a carbon monoxide partial pressure of 0.4 mmHg is equivalent to a PO_2 of 92 mm Hg).

   a. **Chemoreceptors** that increase alveolar ventilation are not stimulated by carbon monoxide because the PaO_2 remains normal.

   b. Most victims of fires die from acute carbon monoxide poisoning (cigarette smoking is a source of carboxyhemoglobin).

   c. The only treatment of carbon monoxide poisoning is administration of oxygen (hyperbaric chamber a consideration) that produces a high PaO_2 to displace carbon monoxide from hemoglobin.

7. **Cyanosis** is caused by excessive amounts of reduced hemoglobin (more than 5 g) in cutaneous capillaries.

   a. **Anemic patients** may lack sufficient hemoglobin to cause cyanosis, even in the presence of profound hypoxemia, whereas patients with **polycythemia** may appear cyanotic despite adequate arterial concentrations of oxygen.

   b. The degree of cyanosis is influenced by the rate of blood flow through the skin, as reflected by peripheral cyanosis in cold weather.

E. **Blood Transport of Carbon Dioxide**

1. Carbon dioxide formed as a result of metabolic processes in cells readily diffuses across cell membranes into capillary blood (rapid diffusion reflects high solubility as the partial pressure difference between tissues and blood is only 1 to 6 mm Hg).

   a. Carbon dioxide is transported in the blood as dissolved carbon dioxide ($PvCO_2$ is being increased approximately 5 mmHg compared with the $PaCO_2$), bicarbonate ions (HCO_3^-), and carbamino-hemoglobin.

  b. The ratio of dissolved carbon dioxide to HCO_3^- is normally 20:1.
  c. Carbon dioxide that enters erythrocytes reacts with water to form carbonic acid (accelerated by carbonic anhydrase enzyme which is present in erythrocytes but not plasma) which dissociates into H^+ and HCO_3^-.

  2. Haldane effect is the displacement of carbon dioxide from hemoglobin by oxygen that occurs at the lungs.
  3. Body Stores of Carbon Dioxide
  a. In contrast to total body oxygen stores of approximately 1.5 L, there is an estimated 120 L of carbon dioxide dissolved in the body.
  b. In the presence of apneic oxygenation, the $PaCO_2$ increases 5 to 10 mm Hg during the first minute (reflects equilibration of the alveolar gas with the $PvCO_2$) and approximately 3 mm Hg thereafter (reflects metabolic production of carbon dioxide).

F. Respiratory Quotient
  1. The ratio of carbon dioxide output to oxygen uptake is the **respiratory quotient.**
  2. In the resting state, the amount of oxygen added to blood (5 ml·dl^{-1}) exceeds the amount of carbon dioxide that is removed from the blood (4 ml·dl^{-1}), resulting in a respiratory quotient of 0.8.

III. CHANGES ASSOCIATED WITH HIGH ALTITUDE

A. The total partial pressure of all gases in the atmosphere (P_B) decreases progressively as distance above sea level increases (Table 50-3 and Fig. 50-3).
  1. Because the concentration of oxygen remains constant (21%), the decrease in P_B above sea level is associated with a progressive decrease in the ambient PO_2.
  2. The decrease in P_B with increasing altitude is not linear because air is compressible (Fig. 50-3).
B. The pharmacologic effect of inhaled anesthetics is reduced by decreased P_B.
  1. At sea level, 60% inhaled nitrous oxide produces a P_{N_2O} of 456 mm Hg, compared with a P_{N_2O} of 314 mm Hg at 3300 m.

Table 50–3
Effects of Altitude on Respiratory Gases While Breathing Air

Altitude (m/feet)	PB (mm Hg)	PIO$_2$ (mm Hg)	PAO$_2$ (mm Hg)	PACO$_2$ (mm Hg)	SaO$_2$ (%)
Sea level	760	159	104	40	97
3300/10,000	523	110 (436)*	67	36	90
6600/20,000	349	73	40	24	70
9900/30,000	226	47	21	24	20

* Breathing 100% oxygen

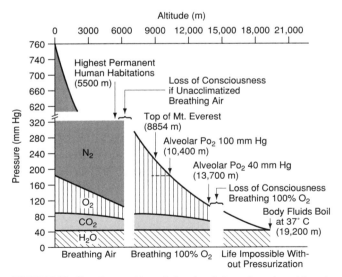

FIGURE 50–3. Composition of alveolar air in patients breathing air (0–6100 m) and 100% oxygen (6100–13700 m). (From Ganong WF. Review of Medical Physiology. Norwalk, CT: Appleton and Lange, 1987; with permission.)

Table 50–4
Compensatory Responses Evoked by Ascent to Altitude

Increased alveolar ventilation
Increased hemoglobin production
Increased 2,3-diphosphoglycerate concentrations
Increased diffusing capacity of the lungs
Increased vascularity of the tissues
Increased cellular use of oxygen

2. The inhaled concentration of nitrous oxide would have to be 87% at 3300 m to produce the same P_{N_2O} (same pharmacologic effect) as the inhalation of 60% N_2O at sea level.

C. **Acclimatization to altitude** reflects compensatory mechanisms (Table 50-4).

1. The initial increase in alveolar ventilation lowers the $PaCO_2$, which blunts the magnitude of the compensatory response.

2. Within a few days, active transport of HCO_3^- returns the cerebrospinal fluid pH to normal and alveolar ventilation again increases despite a low $PaCO_2$.

D. **Acute mountain sickness** is a syndrome of headache, insomnia, dyspnea, and fatigue that is associated with rapid ascent to altitude.

1. Symptoms usually develop 8 to 24 hours after arrival at altitude and last 4 to 8 days.

2. Pulmonary edema and cerebral edema are serious forms of acute mountain sickness.

E. **Chronic mountain sickness** is characterized by polycythemia, pulmonary hypertension, and right ventricular failure.

IV. CHANGES ASSOCIATED WITH EXCESSIVE BAROMETRIC PRESSURE (Table 50-5)

A. The P_B increases by the equivalent of 1 atmosphere for every 10 m below the surface of sea water (10.4 m for fresh water).

1. An important effect of increased P_B below the surface of water is compression of gases in the lungs to smaller volumes.

2. High P_B produces **nitrogen narcosis** when the inhaled gases are air.

Table 50–5
Pressure-Related Diving Side Effects

Pulmonary barotrauma
  Pneumothorax
  Arterial air embolism (stroke, cardiac dysrhythmias)
Middle ear barotrauma
  Conductive hearing loss
  Vertigo
  Tympanic membrane rupture
Paranasal sinus barotrauma
Nitrogen narcosis
  Resembles alcohol intoxication
  Occurs only when diving depth exceeds 30 m
Decompression sickness

---

3. **Decompression sickness** (caisson disease) occurs when sudden decreases in the P_B (as when a diver returns to surface) allow liberation of nitrogen bubbles in body tissues into the circulation, leading to occlusion of arteries and veins (nitrogen bubbles that form in the blood block pulmonary blood flow, manifesting as dyspnea **[chokes]**).

B. **Hyperbaric Oxygen Therapy**
  1. Indications for hyperbaric oxygen therapy are evolving (Table 50–6).
  2. The elimination half-time of carboxyhemoglobin is decreased from 320 minutes in a patient breathing room air to 23 minutes with breathing 100% oxygen at 3 atmospheres.

Table 50–6
Indications for Hyperbaric Oxygen Therapy

Decompression sickness
Air embolism
Carbon monoxide poisoning
Clostridial gangrene
Refractory osteomyelitis
Radiation necrosis
Profound anemia

Table 50–7
Complications of Hyperbaric Oxygen Therapy

Tympanic membrane rupture

Nasal sinus trauma

Pneumothorax

Air embolism

Central nervous system toxicity

Oxygen toxicity

3. Complications of hyperbaric oxygen therapy reflect barometric pressure changes or oxygen toxicity (Table 50-7).
   a. Any air-filled cavity that cannot equilibrate with ambient pressure, such as the middle ear when the eustachian tube is blocked, is subject to barotrauma during hyperbaric oxygen therapy.
   b. Almost all patients show oxygen toxicity after breathing 100% oxygen for 6 hours at 2 atmospheres.

51

Acid-Base Balance

The concentration of hydrogen (H^+) and bicarbonate (HCO_3^-) ions in plasma must be precisely regulated in the presence of enormous variations in dietary intake, metabolic production, and normal excretory losses of these ions. (Updated and revised from Stoelting RK. Acid-base balance. In: Pharmacology and Physiology in Anesthetic Practice. 2nd ed. Philadelphia, JB Lippincott, 1991:745–51.) The H^+ concentration is regulated to maintain the pH between 7.35 and 7.45 as small changes in H^+ concentration from normal can cause marked alterations in enzyme activity and the rates of chemical reactions in cells (Table 51-1).

I. MECHANISMS FOR REGULATION OF HYDROGEN ION CONCENTRATION

A. Regulation of pH over a narrow range is a complex physiologic process that depends on **buffer systems** (rapid but incomplete) plus **ventilatory responses** and **renal responses** (less rapid but nearly complete).

1. **Buffer Systems** (Table 51-2)
2. **Ventilatory Responses**
    a. Alveolar ventilation increases or decreases promptly in response to changes in H^+ concentration.
    b. In the presence of constant carbon dioxide production, the dissolved concentration of carbon dioxide is inversely proportional to alveolar ventilation.
    c. **Degree of ventilatory response** to a metabolic abnormality is incomplete, as the intensity of the stimulus responsible for increases or decreases in alveolar ventilation will begin to diminish as pH returns toward 7.4.
3. **Renal Responses**
    a. Renal responses that regulate H^+ concentration do so by acidification or alkalinization of the urine (excess H^+ or HCO_3^- enters the urine so as to be removed from extracellular fluid).
    b. **Renal tubular secretion of hydrogen ions** (Fig. 51-1).

Table 51–1
Relation of Hydrogen Ion (H^+) Concentration to pH

H^+ ($nmol \cdot L^{-1}$)	pH
80	7.10
63	7.20
50	7.30
42	7.38
40	7.40
38	7.42
32	7.50
25	7.60
20	7.70

Table 51–2
Buffer Systems

Hemoglobin buffering system (reduced hemoglobin combines with H^+)

Protein buffering system (an estimated 75% of buffering occurs intracellularly by virtue of proteins)

Phosphate buffering system (important in renal tubules)

Bicarbonate buffering system

    c. H^+ must combine with buffers in the lumens of renal tubules (ammonia combines with H^+ to form ammonium) to prevent tubular fluid pH from declining below the pH that allows continued secretion of H^+ by the renal tubular epithelial cells (Fig. 51–2).

    d. Degree of renal compensation is complete (pH returns to almost 7.40), but the process is slow (hours).

II. ACID-BASE DISTURBANCES

    A. Acid-base disturbances are categorized as respiratory or metabolic acidosis (pH lower than 7.35) or alkalosis (pH higher than 7.45) (Table 51–3).

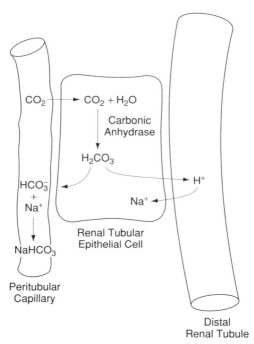

FIGURE 51–1. Schematic depiction of the renal tubular secretion of hydrogen ions (H⁺), which are formed from the dissociation of carbonic acid (H_2CO_3) in renal tubular epithelial cells.

1. An acid-base disturbance that results primarily from changes in alveolar ventilation is described as **respiratory acidosis or alkalosis.**

2. An acid-base disturbance unrelated to changes in alveolar ventilation is designated as **metabolic acidosis or alkalosis.**

3. **Compensation** describes the secondary renal or ventilatory responses that occur as a result of the primary acid-base disturbance in an attempt to return the pH toward a normal value.

4. The principal manifestation of respiratory or metabolic acidosis is **depression of the central nervous system** (coma is characteristic of diabetic acidosis or uremia).

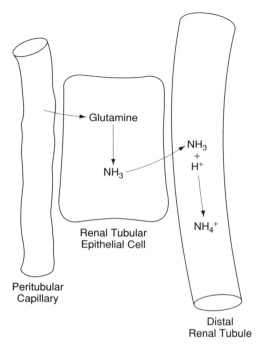

FIGURE 51–2. Ammonia (NH_3) formed in renal tubular epithelial cells combines with hydrogen ions (H^+) in the renal tubules to form ammonium (NH_4^+).

    5. The principal manifestation of respiratory or metabolic alkalosis is increased excitability of the peripheral nervous system **(tetany)** and central nervous system **(seizures).**

  B. **Respiratory acidosis** occurs when a drug or disease decreases alveolar ventilation.

  C. **Respiratory alkalosis** occurs when increased alveolar ventilation (iatrogenic during anesthesia) lowers the $PaCO_2$ and increases pH to higher than 7.45.

  D. **Metabolic acidosis** may reflect renal failure or anaerobic metabolism (inadequate tissue oxygenation) and accumulation of lactic acid.

    1. Metabolic acidosis impairs myocardial contractility (minimally when pH remains higher than 7.2) and

Table 51–3
Classification of Acid-Base Disturbances

	pH	*PaCO₂*	*HCO₃⁻*
Respiratory Acidosis			
Acute	− −	+ + +	+
Chronic	NC	+ + +	+ +
Respiratory Alkalosis			
Acute	+ +	− − −	−
Chronic	NC	− − −	− −
Metabolic Acidosis			
Acute	− − −	−	− − −
Chronic	−	− − −	− − −
Metabolic Alkalosis			
Acute	+ + +	+	+ + +
Chronic	+ +	+ +	+ + +

+, increase; −, decrease; NC, no change from normal

the responses to endogenous or exogenous catechol-amines.

2. Treatment of metabolic acidosis with intravenous sodium bicarbonate requires a concomitant increase in alveolar ventilation to remove the additional carbon dioxide produced from the bicarbonate.

E. **Metabolic alkalosis** occurs in the presence of vomiting or nasogastric suction (loss of hydrochloric acid) and excessive administration of sodium bicarbonate, as may occur during cardiopulmonary resuscitation.

F. **Compensation for Acid Base Disturbances**
   1. Respiratory acidosis is compensated for within 6 to 12 hours by increased renal secretion of H⁺, with a resulting increase in the plasma HCO₃⁻ concentration.
      a. After a few days, the pH will be normal despite persistence of an increased PaCO₂.
      b. Sudden correction of chronic respiratory acidosis (iatrogenic hyperventilation of the lungs) may produce metabolic alkalosis because increased amounts of HCO₃⁻ in the plasma cannot be promptly eliminated by the kidneys.
   2. Respiratory alkalosis is compensated for by decreased reabsorption of HCO₃⁻ from the renal tubules such

that pH returns toward normal despite persistence of a decreased $PaCO_2$.

3. Metabolic acidosis stimulates alveolar ventilation, which causes rapid removal of carbon dioxide from the body and decreases the H^+ concentration toward, but not completely to (partial respiratory compensation), normal.

4. Metabolic alkalosis diminishes alveolar ventilation which, in turn, causes accumulation of carbon dioxide and a subsequent increase in H^+ concentration toward, but not completely to (partial respiratory compensation), normal.

   a. Renal compensation for metabolic alkalosis is by increased reabsorption of H^+ (degree of compensation is limited by the availability of Na^+, K^+, and Cl^-).

   b. The presence of paradoxical aciduria indicates electrolyte depletion (vomiting).

52
Endocrine System

Endocrine glands secrete hormones into the blood for delivery to distant sites where a response is evoked. (Updated and revised from Stoelting RK. Endocrine system. In: Pharmacology and Physiology in Anesthetic Practice. 2nd ed. Philadelphia, JB Lippincott, 1991: 752–68.) Hormone output is typically regulated by a negative feedback system in which increasing circulating plasma concentrations of the hormone reduce its subsequent release from the parent gland. **Unrecognized endocrine dysfunction** is unlikely if it can be established preoperatively that (1) body weight is unchanged, (2) heart rate and blood pressure are normal, (3) glycosuria is absent, (4) sexual function is normal, and (5) there is no history of recent medication pertinent to the endocrine system.

I. MECHANISMS OF HORMONE ACTION

   A. Hormones typically exert their physiologic effects by attaching to specific receptors on plasma cell membranes, leading to production of cyclic adenosine monophosphate (cyclic AMP).

   B. An alternative mechanism of action for hormones is to stimulate formation of intracellular proteins that function as enzymes or carrier proteins.

II. PITUITARY GLAND

   A. The pituitary gland lies in the sella turcica at the base of the brain (physiologically lying outside the blood–brain barrier) and is connected to the hypothalamus by the pituitary stalk.

   1. The **anterior pituitary** (adenohypophysis) stores and secretes six trophic hormones (Table 52-1).

   2. The **posterior pituitary** (neurohypophysis) stores and secretes two hormones that are initially synthesized in the hypothalamus and are subsequently transported to the posterior pituitary.

   3. Hormones designed as **hypothalamic-releasing hormones** and **hypothalamic-inhibitory hor-**

Table 52–1
Pituitary Hormones

Hormone	Cell Type	Principal Action
Anterior Pituitary		
Human growth hormone (HGH, somatotropin)	Somatotrophs	Accelerates body growth
Prolactin	Mammotrophs	Stimulates secretion of milk and maternal behavior, inhibits ovulation
Luteinizing hormone (LH)	Gonadotrophs	Stimulates ovulation in females and testosterone secretion in males
Follicle stimulating hormone (FSH)	Gonadotrophs	Stimulates ovarian follicle growth in females and spermatogenesis in males
Adrenocorticotrophic hormone (ACTH)	Corticotrophs	Stimulates adrenal cortex secretion and growth
Thyroid-stimulating hormone (TSH)	Thyrotrophs	Stimulates thyroid secretion and growth
Beta-lipotropin	Corticotrophs	Precursor of endorphins?
Posterior Pituitary		
Antidiuretic hormone (ADH, vasopressin)	Supraoptic nuclei	Promotes water retention and regulates plasma osmolarity
Oxytocin	Paraventricular nuclei	Causes ejection of milk and uterine contraction

Table 52–2
Hypothalamic Hormones

Hormone	Target Anterior Pituitary Hormone*
Human growth hormone–releasing hormone	HGH
Human growth hormone–inhibiting hormone (somatostatin)	HGH, prolactin, TSH
Prolactin-releasing factor	Prolactin
Prolactin-inhibiting factor	Prolactin
Luteinizing hormone–releasing hormone	LH, FSH
Corticotropin-releasing hormone	ACTH, beta-lipotropin, endorphins
Thyrotropin-releasing hormone	TSH

*See Table 52-1 for an explanation of abbreviations.

mones originating in the hypothalamus control secretions from the anterior pituitary (Table 52-2).

B. Anterior Pituitary

   1. Human growth hormone (HGH) (Tables 52-1 and 52-3)

      a. HGH stimulates linear bone growth (excess secretion results in giantism before epiphyseal closure and acromegaly after closure) and evokes intense metabolic effects (anabolic effect, ketogenic effect, diabetogenic effect).

      b. Many of the activities of HGH require the prior generation of a family of peptides known as **somatomedins**.

   2. Prolactin (Tables 52-1 and 52-4)

   3. Adrenocorticotrophic Hormone (ACTH) (Tables 52-1 and 52-5)

      a. Diurnal variation in ACTH levels results in high plasma cortisol concentrations in the morning and low levels around midnight (plasma cortisol concentrations should be interpreted on the basis of time of measurement).

      b. Hypophysectomy eliminates the secretion of cortisol, but electrolyte changes are minimal because aldosterone secretion continues.

Table 52–3
Regulation of Human Growth Hormone (HGH) Secretion

Stimulation	Inhibition
HGH-releasing hormone	HGH-inhibiting hormone
Stress	HGH
Physiologic sleep	Pregnancy
Hypoglycemia	Hyperglycemia
Free fatty acid decrease	Free fatty acid increase
Amino acid increase	Cortisol
Fasting	Obesity
Estrogens	
Dopamine	
Alpha-agonists	

    c. Pallor is a hallmark of hypopituitarism, whereas **hyperpigmentation** occurs in the presence of primary adrenal disease.

    d. Chronic administration of corticosteroids leads to functional atrophy of the hypothalamic-pituitary axis (supplemental exogenous corticosteroids may be administered preoperatively for fear that stressful events during the perioperative period might

Table 52–4
Regulation of Prolactin Secretion

Stimulation	Inhibition
Prolactin-releasing factor	Prolactin-inhibiting factor
Pregnancy	Prolactin
Suckling	Dopamine
Stress	L-dopa
Physiologic sleep	
Metoclopramide	
Cimetidine	
Opioids	
Alpha-methyldopa	

Table 52–5
Regulation of Adrenocorticotrophic Hormone (ACTH) Secretion

Stimulation	*Inhibition*
Corticotropin-releasing hormone	ACTH
Cortisol decrease	Cortisol increase
Stress	Opioids
Sleep-wake transition	
Hypoglycemia	
Sepsis	
Trauma	
Alpha-agonists	
Beta-antagonists	

      evoke life-threatening hypotension in the absence of adequate circulating concentrations of cortisol).

  4. Thyroid Stimulating Hormone (TSH) (Tables 52-1 and 52-2)

    a. Hypothyroidism, with increased plasma concentrations of TSH, indicates a primary defect at the thyroid gland and an attempt by the anterior pituitary to stimulate hormonal output by release of TSH.

    b. A defect at the hypothalamus or anterior pituitary is indicated by low circulating concentrations of both TSH and thyroid hormones.

C. Posterior Pituitary

  1. Antidiuretic hormone (ADH) (Tables 52-1 and 52-6)

    a. Hydration and establishment of an adequate blood volume before induction of anesthesia serve to maintain urine output, presumably by blunting the release of ADH associated with painful stimulation or fluid deprivation prior to surgery.

    b. Administration of morphine, and presumably other opioids, in the absence of painful stimulation does not evoke the release of ADH.

    c. Fluoride resulting from the metabolism of certain volatile anesthetics (enflurane, sevoflurane) could theoretically interfere with normal receptor re-

Table 52–6
Regulation of Antidiuretic Hormone (ADH) Secretion

Stimulation	*Inhibition*
Increased plasma osmolarity	Decreased plasma osmolarity
Hypovolemia	Ethanol
Pain	Alpha-agonists
Hypotension	Cortisol
Stress	Hypothermia
Hyperthermia	
Nausea and vomiting	
Opioids (?)	

sponses to ADH, resulting in a high-volume output of dilute urine.

   d. Diabetes insipidus results when there is destruction of neurons in the hypothalamus or in association with pituitary surgery (transient).

   2. Oxytocin (Table 52–1)

III. THYROID GLAND

   A. The thyroid gland is responsible for maintaining the optimal level of metabolism in tissues via the secretion of thyroxine (T_4) and triiodothyronine (T_3).

   1. Thyroid hormones increase minute oxygen consumption in nearly all tissues except the brain (minimum alveolar concentration [MAC] of anesthetic is not altered by hyperthyroidism or hypothyroidism).

   2. Thyroid hormones stimulate all aspects of carbohydrate metabolism and facilitate the mobilization of free fatty acids.

   3. The plasma concentration of T_4 is the standard screening test for thyroid gland function.

   B. Mechanism of Action

   1. Thyroid hormones probably exert most of their effects through control of protein synthesis, including enzymes.

   2. Sympathomimetic effects that accompany thyroid hormone stimulation most likely reflect an increased number and sensitivity of beta receptors in response to release of T_4 and T_3.

3. Increased metabolism produced by thyroid hormones causes vasodilation in tissues to provide the required blood flow to deliver necessary oxygen and carry away metabolites and heat.

4. Excess protein catabolism associated with increased secretion of thyroid hormones is the presumed mechanism for the skeletal muscle weakness that is characteristic of hyperthyroidism.

C. **Calcitonin** is a polypeptide hormone secreted by the thyroid gland that evokes a decrease in the plasma concentration of calcium ions (Ca^{2+}) (due to a decrease in activity of osteoclasts and an increase in osteoblastic activity).

IV. PARATHYROID GLANDS

A. The **four parathyroid glands** secrete parathyroid hormone in (inversely related to the plasma ionized Ca^{2+} concentrations), which is responsible for regulating the plasma concentration of Ca^{2+}.

B. The most prominent effect of parathyroid hormone is to promote mobilization of Ca^{2+} from bone, reflecting stimulation of osteoclastic activity.

V. ADRENAL CORTEX

A. The two major classes of corticosteroids are **mineralocorticoids** (aldosterone) and **glucocorticoids** (cortisol) (Table 52-7).

B. **Mineralocorticoids**
1. **Physiologic effects** of aldosterone are absorption of sodium ions (Na^+) and simultaneous secretion of potassium ions (K^+) by the renal tubules.
2. **Regulation of secretion** of aldosterone is principally determined by the plasma K^+ concentration (an increase in plasma K^+ of less than 1 mEq·L^{-1} will triple the rate of aldosterone secretion).

C. **Glucocorticoids**
1. **Cortisol** is responsible for at least 95% of glucocorticoid activity and is one of the few hormones essential for life.
2. **Physiologic Effects** (Table 52-8)
3. **Regulation of secretion** of cortisol (basal rate is 20 mg daily, which may increase to 150 mg daily with maximum stress) is principally determined by re-

TABLE 52-7
Physiologic Effects of Endogenous Corticosteroids (mg)

	Daily Secretion	Sodium Retention*	Glucocorticoid Effect*	Antiinflammatory Effect*
Aldosterone	0.125	3000	0.3	Insignificant
Desoxycorticosterone		100	0	0
Cortisol	20	1	1	1
Corticosterone	Minimal	15	0.35	0.3
Cortisone	Minimal	0.8	0.8	0.8

*Relative to cortisol

Table 52–8
Physiologic Effects of Cortisol Gluconeogenesis (Adrenal Diabetes)

Protein catabolism (skeletal muscle weakness)

Fatty acid mobilization ("buffalo-like torso")

Antiinflammatory effects
  Stabilization of lysosomal membranes
  Reduced migration of leukocytes
  Decreased capillary permeability
  Decreased immunity against bacterial and viral infection
  Decreased likelihood of immunologic rejection of transplanted
    tissues

lease of ACTH from the anterior pituitary (Table 52–5).

VI. REPRODUCTIVE GLANDS

- **A. Testes** secrete male sex hormones (androgens), of which testosterone is the most important (development of male sex characteristics).
- **B. Ovaries** secrete estrogen (development of female sexual characteristics) and progesterone (preparation of the uterus for pregnancy and breasts for lactation) in response to luteinizing hormone (LH) and follicle stimulating hormone (FSH) (Table 52–1).
    1. **Menstruation** consists of three phases which recur every 21 to 35 days: follicular (onset of menstrual bleeding reflecting a decrease in the plasma concentration of progesterone), ovulating (body temperature increases about 0.5°C with ovulation), and luteal (development of corpus luteum).
    2. **Pregnancy** is initially confirmed by the presence of the placental hormone, **chorionic gonadotropin,** which appears in the maternal plasma and urine (basis for pregnancy tests) within 9 days following conception.
        a. Increased plasma concentrations of progesterone are associated with sedative effects (decreased anesthetic requirements [MAC]) and stimulation of ventilation (increased alveolar ventilation).
        b. The parturient with asthma may experience unpredictable changes in airway reactivity.

C. **Menopause** occurs between the ages of 45 and 55 years as the ovaries gradually become unresponsive to LH and FSH.
   1. Sensations of warmth spreading from the trunk to the face (hot flashes) coincide with surges of LH secretion.
   2. Exogenous administration of estrogens prevents hot flashes.

VII. PANCREAS

A. The pancreas secretes digestive substances into the duodenum and hormones, including insulin (secreted by beta cells of the islets of Langerhans) and glucagon.
B. **Insulin** is an anabolic hormone promoting the storage of glucose, fatty acids, and amino acids (Fig. 52-1).
   1. The amount of insulin secreted daily is equivalent to approximately 40 units.
      a. Insulin binds to receptor proteins in cell membranes, leading to activation of the glucose transport system.
      b. In the circulation, insulin has an elimination half-time of about 5 minutes, with more than 80% being degraded in the liver and kidneys.
   2. **Regulation of insulin secretion** is via a negative feedback effect of blood glucose concentration on the pancreas (Table 52-9).
      a. Virtually no insulin is secreted when the blood glucose concentration is lower than 50 mg·dl^{-1}, and maximum stimulation occurs when the blood glucose concentration is higher than 300 mg·dl^{-1}.
      b. The pancreas is richly innervated by the autonomic nervous system (beta stimulation facilitates release, whereas alpha stimulation inhibits release of insulin).
      c. Glycosuria is more likely after intravenous administration of glucose than after oral administration, emphasizing that oral glucose is a more potent stimulus to the release of insulin.
   3. **Physiologic effects** of insulin include promoting the use of carbohydrates for energy (facilitates glucose uptake and storage in the liver by its effects on specific enzymes [glucokinase, phosphorylase]) while depressing the use of fats (inhibits lipase) and amino acids.

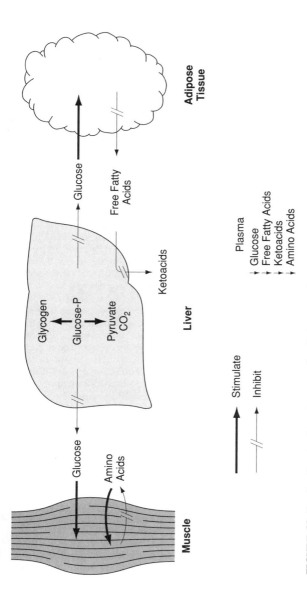

FIGURE 52-1. Insulin stimulates tissue uptake of glucose and amino acids, whereas release of fatty acids is inhibited. As a result, the plasma concentrations of glucose, free fatty acids, amino acids, and ketoacids decrease. (From Berne RM, Levy MN. Physiology, 2nd ed. St. Louis: CV Mosby, 1988; with permission.)

Adipose Tissue

Glucose

Free Fatty Acids

Liver

Glycogen ⇄ Glucose-P ⇄ Pyruvate
CO_2

Ketoacids

Muscle

Glucose

Amino Acids

Plasma

↓ Glucose
↓ Free Fatty Acids
↓ Ketoacids
↓ Amino Acids

Stimulate

Inhibit

599

Table 52–9
Regulation of Insulin Secretion

Stimulation	*Inhibition*
Hyperglycemia	Hypoglycemia
Beta-agonists	Beta-antagonists
Acetylcholine	Alpha-agonists
Glucagon	Somatostatin
	Diazoxide
	Thiazide diuretics
	Volatile anesthetics
	Insulin

   a. Resting skeletal muscle is almost impermeable to glucose except in the presence of insulin.
   b. Brain cells are unique in that the permeability of these cells' membranes to glucose is not dependent on the presence of insulin (crucial because brain cells use only glucose for energy).
4. **Diabetes mellitus** is characterized by an absolute or relative lack of insulin manifesting as hyperglycemia.
   a. Increased free fatty acid concentrations in the plasma of diabetic patients reflects loss of insulin-induced inhibition of the lipase enzyme system such that mobilization of fatty acids proceeds unopposed (even low concentrations of insulin that do not prevent hyperglycemia will block lipolysis).
   b. The insulin-deficient liver is likely to use fatty acids to produce ketones, which can serve as an energy source for skeletal muscles and cardiac muscles.
   c. Production of ketones can lead to ketoacidosis, whereas urinary excretion of these anions contributes to depletion of electrolytes, especially K^+ (hypokalemia may not be apparent because intracellular K^+ is exchanged for extracellular K^+ to compensate for the acidosis).
   d. **Ketosis** can reliably be prevented by providing glucose and insulin, a fact that is uniquely important in the perioperative period when nutritional uptake is altered.
5. **Glucagon** is a catabolic hormone acting to mobilize glucose, fatty acids, and amino acids into the circulation (Fig. 52–2).

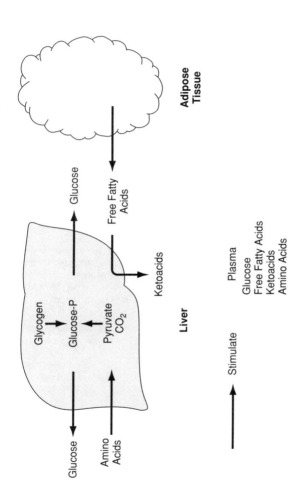

FIGURE 52-2. Glucagon stimulates tissue release of glucose, free fatty acids, and ketoacids, as well as hepatic uptake of amino acids. (From Berne RM, Levy MN. Physiology, 2nd ed. St. Louis: CV Mosby, 1988; with permission.)

601

Table 52–10
Regulation of Glucagon Secretion

Stimulation	*Inhibition*
Hypoglycemia	Hyperglycemia
Stress	Somatostatin
Sepsis	Insulin
Trauma	Free fatty acids
Beta-agonists	Alpha-agonists
Acetylcholine	
Cortisol	

- a. The responses elicited by glucagon are reciprocal to the effects of insulin, emphasizing that these two hormones are also reciprocally secreted (Table 52-10).
- b. The principal stimulus for secretion of glucagon is hypoglycemia.
- c. Glucagon is able to increase the blood concentrations of glucose abruptly by stimulating glycogenolysis in the liver (reflects activation of adenylate cyclase and subsequent formation of cyclic AMP, the metabolic effects of which are identical to those of epinephrine).

Chapter

53
Kidneys

The principal function of the kidneys is to stabilize the composition of the extracellular fluid, as reflected by electrolyte and hydrogen ion (H^+) concentrations. (Updated and revised from Stoelting RK. Kidneys. In: Pharmacology and Physiology in Anesthetic Practice. 2nd ed. Philadelphia, JB Lippincott, 1991:769–81.) End-products of protein metabolism (urea) are excreted and essential body nutrients (amino acids, glucose) are retained. The kidneys also secrete hormones for the regulation of blood pressure (angiotensin II, prostaglandins, kinins) and the production of erythrocytes (erythropoietin).

I. NEPHRON

A. The functional unit of the kidney is the nephron (1.2 million per kidney), which is composed of the **glomerulus** and **renal tubule** (Fig. 53-1).

B. **Glomerulus** is formed by a tuft of capillaries that invaginate into the dilated blind end of the renal tubule known as **Bowman's capsule.**

    1. Glomerular capillaries are unique anatomically in that they are interposed between two sets of arterioles (afferent and efferent).

    2. Pressure in glomerular capillaries causes water and low-molecular-weight substances to filter into Bowman's capsule, which is in direct continuity with the proximal renal tubule.

C. **Renal tubule** provides the pathway for glomerular filtrate to be delivered to the renal pelvis as urine.

    1. As the glomerular filtrate travels along the renal tubules, most of its water and varying amounts of solutes are reabsorbed from the renal tubular lumens into peritubular capillaries (Table 53-1).

    2. Unwanted metabolic waste products (urea) are filtered through the glomerular capillaries but, unlike water and electrolytes, are not reabsorbed as the glomerular filtrate progresses through the renal tubules (Table 53-1).

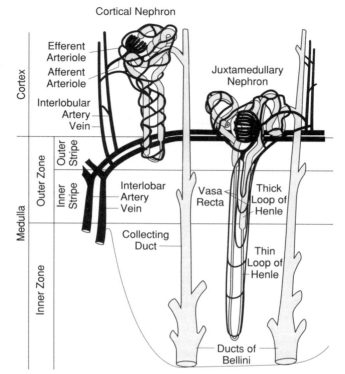

FIGURE 53–1. Schematic depiction of the nephron and accompanying blood supply. (From Pitts RF. Physiology of the Kidney and Body Fluids, 3rd ed. Chicago: Year Book Medical Publishers, 1974; with permission.)

II. RENAL BLOOD FLOW

    A. Renal blood flow (20% to 25% of the resting cardiac output) may be decreased by anesthetics (decreased cardiac output) or sympathetic nervous system stimulation (increased renal vascular resistance).

        1. Glomerular capillaries separate the afferent arteriole from the efferent arteriole (Fig. 53–2).

        2. Peritubular capillaries accept blood flow from efferent arterioles and subsequently function in much the same way as the venous ends of tissue capillaries.

Table 53-1
Magnitude and Site of Solute Reabsorption or Secretion in the Renal Tubules

	Filtered (24 b)	Reabsorbed (24 b)	Secreted (24 b)	Excreted (24 b)	Percent Reabsorbed	Location
Water (L)	180	179		1	99.4	P,L,D,C
Na$^+$ (mEq)	26,000	25,850		150	99.4	P,L,D,C
K$^+$ (mEq)	600	560	50	90	93.3	P,L,D,C
Cl$^-$ (mEq)	18,000	17,850		150	99.2	P,L,D,C
HCO$_3$$^-$ (mEq)	4900	4900		0	100	P,D
Urea (mM)	870	460		410	53	P,L,D,C
Uric acid (mM)	50	49	4	5	98	P
Glucose (mM)	800	800		0	100	P

P, proximal tubule; *L*, loop of Henle; *D*, distal tubule; *C*, convoluted tubule.

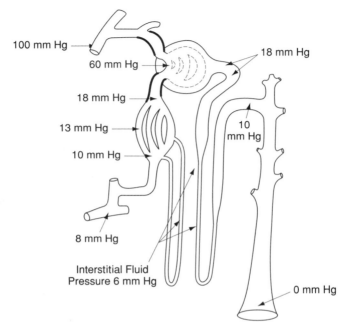

100 mm Hg

60 mm Hg

18 mm Hg

18 mm Hg

13 mm Hg

10 mm Hg

10 mm Hg

8 mm Hg

Interstitial Fluid
Pressure 6 mm Hg

0 mm Hg

FIGURE 53–2. Intravascular pressures in the renal circulation. (From Guyton AC. Textbook of Medical Physiology, 7th ed. Philadelphia: WB Saunders, 1986; with permission.)

    a. Fluid from the renal tubules is absorbed into low-pressure peritubular capillaries.

    b. Of the 180 L of fluid filtered daily through the glomerular capillaries, all but approximately 1.5 L is reabsorbed from the renal tubules back into peritubular capillaries, which eventually empty into the inferior vena cava.

B. Vasa recta represent a specialized portion of the peritubular capillaries that are important in the formation of concentrated urine **(countercurrent system).**

C. Autoregulation of Renal Blood Flow

    1. Changes in mean arterial pressure between 60 and 160 mmHg autoregulate renal blood flow and glomerular filtration rate (Fig. 53–3).

        a. Autoregulation of renal blood flow is due to an

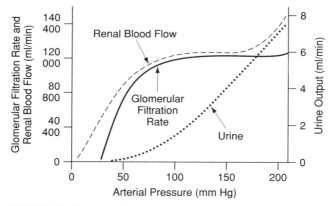

FIGURE 53–3. Renal blood flow and glomerular filtration rate, but not urine output, are autoregulated between a mean arterial pressure of approximately 60 and 160 mmHg. (From Guyton AC. Textbook of Medical Physiology, 7th ed. Philadelphia: WB Saunders, 1986; with permission.)

intrinsic mechanism that results in vasodilation or vasoconstriction of afferent renal arterioles.

b. The impact of anesthetic drugs on autoregulation has not been extensively studied (autoregulation remained intact during administration of halothane to an animal model).

c. Prostaglandins may participate in the autoregulation of renal blood flow and glomerular filtration rate, and also influence the tubular transport of ions and water (may be impaired by nonsteroidal antiinflammatory drugs; see Chapter 11).

d. In well-hydrated patients with normal renal function, prostaglandins play no apparent role in regulation of renal blood flow or fluid and electrolyte excretion.

2. Juxtaglomerular apparatus is the anatomic site in the distal renal tubules where cells in the renal arterioles release renin into the circulation (hypotension, renal ischemia, sympathetic nervous system stimulation) in an attempt by the kidneys to maintain a normal renal blood flow and glomerular filtration rate.

III. GLOMERULAR FILTRATE

A. Fluid that filters across glomerular capillaries into the renal tubules is designated glomerular filtrate.

B. **Glomerular filtration rate** is the amount of glomerular filtrate formed each minute by all the nephrons (normal rate is 125 ml·min^{-1}, 99% of which is reabsorbed, resulting in a daily urine output of 1 to 2 L).

C. **Mechanism of Glomerular Filtration**

  1. Pressure inside glomerular capillaries causes filtration of fluid through capillary membranes into the renal tubules.

  2. Filtration pressure responsible for glomerular filtration rate is influenced by **mean arterial pressure** (impact is blunted by autoregulation), **cardiac output** (parallels renal blood flow), and **sympathetic nervous system activity** (produces preferential constriction of afferent renal arterioles and urine output may approach zero).

IV. RENAL TUBULAR FUNCTION

A. Glomerular filtrate flows through renal tubules and collecting ducts, during which time substances are either selectively reabsorbed from tubules into peritubular capillaries or secreted (potassium ions [K^+], H^+) into tubules by tubular epithelial cells.

  1. An estimated two thirds of all reabsorptive and secretory processes take place in proximal renal tubules.

  2. The major physiologic determinants of the reabsorption of sodium ions (Na^+) and water are **aldosterone** (promotes reabsorption of Na^+ and secretion of H^+ and K^+ at the distal convoluted tubules), **antidiuretic hormone** (ADH promotes reabsorption of water into peritubular capillaries), **renal prostaglandins,** and **atrial natriuretic factor.**

   a. **Painful stimulation** may evoke the release of ADH.

   b. Anesthetic drugs and opioids, in the absence of surgical stimulation, do not predictably cause the release of ADH.

B. **Countercurrent system** in the kidneys is provided by the U-shaped anatomic arrangement of the peritubular capillaries (vasa recta) to those loops of Henle that extend into the medulla. This system makes it possible for the kidneys to eliminate solutes with minimal excretion of water.

V. **TUBULAR TRANSPORT MAXIMUM** (Tm) is the maximal amount of a substance that can be actively reabsorbed (depends on carrier substance and enzymes) from the lumens of renal tubules each minute (for glucose, the Tm is approximately 220 mg·min^{-1}).

VI. REGULATION OF BODY FLUID CHARACTERISTICS

A. The kidneys are the most important organs for regulating the characteristics of body fluids (Table 53–2).
B. **Thirst reflex** is most likely a response to an increased concentration of Na$^+$ in the extracellular fluid.

VII. ATRIAL NATRIURETIC FACTOR

A. This hormone is secreted by the cardiac atria and produces a dose-dependent increase in urine volume and Na$^+$ excretion, primarily by increasing glomerular filtration rate.
B. Blood pressure decreases and renal artery vasodilation reflect the role of this hormone as a potent vasodilator.
C. Circulating plasma concentrations of atrial natriuretic factor are linearly related to right and left atrial pressure.
D. Inhibition of hormone release (positive end-expiratory pressure, hypothermic cardiopulmonary bypass) diminishes urine output and urinary Na$^+$ excretion.

Table 53–2
Regulation of Body Fluid Characteristics by the Kidneys

Blood volume

Extracellular fluid volume

Osmolarity of body fluids (determined almost exclusively by extracellular fluid concentration of sodium)

Plasma concentration of ions
  Potassium (aldosterone)
  Sodium (aldosterone)
  Hydrogen (exchange with sodium)
  Calcium
  Magnesium

Urea

Table 53-3
Causes of Acute Renal Failure

Acute glomerulonephritis (antibodies against streptococcal antigen
  become entrapped in the basement membrane of the glomerular
  capillaries)
Acute tubular necrosis
  Nephrotoxins
  Ischemia (hemorrhage, hypotension, transfusion reaction)

VIII. ACUTE RENAL FAILURE (Table 53-3)

A. There is concern that decreased intraoperative urine
   output may be followed by postoperative acute renal
   failure (common practice is to treat low urine output
   intraoperatively with intravenous infusion of crystalloid solutions and, possibly, diuretics [mannitol, furose-
   mide]).
B. Low urine output intraoperatively does not predict postoperative renal function if intravascular fluid volume is
   maintained (Fig. 53-4).

IX. CHRONIC RENAL FAILURE

A. Despite different causes (chronic glomerulonephritis or
   pyelonephritis), the common denominators in patients
   who develop chronic renal failure are **progressive loss
   of nephron function** and a **decline in glomerular
   filtration rate** (Table 53-4).
B. **Manifestations of Chronic Renal Failure** (Tables 53-
   5 and 53-6)
   1. Renal failure may influence drug metabolism.
      a. Drug-metabolizing enzymes present in the liver
         may also be present in the renal cortex.
      b. There may be an accumulation of metabolites that
         undergo renal excretion.
      c. In uremic patients, the binding of many acidic
         drugs to albumin is decreased (basic drugs bind
         more commonly to alpha-1 acid glycoprotein).
   2. Specific gravity of the urine approaches that of the
      glomerular filtrate (approximately 1.008) as progres-
      sively more nephrons are lost and the countercurrent
      system fails.
   3. The inability of diseased kidneys to excrete K^+ has
      important anesthetic implications, especially with

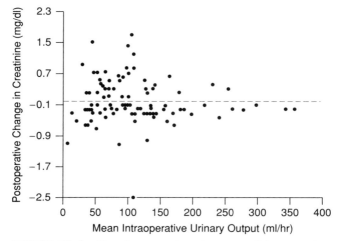

FIGURE 53–4. Mean intraoperative urine output did not correlate with postoperative changes in the plasma concentration of creatinine. (Alpert RA, Roizen MF, Hamilton WK, et al. Intraoperative urinary output does not predict postoperative renal function in patients undergoing abdominal aortic revascularization. Surgery 1984;95:707–11; with permission.)

respect to cardiac rhythm and responses at the neuromuscular junction.

4. Dialysis is useful in correcting electrolyte, fluid (hypertension), and platelet function (an analogue of vasopressin, DDAVP, is also effective in shortening bleeding time).

C. **Dialytic therapy** (hemodialysis or peritoneal dialysis) is associated with multiple side effects (Table 53–7).

1. The need to maintain chronic vascular access via a surgically created arteriovenous fistula is a major cause of morbidity in patients with chronic renal failure.

2. Peritonitis is the major complication associated with peritoneal dialysis.

X. NEPHROTIC SYNDROME

A. Nephrotic syndrome is characterized by the loss of large amounts of protein into the urine, which causes a de-

(text continues on page 614)

Table 53-4
Stages of Chronic Renal Failure

	Estimated Number of Nephrons (% of Total)	Glomerular Filtration Rate (ml·min⁻¹)	Signs	Laboratory Changes
Normal		125	None	None
Decreased renal reserve	40	50-80	None	None
Renal insufficiency	10-40	12-50	Polyuria Nocturia	Increased blood urea nitrogen Increased creatinine
Uremia	10	<12	See Table 53-5	See Table 53-5

Table 53–5
Manifestations of Chronic Renal Failure

Accumulation of metabolic waste products in the blood
Excretion of fixed specific gravity urine
Metabolic acidosis
Hyperkalemia
Anemia (treated with erythropoietin)
Platelet dysfunction
Fluid overload and hypertension
Nervous system dysfunction
Osteomalacia

Table 53–6
Renal Function Tests

	Normal Value	*Factors Influencing Interpretation*
Blood urea nitrogen	$8-20$ mg·dl^{-1}	Dehydration Variable protein intake Gastrointestinal bleeding Catabolism
Creatinine	$0.5-1.2$ mg·dl^{-1}	Age Skeletal muscle mass Catabolism
Creatinine clearance	120 ml·min^{-1}	Accurate urine volume measurement

Table 53–7
Complications of Dialytic Therapy

Dementia
Hypotension
Hypoxemia
Skeletal muscle cramping
Protein depletion
Infection
Anticoagulation
Access failure

crease in colloid osmotic pressure (edema, ascites, pericardial effusion).

B. Glucocorticoids may be efficacious in nephrotic syndrome secondary to lipoid nephrosis.

XI. TRANSPORT OF URINE TO THE BLADDER

A. Urine is transported to the bladder through the ureters (parasympathetic nervous system stimulation increases peristalsis in the ureters).

B. Obstruction of a ureter by a stone causes intense reflex constriction and pain.

Chapter

54

Liver and Gastrointestinal Tract

The liver is the largest gland in the body (2% of adult body weight), and hepatocytes represent approximately 80% of the cytoplasmic mass within the liver. (Updated and revised from Stoelting RK. Liver and gastrointestinal tract. In: Pharmacology and Physiology in Anesthetic Practice. 2nd ed. Philadelphia, JB Lippincott, 1991:782–94). The primary function of the gastrointestinal tract is to provide the body with a continual supply of water, electrolytes, and nutrients.

I. LIVER

A. Anatomy

1. The liver is divided into four lobes consisting of 50,000 to 100,000 individual hepatic lobules (Fig. 54–1).

    a. Hepatic lobules are lined by Kupffer's cells, which phagocytize 99% or more of bacteria in the portal venous blood.

    b. Approximately one third to one half of all the lymph is formed in the liver.

    c. Hepatocyte plasma membranes contain adrenoceptors (alpha-1, alpha-2, beta-2) whose activity may be influenced by volatile anesthetics.

    d. The common hepatic duct and cystic duct from the gallbladder join to form the common bile duct, which enters the duodenum at a site surrounded by the sphincter of Oddi (Fig. 54–2).

B. Hepatic Blood Flow

1. The liver receives a **dual afferent blood supply** (1450 ml·mm^{-1}) from the hepatic artery (25% of total flow and 45% to 50% of hepatic oxygen delivery) and portal vein (Fig. 54–3).

2. **Control of Hepatic Blood Flow**

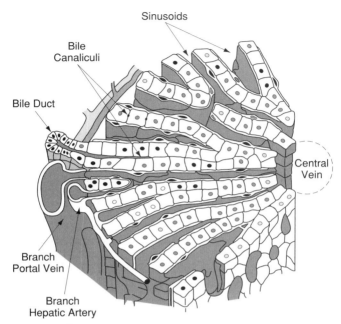

FIGURE 54–1. Schematic depiction of a hepatic lobule with a central vein and plates of hepatic cells extending radially. Blood from peripherally located branches of the hepatic artery and vein perfuses the sinusoids. Bile ducts drain the bile canaliculi that pass between the hepatocytes. (From Bloom W, Fawcell DW. A Textbook of Histology, 10th ed. Philadelphia: WB Saunders, 1975; with permission.)

    a. Portal vein blood flow parallels cardiac output, and autoregulation (limited) of hepatic blood flow occurs only via the hepatic artery to offset the effects of decreased cardiac output.

    b. Autoregulation of hepatic blood flow is better maintained in the presence of isoflurane than halothane anesthesia (see Fig. 2–11).

    c. Portal vein blood flow is decreased by hepatic cirrhosis (fibrotic constriction increases resistance to blood flow), congestive heart failure (increased central venous pressure transmitted to hepatic veins), and positive pressure ventilation of the lungs.

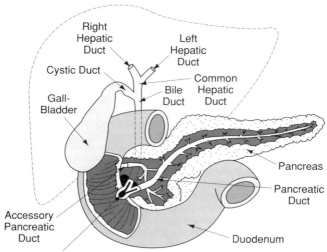

FIGURE 54–2. Connections of the ducts of the gallbladder, liver, and pancreas. (From Bell GH, Emslie-Smith D, Paterson CR. Textbook of Physiology and Biochemistry, 9th ed. New York: Churchill-Livingstone; 1976; with permission.)

    d. The greatest decreases in hepatic blood flow occur during intraabdominal operations near the liver, presumably owing to the mechanical interference with blood flow that is produced by surgical retraction in the operative area, as well as the release of vasoconstricting substances, such as catecholamines.

  3. Reservoir Function

    a. The liver normally contains about 500 ml of blood, or approximately 10% of the total blood volume (may increase to 1 L when right atrial pressure is increased, as occurs in the presence of congestive heart failure).

    b. The liver is the single most important source of additional blood during strenuous exercise or acute hemorrhage.

C. Bile Secretion

  1. Hepatocytes continually form bile (500 ml daily) and

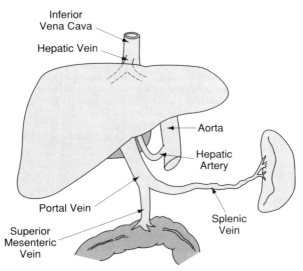

FIGURE 54–3. Schematic depiction of the dual afferent blood supply to the liver provided by the portal vein and hepatic artery.

then secrete it into bile canaliculi, which empty into progressively larger ducts, ultimately reaching the common bile duct (Fig. 54-2).

2. The most potent stimulus for emptying the gallbladder is the presence of fat in the duodenum, which evokes the release of the hormone cholecystokinin by the duodenal mucosa (causes selective contraction of gallbladder smooth muscle).

3. **Bile salts** are necessary for absorption of fat-soluble vitamins.

4. **Bilirubin** is formed from hemoglobin that is released from ruptured erythrocytes (Fig. 54-4).

   a. **Jaundice** is present when bilirubin concentrations increase to about three times normal.

   b. The most common types of jaundice are hemolytic jaundice owing to increased destruction of erythrocytes and obstructive jaundice owing to obstruction of bile ducts.

5. Cholesterol accounts for 85% of the gallstones that develop in 10% to 20% of the adult population (chemodeoxycholic acid may hasten dissolution).

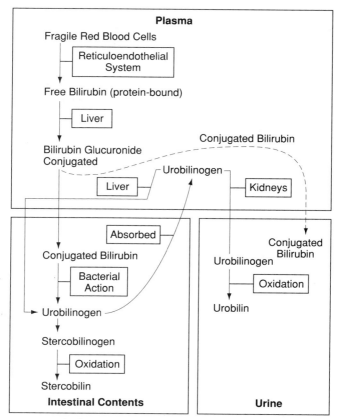

FIGURE 54–4. Schematic depiction of bilirubin formation and excretion. (From Guyton AC. Textbook of Medical Physiology, 7th ed. Philadelphia: WB Saunders, 1986; with permission.)

D. Metabolic Functions

1. Metabolism of carbohydrates, lipids, and proteins is dependent on normal hepatic function.
2. **Carbohydrates**
   a. When hyperglycemia is present, glycogen is deposited in the liver.
   b. When hypoglycemia occurs, **glycogenolysis** pro-

vides glucose and amino acids that can be converted to glucose by **gluconeogenesis.**

3. **Lipids** undergo beta oxidation to acetoacetic acid in the liver.

4. **Proteins**
   a. The most important liver functions in protein metabolism are deamination of amino acids, formation of urea for removal of ammonia, and formation of plasma proteins.
   b. Hepatic coma occurs with accumulation of ammonia.

II. GASTROINTESTINAL TRACT

A. The contents of the gastrointestinal tract must move through the entire system at an appropriate rate for digestive and absorptive functions to occur.
   1. Approximately 9 L of fluid and secretions enters the gastrointestinal tract daily, and all but approximately 100 ml is absorbed by the small intestine and colon (Fig. 54–5).
   2. The pH of gastrointestinal secretions varies widely (Table 54–1).

B. **Anatomy**
   1. The smooth muscle of the gastrointestinal tract is a syncytium such that electrical signals originating in one smooth muscle fiber are easily propagated from fiber to fiber.
   2. Mechanical activity of the gastrointestinal tract is enhanced by distension of the lumen and parasympathetic nervous system stimulation, whereas sympathetic nervous system stimulation reduces mechanical activity to almost zero.

C. **Blood Flow**
   1. Blood flow parallels the digestive activity of the gastrointestinal tract (approximately 80% of portal vein blood flow originates from the stomach and gastrointestinal tract).
   2. Stimulation of the sympathetic nervous system causes vasoconstriction of the arterial blood supply to the gastrointestinal tract.
   3. **Portal Venous Pressure**
      a. The gradual increase in resistance to portal vein blood flow produced by cirrhosis of the liver causes large collaterals to develop between the portal vein and the systemic veins (esophageal varices).

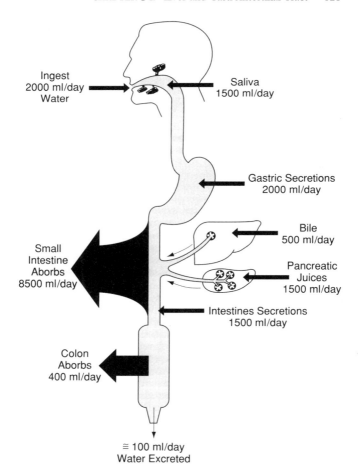

FIGURE 54–5. Overall fluid balance in the human gastrointestinal tract. Approximately 2 L of water is ingested each day, and approximately 7 L of various secretions enters the gastrointestinal tract. Of this 9 L, 8.5 L is absorbed from the small intestine. Approximately 0.5 L passes to the colon, which normally absorbs 80% to 90% of the water presented to it. (From Berne RM, Levy MN. Physiology, 2nd ed. St. Louis: CV Mosby, 1988; with permission.)

Table 54–1
pH of Gastrointestinal Secretions

Secretion	pH
Saliva	6–7
Gastric fluid	1–3.5
Bile	7–8
Pancreatic fluid	8–8.3
Small intestine	6.5–7.5
Colon	7.5–8

    b. In the absence of the development of adequate collaterals, sustained increases in portal vein pressure may cause protein-containing fluid to escape from the surface of the liver and gastrointestinal tract, resulting in **ascites.**

  4. Splenic Circulation

    a. A small amount of blood (150 to 200 ml) is stored in the splenic venous sinuses and can be released by sympathetic nervous system stimulation (increases the hematocrit by 1% to 2%).

    b. The spleen functions to remove fragile erythrocytes from the circulation, and the resulting hemoglobin is ingested by reticuloendothelial cells of the spleen.

D. Innervation

  1. The gastrointestinal tract receives innervation from both divisions of the autonomic nervous system and an intrinsic nervous system (myenteric plexus and submucous plexus).

    a. The cranial component of parasympathetic nervous system innervation to the gastrointestinal tract (esophagus to the level of the transverse colon) is by way of the vagus nerves.

    b. The distal portion of the colon is richly supplied by the sacral parasympathetics via the pelvic nerves from the hypogastric plexus.

    c. Fibers of the sympathetic nervous system destined for the gastrointestinal tract pass through ganglia, such as the celiac ganglia.

  2. A large number of neuromodulatory substances act on the gastrointestinal tract.

E. Motility

1. The two types of gastrointestinal motility are mixing contractions and propulsive movements **(peristalsis).**

   a. The usual stimulus for peristalsis is distention.

   b. Peristalsis is decreased by parasympathetic nervous system activity and anticholinergic drugs.

2. Ileus follows trauma to the intestine or irritation of the peritoneum.

   a. Peristalsis returns to the small intestine within 6 to 8 hours, but colonic peristalsis may take 2 to 3 days.

   b. Adynamic ileus can be relieved by placing a tube into the small intestine and aspirating fluid and gas until peristalsis returns.

F. Salivary glands (parotid and submaxillary glands) produce 0.5 to 1 ml·min^{-1} of saliva, largely in response to parasympathetic nervous system stimulation.

G. Esophagus serves as a conduit for passage of food from the pharynx to the stomach (swallowing inhibits breathing).

1. **Lower esophageal sphincter** is difficult to identify anatomically, but the lower 1 to 2 cm of the esophagus functions as a sphincter, with a resting pressure of approximately 30 mmHg.

   a. Anticholinergic drugs and pregnancy decrease lower esophageal sphincter tone, whereas gastrin and metoclopramide increase the tone.

   b. The influence, if any, of changes in lower esophageal sphincter tone and barrier pressure (lower esophageal sphincter pressure minus gastric pressure) and subsequent inhalation of gastric fluid during anesthesia remains undocumented.

2. Chronic incompetence of the lower esophageal sphincter permits reflux of gastric contents into the esophagus, with associated esophagitis.

H. Stomach is a specialized organ of the digestive tract that stores and processes food for absorption by the gastrointestinal tract (Fig. 54–6).

1. **Gastric secretions** may include up to 50 ml·h^{-1} of highly acidic gastric fluid and mucus **(prolonged preoperative fasting does not ensure an empty stomach).**

   a. **Parietal cells** secrete hydrochloric acid (kills bacteria, aids protein digestion) in response to stimula-

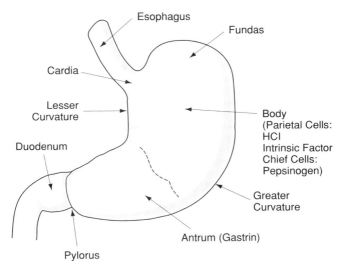

FIGURE 54–6.   Anatomy of the stomach, indicating the site of production of secretions. Mucus is secreted in all parts of the stomach.

tion by histamine, acetylcholine (vagal stimulation), and gastrin (see Chapter 21).

b. Intrinsic factor, which is essential for absorption of vitamin B_{12}, is secreted by parietal cells.

c. **Chief cells** secrete pepsinogens that undergo cleavage to pepsins, which serve as proteolytic enzymes for the digestion of proteins.

d. **G cells** secrete gastrin into the circulation for delivery to parietal cells.

e. The stomach is richly innervated by the vagus nerves and celiac plexus.

2. Gastric Fluid Volume and Rate of Gastric Emptying

a. Neural mechanisms (parasympathetic nervous system stimulation enhances gastric fluid secretion and motility) and humoral mechanisms influence gastric fluid volume and emptying time.

b. Foods pass through the stomach at different rates (carbohydrates pass faster than proteins, which pass faster than fat).

    c. Clear liquids leave the stomach in about 30 minutes, such that their ingestion (as with oral medications) up until about 2 hours before the time of scheduled surgery does not increase gastric fluid volume at the induction of anesthesia.

    d. Events that predictably slow gastric emptying for solids include enhanced sympathetic nervous system activity (fear or pain), active labor, and administration of opioids.

  3. Absorption from the stomach is poor, and only highly lipid-soluble liquids, such as ethanol, and drugs, such as aspirin, can be significantly absorbed from the stomach.

I. Small intestine consists of the duodenum (pylorus to ligament of Treitz), jejunum, and ileum (ends at the ileocecal valve).

  1. The small intestine is the site of most of the digestion and absorption (surface area of about 250 m^2) of proteins, fats, and carbohydrates (Table 54–2).

    a. Malnutrition is likely when more than 50% of the small intestine is resected.

    b. Chyme, 1 to 2 L daily, takes 3 to 5 hours to pass from the pylorus to ileocecal valve.

Table 54–2
Sites of Absorption

	Duodenum	*Jejunum*	*Ileum*	*Colon*
Glucose	++	+++	++	0
Amino acids	++	+++	++	0
Fatty acids	+++	++	+	0
Bile salts	0	+	+++	0
Water-soluble vitamins	+++	++	0	0
Vitamin B_{12}	0	+	+++	0
Sodium	+++	++	+++	+++
Potassium	0	0	+	++
Hydrogen	0	+	++	++
Chloride	+++	++	+	+
Calcium	+++	++	+	?

0, none; +, minimal; ++, moderate; +++, maximal

   2. **Secretions of the small intestine** include mucus to
      protect the duodenal wall from damage by acidic gas-
      tric fluid and digestive enzymes.
   3. **Absorption from the Small Intestine** (Table
      54–2)
J. **Colon** functions as the site for absorption of water and
   electrolytes from chyme and for storage of feces (Fig.
   54–7).
   1. Vagal stimulation causes contractions of the proximal
      colon (inhibited by sympathetic nervous system stimu-
      lation), and stimulation of the pelvic nerves causes
      expulsive movements.
   2. Bacteria are predictably present in the colon.
   3. **Secretions of the colon** are almost exclusively alka-
      line mucus (bicarbonate), which protects the mucosa
      against trauma.
      a. Irritation of a segment of the colon, as occurs with
         bacterial infection, causes the mucosa to secrete
         large quantities of water and electrolytes.

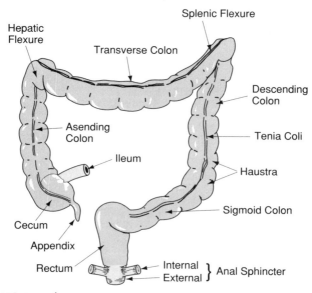

FIGURE 54–7. Anatomy of the colon.

b. The resulting diarrhea may result in dehydration and cardiovascular collapse.

III. PANCREAS

A. The pancreas serves as both an endocrine (insulin or glucagon) and exocrine (bicarbonate to neutralize duodenal contents and digestive enzymes) gland.

B. Regulation of Pancreatic Secretions

1. **Secretin,** released by the duodenal mucosa in response to hydrochloric acid, enters the circulation to cause the pancreas to secrete large amounts of alkaline fluid.

2. **Cholecystokinin** is released by the duodenum and enters the circulation to cause the pancreas to secrete digestive enzymes (trypsins, amylase, lipases).

3. Damage to the pancreas or blockage of the pancreatic duct may cause pooling of proteolytic enzymes, resulting in acute pancreatitis owing to autodigestion by these enzymes.

4. Pancreatic secretions are stimulated by the parasympathetic nervous system and inhibited by the sympathetic nervous system.

55

Skeletal and Smooth Muscle

Skeletal muscle (250 million cells in more than 400 skeletal muscles, comprising 40% of body mass) is responsible for voluntary actions whereas smooth muscle and cardiac muscle are responsible for involuntary actions. (Updated and revised from Stoelting RK. Skeletal and smooth muscle. In: Pharmacology and Physiology in Anesthetic Practice. 2nd ed. Philadelphia, JB Lippincott, 1991:795–800). Inappropriate activity of smooth muscle is involved in many illnesses, including hypertension, atherosclerosis, asthma, and disorders of the gastrointestinal tract.

I. SKELETAL MUSCLE

A. Skeletal muscle is made up of individual muscle fibers.

1. Each muscle fiber is composed of thousands of **myofibrils** that consist of contractile proteins (myosin, actin tropomyosin, and troponin).

   a. Myofibrils are suspended in **sarcoplasm,** which contains ions and an extensive endoplasmic reticulum **(sarcoplasmic reticulum).**

   b. The cell membrane of the muscle fiber is known as the **sarcolemma.**

   c. At the end of skeletal muscle fibers, surfaces of the sarcolemma fuse with tendon fibers that insert into bones.

2. **Hypertrophy** is synthesis of new myofibrils, whereas **hyperplasia** is formation of more cells.

B. **Excitation-Contraction Coupling**

1. The process by which depolarization of the sarcolemma and propagation of an action potential initiates skeletal muscle contraction is described as excitation-contraction coupling.

   a. An action potential reflects opening of fast channels in the skeletal muscle membrane, allowing rapid inward movement of sodium ions (Na^+) which is followed by outward movement of potassium ions (K^+) and repolarization.

  b. Action potentials cause the sarcoplasmic reticulum to release calcium ions (Ca^{2+}) which bind to troponin, thus abolishing the inhibitory effect of troponin on the interaction between myosin and actin **(cross-bridging leads to contraction).**

2. Shortly after releasing Ca^{2+}, the sarcoplasmic reticulum begins to reaccumulate this ion such that cross-bridging between myosin and actin ceases and skeletal muscle relaxes.

  a. Failure of this Ca^{2+} pump results in sustained skeletal muscle activity and increases in heat production **(malignant hyperthermia).**

  b. A mutation of the gene for the Ca^{2+} channel **(ryanodine receptor)** is thought to be responsible for malignant hyperthermia susceptibility.

C. **Neuromuscular Junction** (see Fig. 8-4)

  1. **Mechanism of Acetylcholine Effects** (see Fig. 8-5)

  2. **Altered Responses to Acetylcholine**

  a. Anticholinesterase drugs inhibit acetylcholinesterase enzyme, allowing accumulation of acetylcholine at receptors and subsequent displacement of nondepolarizing neuromuscular blocking drugs from alpha subunits.

  b. **Myasthenia gravis** is characterized by a decrease in the number of nicotinic acetylcholine receptors.

  3. **Blood Flow**

  a. Skeletal muscle blood flow can increase more than 20 times (a greater increase than in any other tissue in the body) during strenuous exercise.

  b. Skeletal muscle blood flow at rest is 3 to 4 ml·100 $g^{-1}·min^{-1}$.

D. **Innervation**

  1. Skeletal muscles are innervated by large myelinated nerve fibers that originate from the ventral (anterior) horn of the spinal cord and subsequently reach the muscle through a mixed peripheral nerve.

  2. **Denervation hypersensitivity** is the development of abnormal excitability of the denervated skeletal muscle to its neurotransmitter, acetylcholine (spread of cholinergic receptors over the entire skeletal muscle membrane occurs 3 to 5 days after denervation).

  3. **Electromyogram** is the recording from skin electrodes of the electrical current that spreads from skele-

tal muscles to skin during simultaneous contraction of numerous skeletal muscle fibers.

II. SMOOTH MUSCLE

A. Smooth muscle is categorized as either **multiunit** (which contraction is controlled almost exclusively by nerve signals and spontaneous contractions rarely occur) or **visceral** (forms a functional syncytium that often undergoes spontaneous contraction in the absence of nerve stimulation; prominent in tubular structures).

1. Visceral smooth muscle is unique in its sensitivity to hormones or local tissue factors.
2. Drugs relax smooth muscle by increasing the intracellular concentration of cyclic adenosine monophosphate or cyclic guanosine monophosphate.

B. Mechanism of Contraction

1. In contrast to skeletal muscles, in smooth muscle, the calcium-calmodulin complex (lack troponin) activates the enzyme necessary for actin to slide on myosin to produce contraction.

   a. Sarcoplasmic reticulum of smooth muscle is poorly developed, and Ca^{2+} that causes contraction of smooth muscles enters from extracellular fluid (takes 50 times longer than for skeletal muscle).

   b. Relaxation of smooth muscle occurs when Ca^{2+} is pumped back into the extracellular fluid (proceeds slowly, so the duration of smooth muscle contraction is often seconds rather than milliseconds, as is characteristic of skeletal muscles).

2. Smooth muscles, unlike skeletal muscles, do not atrophy when denervated, but they do become hyperresponsive to the usual neurotransmitter.

C. Neuromuscular Junction

1. A neuromuscular junction similar to that of skeletal muscles does not occur in smooth muscles.
2. Nerve fibers branch diffusely on top of a sheet of smooth muscle fibers without making actual contact.

   a. These nerve fibers secrete acetylcholine or norepinephrine, which function as excitatory or inhibitory neurotransmitters, depending on the characteristic of the corresponding receptor.

   b. When the neurotransmitter interacts with an inhibitory receptor instead of an excitatory receptor, the membrane potential of the muscle fiber becomes more negative (hyperpolarized).

D. Uterine smooth muscle is characterized by a high degree of spontaneous electrical (unlike the heart, there is no predominant pacemaker) and contractile activity.

   1. The contraction process spreads from one cell to another at a rate of 1 to 3 $cm \cdot sec^{-1}$.

   2. Alpha and beta inhibitory receptors are also present in the myometrium.

Chapter

56

Erythrocytes and Leukocytes

Erythrocytes (red blood cells [RBCs]) are the most abundant of all cells in the body (comprising 25 trillion of the estimated 75 trillion cells), emphasizing their irreplaceable role in delivery of oxygen to tissues. (Updated and revised from Stoelting RK. Erythrocytes and leukocytes. In: Pharmacology and Physiology in Anesthetic Practice. 2nd ed. Philadelphia, JB Lippincott, 1991:801–12.)

I. ERYTHROCYTES

A. The major function of RBCs is to transport hemoglobin, which, in turn, carries oxygen from the lungs to tissues.

1. In addition to transporting hemoglobin, RBCs contain large amounts of **carbonic anhydrase,** which makes it possible to efficiently transport carbon dioxide from tissues to the lungs.

2. Hemoglobin provides approximately 70% of the buffering capacity of whole blood.

B. **Anatomy**

1. RBCs are biconcave disks with a mean diameter of 8 μm.

2. The average number of RBCs in each milliliter of plasma varies among individuals and is influenced by barometric pressure (Table 56–1).

3. Each gram of hemoglobin is capable of combining with 1.34 ml of oxygen.

C. **Bone Marrow**

1. In the adult, RBCs, platelets, and many of the leukocytes are formed in the bone marrow (one of the largest organs in the body, approaching the size and weight of the liver).

2. The marrow of almost all bones produces RBCs until about 5 years of age; after 20 years of age, most RBCs are produced in the marrow of membranous bones (vertebrae, sternum, ribs, pelvis).

Table 56–1
Erythrocytes in the Plasma

	Content
Erythrocytes (ml)	
Male	$4.3-5.9 \times 10^6$
Female	$3.5-5.5 \times 10^6$
Hematocrit (percent)	
Male	39–55
Female	36–48
Hemoglobin ($g \cdot dl^{-1}$)	
Male	13.9–16.3
Female	12.0–15.0

3. **Control of Production**
   a. The total mass of RBCs in the circulation is regulated within narrow limits to provide optimal oxygenation without excessive viscosity (Fig. 56–1).
   b. Any event that decreases tissue oxygen delivery (anemia, chronic pulmonary disease, cardiac failure) will stimulate production of RBCs by the bone marrow.
   c. **Erythropoietin** is synthesized in response to arterial hypoxemia (kidneys release renal erythropoietic factor that acts in the circulation to split away the erythropoietin molecule) and acts to stimulate RBC production in the bone marrow.
   d. **Vitamins necessary for formation of RBCs** include **vitamin B_{12}** (failure of nuclear maturation) and **folic acid** (macrocytic anemia).
4. **Destruction** of RBCs normally occurs about 120 days after they leave the bone marrow. Released hemoglobin is rapidly phagocytized by reticuloendothelial cells (Fig. 56–1).

II. BLOOD GROUPS

A. Genetically determined antigens (A, B, and Rh are the most antigenic) are present on the cell membranes of RBCs.
B. **ABO Antigen System**

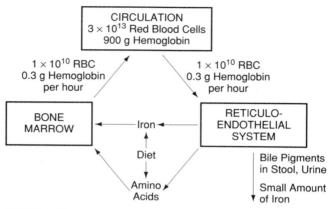

FIGURE 56–1. Erythrocyte formation and destruction. (From Ganong WF. Review of Medical Physiology, 13th ed. Norwalk, CT: Appleton and Lange, 1987; with permission.)

1. Blood is grouped for transfusion as A, B, AB, and O on the basis of the antigens present on RBC membranes (Table 56–2).
   a. In the absence of the A or B antigen, the opposite antibody (agglutinin) is present in the circulation (Table 56–2).
   b. It seems paradoxical that antibodies are produced in the absence of the respective antigen (likely that small amounts of A and B antigen enter by way of food or bacteria).
2. **Blood typing** is the in vitro mixing of a small amount

Table 56–2
ABO Antigen System

Blood Type	Incidence (percent)	Genotype	Antigens (Allutinogens)	Antibodies (Agglutinins)
O	47	OO		Anti-A, Anti-B
A	41	OA, AA	A	Anti-B
B	9	OB, BB	B	Anti-A
AB	3	AB	A, B	

of the patient's blood with plasma containing antibodies against the A or B antigen, followed by determination of the presence or absence of agglutination.

   a. Using this procedure, blood can be typed as O, A, B, or AB (also Rh-positive or Rh-negative).
   b. Cross-matching is the procedure that determines compatibility of the patient's blood with the donor's RBCs and plasma.

3. Rh blood types are determined by six common types of antigens that are collectively known as the Rh factor.

   a. An individual who is Rh-negative develops anti-Rh antibodies upon exposure to Rh-positive blood during transfusion, or during pregnancy when an Rh-negative mother is sensitized to the Rh-positive factor in her child.
   b. If an Rh-negative individual is transfused with Rh-positive blood, there is often no immediate reaction (may be a delayed and usually mild transfusion reaction).
   c. Destruction of Rh antigens in the first few days following delivery before an anti-Rh antibody response occurs is possible by injecting immune globulin against the antigen.

C. Hemolytic Transfusion Reactions

1. Transfusion of ABO type blood that is different than that of the recipient results in agglutination of the transfused RBCs by antibodies present in the plasma of the recipient, as well as hemolysis of the transfused RBCs (activation of the complement system).
2. Acute renal failure often accompanies a severe transfusion reaction.

III. LEUKOCYTES (Table 56-3)

A. Acting together, leukocytes provide an important defense against invading organisms (bacterial, viral, or parasitic) and are necessary for immune responses.

B. Neutrophils are the most numerous leukocytes in the blood and represent the body's first line of defense against bacterial infection (seeking out, ingesting, and killing bacteria [a process termed phagocytosis]).

1. To maintain a normal circulating blood level of neutrophils, it is necessary for the bone marrow to produce more than 100 billion neutrophils daily.

Table 56–3
Classification of Leukocytes

	Cells in Each ml of Plasma (range)	Percent of Total (range)
Granulocytes		
Neutrophils	3000–6000	55–65
Eosinophils	0–300	1–3
Basophils	0–100	0–1
Monocytes (Macrophages)	300–500	3–6
Lymphocytes	1500–3500	25–35
Total Leukocytes	4000–11,000	

    2. In the presence of infection, the need for neutrophils **(leukocytosis)** is even greater because these cells are destroyed in the process of phagocytosis.

  C. **Eosinophils** in the circulation increase in the presence of parasitic infections and during allergic reactions.

  D. **Basophils** in the blood are similar to mast cells in tissues in that both types of cells contain granules that store chemical mediators (histamine, heparin, leukotrienes, tryptase).

    1. **Degranulation** of previously sensitized cells occurs when IgE antibodies selectively attach to cell membranes and alter their permeability.

    2. Release of chemical mediators (especially histamine) from these cells is responsible for the manifestations of allergic reactions.

  E. **Monocytes** enter the circulation from the bone marrow, but after approximately 24 hours, they migrate into tissues to become macrophages (phagocytic) and constitute the reticuloendothelial system (Table 56-4).

Table 56–4
Designation of Macrophages in Different Tissues

Kupffer's cells (hepatic sinuses)

Reticulum cells (lymph nodes)

Alveolar macrophages

Histiocytes (subcutaneous tissues)

Table 56–5
Bacterial Destruction by Leukocytes

Diapedesis (passage of neutrophils and monocytes through pores in blood vessels)

Chemotaxis (phenomenon by which different chemical substances in tissues attract neutrophils and monocytes; may be inhibited by volatile anesthetics)

Opsonization (coating of bacteria by complement proteins to make them susceptible to phagocytosis)

Phagocytosis (ingestion of electropositive foreign materials by neutrophils and monocytes)

    F. Lymphocytes enter the circulation via the lymphatic system and play a prominent role in immunity.

IV. AGRANULOCYTOSIS is the acute cessation of leukocyte production by the bone marrow (ulcers appear in the mouth and colon within 2 to 3 days, reflecting the uninhibited growth of bacteria that normally inhabit these areas).

V. BACTERIAL DESTRUCTION (Table 56–5)

VI. INFLAMMATION is a series of sequential changes (release of histamine, bradykinin, and serotonin; edema, decreased blood flow; phagocytosis) that occur in tissues in response to injury.

VII. IMMUNITY

    A. Humoral immunity (defense against bacteria owing to circulating antibodies) and **cellular immunity** (delayed allergic reactions, rejection of foreign tissue, destruction of early cancer cells) are the two types of immune defense systems (Fig. 56–2).

        1. Lymphocytes responsible for humoral immunity are designated **B lymphocytes** (Fig. 56–2).

            a. Most of the preprocessing of B lymphocytes that prepares them to manufacture antibodies occurs before and shortly after birth.

            b. Most of the preprocessing of T lymphocytes oc-

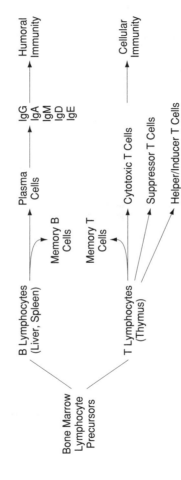

FIGURE 56–2. Schematic depiction of the development of the immune system.

curs in the thymus shortly before and for a few months after birth.

   c. It is believed that, during the processing of B and T lymphocytes, all those clones of lymphocytes capable of destroying the body's own tissues are self-destroyed.

   d. Autoimmune diseases (thyroiditis, rheumatic fever, glomerulonephritis, myasthenia gravis, lupus erythematosus) may be manifestations of diminished immune tolerance to the body's own tissues.

   e. Selective suppression of T lymphocytes, such as with cyclosporine, may interfere with early destruction of cancer cells, manifesting as an increased incidence of cancer in patients who receive chronic immunosuppressive therapy to improve acceptance of organ transplants.

2. The human immunodeficiency virus specifically attacks helper/inducer T lymphocytes (T4 cells), resulting in the eventual loss of immune function and death from cancer or infections due to normally nonpathogenic bacteria.

B. Antigens are foreign proteins or chemicals that evoke the production of antibodies.

C. Antibodies (each of which is specific for a particular antigen) are formed by plasma cells derived from B lymphocytes.

  1. Structure (Table 56-6)

  2. Mechanism of Action

   a. Antibodies act by exerting direct effects on the antigen, by activation of the complement system, or by initiation of an anaphylactic reaction.

   b. Complement system is a group of enzyme precursors that are normally present in the plasma in an inactive form (activation occurs when an antibody binds to an antigen on the cell membrane of mast cells and basophils) (Fig. 56-3).

   c. Hereditary angioedema is periodic swelling owing to decreased functional activity of the C1 esterase inhibitor.

   d. Activation of the alternative pathway occurs via nonimmunologic mechanisms (radiographic contrast media), independent of antibodies.

   e. Anaphylactic reaction occurs when an antigen attaches to IgE antibodies on cell membranes of circulating basophils or tissue mast cells, lead-

Table 56-6
Properties of Immunoglobulins

	IgG	IgA	IgM	IgD	IgE
Location	Plasma, Amniotic Fluid	Plasma, Saliva, Tears	Plasma	Plasma	Plasma
Plasma concentration (mg·dl⁻¹)	600–1500	85–380	50–400	<15	0.01–0.03
Plasma half-time (days)	21–23	6	5	2–8	1–5
Function					
Complement activation	+	–	+	–	–
Degranulation of mast cells	–	–	–	–	+
Bacterial lysis	+	?	+	–	–
Opsonization	+	+	–	–	–
Agglutination	+	+	+	–	–
Virus inactivation	+	+	+	–	–

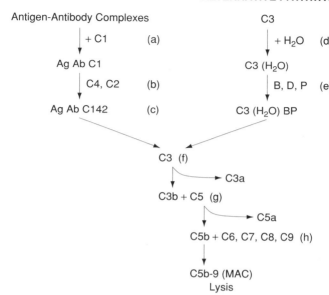

FIGURE 56–3. Diagram depicting the classical and alternative pathways of the complement system. (From Frank MM. Complement in the pathophysiology of human disease. N Engl J Med 1987;316:1525–30; with permission.)

       ing to degranulation and release of chemical mediators (hypotension, bronchoconstriction, edema).

    f. Tryptase, a neutral protease stored in mast cell granules, is liberated into the blood only if mast cell degranulation occurs (measurement of plasma tryptase 1 to 2 hours after an allergic reaction serves as a biochemical marker for the occurrence of an anaphylactic reaction).

VIII. TISSUE TYPING, much like blood typing, is accomplished by determining the types of antigens on the recipient's lymphocyte membranes (human leukocyte antigens [HLA]).

Chapter

57

Hemostasis and Blood Coagulation

Hemostasis in the presence of loss of blood vessel integrity is achieved by several different mechanisms (Table 57-1). (Updated and revised from Stoelting RK. Hemostasis and blood coagulation. In: Pharmacology and Physiology in Anesthetic Practice. 2nd ed. Philadelphia, JB Lippincott, 1991:813-17.)

I. HEMOSTASIS (Table 57-2)

II. BLOOD COAGULATION (Fig. 57-1)

- **A.** More than 30 different substances that promote **(procoagulants)** or inhibit **(anticoagulants)** coagulation have been identified in blood and tissues.
  - **1.** Normally, anticoagulants predominate, and blood does not coagulate.
  - **2.** When a blood vessel is transected or damaged, activity of the procoagulants in this area of damage becomes predominant and clot formation occurs.
    - **a.** Platelets are necessary for clot retraction to occur.
    - **b.** As the blood clot retracts, the edges of the broken blood vessel are pulled together, restoring the integrity of the vascular lumen.
- **B.** **Initiation of coagulation** requires activation of prothrombin by mechanisms that are stimulated by traumatic injury to tissues or to walls of blood vessels (Fig. 57-1).
  - **1.** **Extrinsic coagulation pathway** is stimulated to form prothrombin activator when blood comes into contact with traumatized vascular walls or extravascular tissues (prothrombin time reflects the integrity of the extrinsic pathway).

Table 57–1
Mechanisms of Hemostasis

Vascular spasm (less intense in sharply cut vessels, as with surgery)

Platelet plug (adhesion and aggregation)

Clot formation (conversion of fibrinogen to fibrin by thrombin)

Growth of fibrous tissue (conversion of clot to fibrous tissue is complete in 7 to 10 days)

2. **Intrinsic coagulation pathway** is stimulated to form prothrombin activator when there is trauma to the vascular walls that exposes collagen to circulating platelets and factor XII (partial thromboplastin time reflects the integrity of the intrinsic pathway).

C. **Factor VIII** consists of **von Willebrand factor** (enhances platelet adhesion) and **factor VIII:C** (deficient or absent in patients with hemophilia A).

D. **Conversion of prothrombin to thrombin** is preceded by formation of factors II, VII, IX and X in the liver (vitamin K is required).

Table 57–2
Nomenclature of Blood Clotting Factors

Factor	Synonyms	Plasma Concentration ($\mu g \cdot ml^{-1}$)	Half-time (h)	Stability in Stored Whole Blood
I	Fibrinogen	2000–4000	95–120	No change
II	Prothrombin	150	65–90	No change
III	Thromboplastin			
IV	Calcium			
V	Proaccelerin	10	15–24	Labile
VII	Proconvertin	0.5	4–6	No change
VIII	Antihemophilic factor	50–100	10–12	Labile
	VIII:vWF	50–100		
	VIII:C	0.05–0.1		
IX	Christmas factor	3	18–30	No change
X	Stuart-Prower factor	15	40–60	No change
XI	Plasma thromboplastin factor	5	45–60	Labile

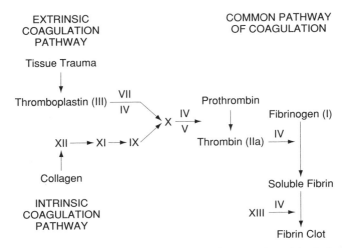

FIGURE 57–1. Schematic depiction of the extrinsic and intrinsic coagulation pathways culminating in the formation of a fibrin clot.

E. **Conversion of fibrinogen to fibrin** is responsible for formation of the reticulum of the clot.
F. **Impact of Progressive Blood Loss**
   1. It is likely that stress, tissue trauma, and increased plasma concentrations of catecholamines offset any hypocoagulable tendency resulting from hemodilution and loss of coagulation factors during progressive blood loss.
   2. These offsetting factors are probably responsible for the increase in coagulability seen in many surgical patients.
G. **Endogenous Control of Coagulation and Clot Formation**
   1. Intrinsic initiation of the clotting process is normally prevented by the smoothness of the vascular endothelium and a monomolecular layer of negatively charged protein on the vascular endothelium that repels clotting factors and platelets.
   2. **Endogenous Anticoagulants**
      a. Antithrombin III binds to thrombin and prevents conversion of thrombin to fibrin (binding is greatly facilitated by heparin).

    b. Heparin is not an effective anticoagulant when administered to patients with deficient circulating antithrombin III levels.

    c. Protein C inhibits the activity of factors V and VIII: C, and **protein S** enhances the effects of protein C.

    d. There is an increased incidence of thrombosis in patients with deficient amounts of endogenous anticoagulants.

  3. Endogenous Lysis of Clots

    a. Blood has the capacity to redissolve fibrin clots via a plasma proteolytic enzyme, **plasmin,** which is generated from its inactive precursor, **plasminogen.**

    b. Plasminogen activators (urokinase [secreted by the kidneys] and streptokinase [secreted by streptococci]) may be used therapeutically to dissolve intravascular clots as may be present in coronary arteries.

H. Thromboembolism occurs when a clot forms in a blood vessel **(thrombus)** and a fragment of this clot breaks off **(embolus)** and travels in the blood until it lodges at a site of vascular narrowing.

  1. An embolus originating in an artery usually occludes a more distal smaller artery, whereas an embolus originating in a vein commonly lodges in the lungs.

  2. Thromboembolism is likely to occur at the site of a roughened endothelial vessel wall (arteriosclerosis, infection, trauma) or in the presence of sluggish blood flow such that clotting factors are not diluted (pregnancy, postoperative immobilization).

I. Disseminated Intravascular Coagulation (DIC)

  1. Events that cause widespread thrombosis in small blood vessels include shock, sepsis, cancer, incompatible blood transfusions, and complications of pregnancy.

  2. Manifestations of DIC include spontaneous hemorrhage, decreased circulating platelets and clotting factors, and hypofibrinogenemia.

Chapter

58

Metabolism of Nutrients

Metabolism refers to all the chemical and energy transformations that occur in the body. (Updated and revised from Stoelting RK. Metabolism of nutrients. In: Pharmacology and Physiology in Anesthetic Practice. 2nd ed. Philadelphia, JB Lippincott, 1991:818–24.) The most important high-energy phosphate bond is adenosine triphosphate (ATP), which provides the energy necessary for most physiologic processes and chemical reactions (skeletal muscle contraction, transport of ions). In the resting state, energy-requiring tasks essential for life require the use of 200 to 250 $ml \cdot min^{-1}$ of oxygen. Activities increase caloric requirements in proportion to the energy expenditure required (Table 58–1).

I. CARBOHYDRATE METABOLISM

   A. At least 99% of all the energy derived from carbohydrates (predominantly glucose) is used to form ATP in cells.

   1. Glucose is dependent on carrier-mediated diffusion (enhanced by insulin) to gain access to cellular cytoplasm.

      a. Immediately upon entering cells, glucose is converted to glucose-6-phosphate under the influence of glucokinase.

      b. This phosphorylation of glucose prevents its escape from cells back into the circulation.

   2. Newborn infants are vulnerable to hypoglycemia because glycogen stores are limited, as is their ability to form glucose by gluconeogenesis.

   B. Glycogen is a storage form of glucose in the liver and skeletal muscles.

   1. The ability to form glycogen makes it possible to store substantial quantities of carbohydrates without significantly altering the osmotic pressure of intracellular fluids.

   2. Glycogen breakdown is catalyzed by activation of

Table 58–1
Estimates of Energy Expenditure in Adults

Activity	Calorie Expenditure $(kcal\cdot min^{-1})$
Basal	1.1
Sitting	1.8
Walking (2.5 miles·h^{-1})	4.3
Walking (4 miles·h^{-1})	8.2
Climbing stairs	9.0
Swimming	10.9
Bicycling (13 miles·h^{-1})	11.1

      phosphorylase in the liver and skeletal muscles and
      by the action of epinephrine on beta receptors.

C. **Gluconeogenesis** is the formation of glucose from amino
    acids and the glycerol portion of fat (stimulated by hypo-
    glycemia, cortisol release, and thyroxine).

D. **Energy Release from Glucose**

  1. For each mole of glucose that is completely degraded
     to carbon dioxide and water, a total of 38 mol of ATP
     is formed.

  2. The most important means by which energy is released
     from the glucose molecule is **glycolysis** and the subse-
     quent oxidation of the end products of glycolysis.

  3. **Oxidative phosphorylation** occurs only in the mito-
     chondria (citric acid cycle) in the presence of adequate
     amounts of oxygen.

  4. **Anaerobic glycolysis** is the release of a small amount
     of energy from glucose in the absence of adequate
     amounts of oxygen.

    a. Carbohydrates are the only nutrients that can form
      ATP without oxygen (may be lifesaving for a few
      minutes when oxygen becomes unavailable).

    b. During anaerobic glycolysis, most pyruvic acid is
      converted to lactic acid.

II. LIPID METABOLISM

A. Lipids include phospholipids, triglycerides (used to pro-
    vide energy for metabolic processes similar to carbohy-
    drates), and cholesterol (component of cell membranes

which is used for synthesis of corticosteroids and sex hormones).

B. Lipoproteins, which are synthesized principally in the liver, are mixtures of phospholipids, triglycerides, cholesterol, and proteins (Table 58-2).

1. The presumed function of lipoproteins is to provide a mechanism of transport for lipids throughout the body.

2. All the cholesterol in plasma is in lipoprotein complexes.

3. An intrinsic feedback control system increases the endogenous production of cholesterol (blocked with drugs) when exogenous intake is decreased (explaining the relatively modest lowering effect on plasma cholesterol concentrations produced by low-cholesterol diets).

C. Almost all cells, except brain cells, can use fatty acids interchangeably with glucose for energy (Fig. 58-1).

1. In the absence of adequate carbohydrate metabolism (starvation, uncontrolled diabetes mellitus), large quantities of acetoacetic acid, beta-hydroxybutyric acid, and acetone accumulate in the blood to produce **ketosis.**

2. A major function of adipose tissue is to store triglycerides until they are needed for energy.

   a. In contrast to glycogen, large amounts of lipid can be stored in adipose tissue and in the liver.

   b. Catecholamines activate triglyceride lipase in cells, leading to mobilization of fatty acids.

III. PROTEIN METABOLISM

A. Approximately 75% of the solid constituents of the body are proteins (Table 58-3).

B. All proteins are composed of amino acids connected by peptide linkages, and several of these amino acids must be supplied in the diet because they cannot be formed endogenously (essential amino acids) (Table 58-4).

1. Complex proteins may have as many as 100,000 amino acids.

2. The type of protein formed by the cell is genetically determined.

3. Passage of amino acids into cells requires active transport mechanisms.

Table 58-2
Composition of Lipids in the Plasma

	Phospholipid (percent)	Triglyceride (percent)	Free Cholesterol (percent)	Cholesterol Esters (percent)	Protein (percent)	Density
Chylomicrons	3	90	2	3	2	0.94
LDL	21	6	7	46	20	1.019-1.063
HDL	25	5	4	16	50	1.063-1.21
IDL	20	40	5	25	10	1.006-1.019
VLDL	17	55	4	16	8	0.94-1.006

LDL, low density lipoproteins; HDL, high density lipoproteins; IDL, intermediate density lipoproteins; VLDL, very density lipoproteins.

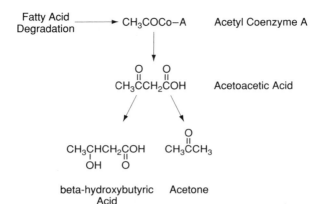

FIGURE 58–1. Fatty acid degradation in the liver leads to the formation of acetyl-CoA. Two molecules of acetyl-CoA combine to form acetoacetic acid, which, in large part, is converted to beta-hydroxybutyric acid, and in lesser amounts, to acetone.

Table 58–3
Types of Proteins

Globular	Fibrous	Conjugated
Albumin	Collagen	Mucoprotein
Globulin	Elastic fibers	Structural components of cells
Fibrinogen	Keratin	
Hemoglobin	Actin	
Enzymes	Myosin	
Nucleoproteins		

C. Storage of Amino Acids
   1. Immediately after entry into cells, amino acids are converted into cellular proteins.
   2. These proteins can be rapidly decomposed into amino acids for transport into the blood.
D. Plasma proteins are represented by albumin (colloid osmotic pressure), globulins (immunity), and fibrinogen (coagulation).
   1. Plasma albumin and fibrinogen and 60% to 80% of the

Table 58—4
Amino Acids

Essential	Nonessential
Arginine	Alanine
Histidine	Asparagine
Isoleucine	Aspartic acid
Leucine	Cysteine
Lysine	Glutamic acid
Methionine	Glutamine
Phenylalanine	Glycine
Threonine	Proline
Tryptophan	Serine
Valine	Tyrosine

      globulins are formed in the liver (remainder of the globulins are formed by the reticuloendothelial system).

  2. Synthesis rate of plasma proteins by the liver depends on the blood concentrations of amino acids.

E. Use of Proteins for Energy

  1. After cells contain a maximal amount of protein, any additional amino acids can be converted to glucose or glycogen (gluconeogenesis) or fatty acids (ketogenesis).

  2. In the absence of protein intake, endogenous proteins are degraded into amino acids.

  3. Growth hormone and insulin promote the synthesis rate of cellular proteins, whereas testosterone increases protein deposition in tissues, particularly the contractile proteins of skeletal muscle.

Drug Index

Index

ONE INDISPENSABLE RESOURCE

From doses to drug interactions, from today's most popular agents to the drugs of the future—this convenient handbook brings together the pharmacologic and physiologic fundamentals of anesthesia and applies them directly to your clinical practice.

With chapter and section headings keyed directly to Stoelting's *Pharmacology and Physiology in Anesthetic Practice, Second Edition,* this unique resource gives you...

- **Complete coverage** of perioperative anesthetic care that combines background information and current practice standards with the newest breakthroughs in the field

- **An easy-to-use outline format** that follows the structure of the parent text and provides key facts at a glance

- **Hundreds of illustrations and tables** that enhance your understanding of drug structure, drug-induced responses, and physiologic mechanisms

- **Current information** on the actions, benefits, and risks of anesthetic agents you use in your daily practice

- **Authoritative views** from a recognized leader in the field

GET THE ANSWERS TO YOUR TOUGHEST CLINICAL CHALLENGES NOW WITH THE WINNING TEAM IN ANESTHETIC MANAGEMENT...

Stoelting's *Handbook of Pharmacology and Physiology in Anesthetic Practice* and *Pharmacology and Physiology in Anesthetic Practice, Second Edition*

ISBN 0-397-51498-0

90000>

9 780397 514984